# Molecular Pathogenesis and Treatment of Chronic Myelogenous Leukemia

Masahiro Kizaki
Editor

# Molecular Pathogenesis and Treatment of Chronic Myelogenous Leukemia

Springer

*Editor*
Masahiro Kizaki
Department of Hematology, Saitama Medical Center
Saitama Medical University
Kawagoe, Saitama
Japan

ISBN 978-4-431-55713-5 ISBN 978-4-431-55714-2 (eBook)
DOI 10.1007/978-4-431-55714-2

Library of Congress Control Number: 2015954659

Springer Tokyo Heidelberg New York Dordrecht London


Printed on acid-free paper

Springer Japan KK is part of Springer Science+Business Media (www.springer.com)

# Preface

Advances in treatment of chronic myeloid leukemia (CML) have been made over the past two decades thanks to research that has furthered our understanding of its molecular pathogenesis. CML is a clonal hematopoietic stem cell disorder characterized by the abnormal proliferation of myeloid cell lineages, which progresses through the chronic phase (CP) to the accelerated and blastic phases. CML is caused by the presence of the Philadelphia (Ph) chromosome in hematopoietic stem cells, which arises from the reciprocal translocation of chromosomes 9 and 22, t(9;22)(q34;q11), resulting in the development of the *bcr-abl* chimeric gene. This chimeric gene produces the BCR-ABL fusion protein that has oncogenic activity. The BCR-ABL fusion protein has constitutive tyrosine kinase (TK) activity that is stronger than that of the naïve ABL protein, conferring a proliferative advantage and aberrant differentiation capacity to affected hematopoietic stem cells, resulting in the oncogenic event of leukemia development. Therefore, formation of the *bcr-abl* chimeric gene and its encoded protein is a primary and central event in the molecular pathogenesis of CML.

Until 2000, drug therapy for CML was limited to non-specific cytotoxic drugs such as busulfan and hydroxyurea, and then interferon (IFN)-α was introduced to regress disease activity, which had a survival benefit. Allogeneic hematopoietic stem cell transplantation (allo-SCT) for CML-CP frequently was a curative therapeutic approach for patients with good performance status and an appropriate stem cell donor, but it also was associated with a high incidence of early morbidity and mortality. Understanding of the molecular pathogenesis of CML resulted in rapid development of new therapeutic agents, including various BCR-ABL specific tyrosine kinase inhibitors (TKIs) such as imatinib, nilotinib, and dasatinib. Current clinical guidelines endorse use of any of these three TKIs for initial management of CML-CP. Molecular-targeted therapy with these TKIs was shown to dramatically improve clinical outcomes of CML patients, increasing the 10-year overall survival (OS) from 20 to 80–90 %. As shown in many clinical studies, CML patients treated with TKIs are expected to live for a long period of time. Thus, identification of appropriate surrogate markers for clinical outcome has become important.

Achieving a more complete and faster molecular response is correlated with good clinical outcome; therefore, improving molecular monitoring techniques for minimal residual disease is crucial. Furthermore, management of TKI-resistant CML and development of new TKIs are also important issues. We now have available multiple TKIs for clinical use, including second- and third-generation agents. In this decade, our goals for the treatment of CML are to optimize the quality of life for patients, to establish the most cost-effective treatment, and to deliver the best treatment and monitoring to each patient anywhere in the world. The ultimate goal for any patient is to discontinue use of TKIs—to achieve treatment-free remission and subsequent cure. In other words, future research into treatment of CML will focus on achieving and maintaining complete molecular remission after discontinuation of TKIs.

This book begins with a discussion of recent advances in basic CML research regarding stem cells and the signaling pathways of leukemic cells; continues by describing various clinical aspects of the use of TKIs in daily clinical practice; and concludes with a discussion of future trials aimed at a cure for this disease. I would like to acknowledge the many excellent colleagues who have contributed to each chapter. In addition, I would like to express my appreciation to the staff of Springer Japan, for all of their efforts in bringing this treatise to publication. It is hoped that this book will encourage implementation of further basic and clinical research projects with the goal of solving the remaining intriguing and important clinical problems of CML treatment.

Kawagoe, Japan Masahiro Kizaki, MD, PhD

# Contents

# Chapter 1
# Identification and Biology of CML Stem Cells

**Hiromi Iwasaki and Koichi Akashi**

**Abstract** Chronic myeloid leukemia (CML) is a typical model to study cancer stem cell biology. CML stem cells reside in the $CD34^{+}CD38^{-}$ fraction coexisting with normal hematopoietic stem cells (HSCs). By acquisition of BCR-ABL, an oncogenic fusion transcript encoding a constitutively active tyrosine kinase, HSCs become CML stem cells and progressively outgrow normal HSCs at the stem cell niche. The majority of CML stem cells is dormant but expands their clones mainly at the myeloid progenitor stage. Therefore, the effective target of tyrosine kinase inhibitor (TKI) is proliferating CML progenitors, and a fraction of CML stem cells persist after long-term TKI treatment. Thus, CML stem cells are heterogeneous, containing a population not addicted to the BCR-ABL kinase signaling. Importantly, those residual CML stem cells express BCR-ABL at a very low level. We hypothesize that the acquisition of BCR-ABL is not sufficient for HSC to become CML stem cells, because BCR-ABL is sometimes detectable in healthy individuals. Such BCR-ABL-expressing HSCs might be pre-CML stem cells, and additional events upregulating BCR-ABL expression might be required for formation of CML stem cells.

**Keywords** Chronic myeloid leukemia • Leukemia stem cell • Oncogene addiction

## 1.1 Cancer Stem Cell Hypothesis in Hematological Malignancies

Cancer stem cells (CSCs) exist and play a critical role in many, but not all, cancer types. Like normal stem cells, CSCs account for a rare cell population and possess self-renewal and differentiation potential to maintain whole cancer tissues [1]. Bonnet and Dick first reported the presence of CSCs in human acute myelogenous

H. Iwasaki (✉)
Center for Cellular and Molecular Medicine, Kyushu University Hospital, 3-1-1 Maidashi, Higashi-ku, Fukuoka 812-8582, Japan
e-mail: iwasakih@med.kyushu-u.ac.jp

K. Akashi
Department of Medicine and Biosystemic Science, Kyushu University Graduate School of Medical Sciences, 3-1-1 Maidashi, Higashi-ku, Fukuoka 812-8582, Japan



M. Kizaki (ed.), *Molecular Pathogenesis and Treatment of Chronic Myelogenous Leukemia*, DOI 10.1007/978-4-431-55714-2_1

leukemia (AML) [2]. Purified $CD34^{+}CD38^{-}$ leukemia cells successfully reconstituted human AML in serially transplanted NOD/SCID mice, whereas neither $CD34^{+}CD38^{+}$ nor $CD34^{-}$ cells were capable of initiating AML development in the immunodeficient mice [2]. This observation clearly demonstrates that leukemia stem cells (LSCs) in human AML exist exclusively within the $CD34^{+}CD38^{-}$ fraction, whose phenotype is similar to normal human hematopoietic stem cells (HSCs) [2]. Subsequently, CSCs have been identified in several types of solid tumors, including breast [3], brain [4], pancreas [5], colon [6], lung [7], and prostate [8]. CSCs are resistant to chemotherapy due to their dormancy and are considered to be a cause of metastasis and/or recurrence of intractable cancers. Thus, eliminating CSCs might be an ultimate strategy of cure for cancers. To achieve this goal, it is necessary to understand the particular biology of CSCs and to identify specific signaling pathways activated in each type of CSCs. Here we discuss the biological significance of chronic myeloid leukemia (CML) stem cells.

## 1.2 The Origin of CML Stem Cell Should Be a HSC with Self-renewal Potential, but Not Myeloid Progenitors

CML is a myeloproliferative neoplasm in which BCR-ABL, an oncogenic fusion transcript encoding a constitutively active tyrosine kinase introduced by a reciprocal translocation between chromosomes 9 and 22, is the hallmark of disease [9–11]. The leukemic transformation in CML is considered to occur at a primitive stem/progenitor stage because BCR-ABL transcripts are detectable not only in myeloid cells but also in lymphoid cells [12, 13]. Recent studies have shown that BCR-ABL fusion is found in the highly purified $CD34^{+}CD38^{-}$ human HSC fraction of CML patients by fluorescence in situ hybridization (FISH) analyses [14].

In mouse models, the retroviral transduction with BCR-ABL successfully transforms normal HSCs into LSCs, but myeloid progenitors including common myeloid progenitors (CMPs) and granulocyte/macrophage progenitors (GMPs) cannot become LSCs [15]: BCR-ABL-transduced murine HSCs but not CMPs or GMPs can develop a CML-like myeloproliferative neoplasm when transplanted [15]. This phenomenon has been confirmed by using the conditional transgenic mouse model in which BCR-ABL expression is initiated at the HSC stage under the 3′ enhancer of stem cell leukemia (SCL) transcription factor [16, 17]. HSCs purified from this transgenic mouse were capable of reproducing a CML-like disease when transplanted [17], whereas neither CMPs nor GMPs can develop the disease. These observations clearly show that the enforced expression of BCR-ABL is sufficient to transform normal HSCs to LSCs. On another hand, BCR-ABL cannot confer a self-renewal property to committed myeloid progenitors. It is of interest because other leukemic fusion genes such as MOZ-TIF2 [15], MLL-ENL [18], and MLL-AF9 [19] can directly transform GMPs to LSCs.

The gold standard of human CSC assay is a xenotransplant model, as Bonnet and Dick employed in their AML stem cell work [2]. In terms of human CML, several reports demonstrated that $CD34^+$ cells purified from chronic-phase patients' bone marrow can reproduce the CML hematopoiesis in vivo [20], suggesting that human CML stem cells reside in the primitive stem/progenitor cell population like AML stem cells. However, the human cell chimerisms were always very low in these experiments, and these cells could not re-reconstitute secondary xenogeneic recipients. Therefore, the formal biological proof for chronic-phase CML stem cells has not yet been obtained in xenograft model. Technical improvement of xenograft system might be necessary to assess human CML stem cells, especially for chronic phase. Perhaps, the attenuation of innate immunity and/or the modification of microenvironment mimicking human bone marrow environment might provide an efficient assay system to provide direct proof for CML stem cell self-renewal in vivo [21–23].

## 1.3 The Upregulation of BCR-ABL Might Be a Critical Step to Clinically Significant Cell Expansion in Chronic Phase of CML

Previous mouse CML models have shown that the enforced expression of BCR-ABL is sufficient for HSCs to transform into LSCs. However, a retroviral gene transduction method and a transgenic mouse model potentially have a serious problem in the expression level of target gene. In general, these methods provide an extremely high expression compared to the physiological level. To overcome this problem, we generated a conditional knock-in mouse strain in which a human p210 BCR-ABL cDNA was inserted into the first exon of bcr gene together with a STOP cassette flanked by loxP sites. By crossing with a Vav-Cre transgenic strain, the STOP cassette is excised and the expression of BCR-ABL is initiated in most hematopoietic cells including HSCs under the physiological control of murine bcr gene expression. We observed these knock-in mice for more than 2 years, but, unexpectedly, a CML-like myeloproliferative neoplasm has never developed (unpublished data). Recently, Foley et al. have reported the similar result by using an independent knock-in strain [24]. These observations raise the possibility that there is a threshold expression level of BCR-ABL to promote leukemic transformation. In other words, there might be a particular mechanism to enhance the expression of BCR-ABL in CML stem/progenitor cells.

This idea is further strengthened by the fact that very low levels of BCR-ABL transcripts are sometimes detectable in healthy individuals [25, 26]. These data suggest the presence of "pre-CML" stem cells possessing a BCR-ABL fusion gene in a fraction of normal individuals. It has also been shown that LSCs purified from chronic-phase CML patients at diagnosis express BCR-ABL at a high level, whereas the expression level per single LSC is attenuated after the successful tyrosine kinase inhibitor (TKI) treatment [27].

We have recently reported a similar phenomenon in t(8;21) AML [28, 29]. In patients achieving long-term remission (>3 years), AML1-ETO transcripts were expressed in a fraction of myeloid/lymphoid progenitors, mature myeloid cells, and B cells. Interestingly, ~1 % of $CD34^{+}CD38^{-}$ HSCs possessed AML1-ETO transcripts whose breakpoints were identical to those determined at diagnosis [30]. Furthermore, these "pre-leukemic" stem cells expressed AML1-ETO transcripts at a quite low level, which was less than 1 % of those expressed in initial LSCs on a per-cell basis [30].

These data strongly suggest that the upregulation of leukemic fusion genes might be a critical step for HSC to transform into LSC, at least in CML and t(8;21) AML. Therefore, it should be critical to elucidate mechanisms of upregulation of leukemia fusion genes in future studies.

## 1.4 Leukemia Stem Cell Burden at the Diagnosis Correlate with Sokal Score, Presumably Reflecting Time Passing from the Initial Acquisition of BCR-ABL

At the very initial stage of CML development, BCR-ABL fusion should be obtained a single HSC in self-renewal activity. This BCR-ABL-expressing HSC should progressively expand to dominate HSC niches to expel normal HSCs. This process is still unknown because it is difficult to find CML patients prior to or at very early phases of disease progression.

Recently, Mustjoki et al. reported the frequency of $BCR\text{-}ABL^{+}$ HSCs in 46 newly diagnosed CML patients with chronic-phase disease [14]. They purified the $CD34^{+}CD38^{-}$ HSC fraction as well as the $CD34^{+}CD38^{+}$ progenitor fraction from diagnostic bone marrow samples by fluorescence-activated cell sorting (FACS) and enumerated $BCR\text{-}ABL^{+}$ cells by FISH analyses [14]. Interestingly, the proportion of $BCR\text{-}ABL^{+}$ HSCs was markedly diversified (median 79 %, range 0.6–100 %). Strikingly, only ~1 % of HSCs had BCR-ABL in some patients. In contrast, the frequencies of $BCR\text{-}ABL^{+}$ cells were significantly high in progenitor populations (median 96 %, range 50–100 %). The initial burden of $BCR\text{-}ABL^{+}$ HSCs correlated with leukocyte count, spleen size, hemoglobin, and blast percentage. Importantly, patients with low percentage of $BCR\text{-}ABL^{+}$ HSCs achieved superior cytogenetic and molecular responses more rapidly compared to patients with high $BCR\text{-}ABL^{+}$ HSC burden [14].

We performed the similar analysis in newly diagnosed Japanese CML patients. Even in patients whose frequencies of $BCR\text{-}ABL^{+}$ HSCs were below 10 %, more than 80 % of CMPs were $BCR\text{-}ABL^{+}$. The percentages of $BCR\text{-}ABL^{+}$ HSCs are positively correlated with Sokal score (unpublished data).

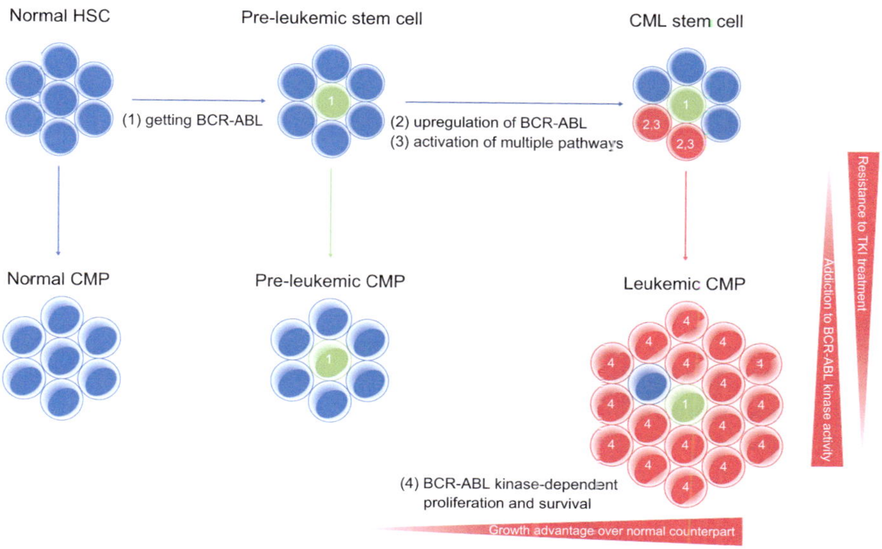


**Fig. 1.1** Clonal expansion of CML hematopoiesis. A reciprocal translocation between chromosomes 9 and 22 occurs at a hematopoietic stem cell (*HSC*) stage. This pre-leukemic stem cell expresses BCR-ABL at a low level and behaves like a normal HSC. To transform into an ultimate leukemia stem cell, the upregulation of BCR-ABL expression should be necessary. However, CML stem cells expressing high BCR-ABL transcripts are not necessarily addictive to the BCR-ABL kinase activity; thus, they are resistant to tyrosine kinase inhibitor (*TKI*) treatment. Instead, CML stem cells can survive by activating multiple BCR-ABL kinase-independent pathways. The massive proliferation of CML clone starts at a common myeloid progenitor (*CMP*) stage but not a stem cell stage. CMPs and their progeny are addictive to the BCR-ABL kinase activity for their survival and thus are sensitive to TKI treatment. It must be necessary to clarify the mechanisms of BCR-ABL upregulation in pre-leukemic stem cells to understand CML pathogenesis

These observations demonstrate that CML stem cells coexist with normal HSCs at an early stage of chronic phase and that myeloid progenitors are responsible for expansion of CML clones (Fig. 1.1). The initial BCR-ABL$^+$ HSC at diagnosis was diversified among patients, and the low BCR-ABL$^+$ HSC burden is associated with low Sokal score. It is reasonable to hypothesize that increment of BCR-ABL$^+$ HSC burden reflects time passing from the first acquisition of BCR-ABL in single HSCs. However, because healthy people sometimes have BCR-ABL at a low level, this process may involve additional gene mutations and/or epigenetic changes that strengthen the survival and self-renewal of CML stem cells or upregulation of BCR-ABL (Fig. 1.1). The analysis of molecular events during these early phases of disease is necessary to understand the CML stem cell biology.

## 1.5 CML Stem Cells Are Not Always Addicted to BCR-ABL Signaling

The constitutively active tyrosine kinase BCR-ABL is detectable in CML patients without exception. CML cells must be addicted to BCR-ABL signaling, because inhibition of BCR-ABL kinase activity by tyrosine kinase inhibitor (TKI) treatment dramatically reduced the leukemic burden of CML [31–33]. It is clear that proliferating CML progenitors are addicted to the BCR-ABL kinase activity. However, CML stem cells are not always addicted to BCR-ABL signaling because the majority of patients relapse after discontinuation of TKI treatment [34].

TKIs exert strong activity of kinase inhibition through binding to the kinase domain of BCR-ABL, and the vast majority of chronic-phase patients treated with TKIs achieve hematological and cytogenetic responses [31–33]. However, even in patients treated with TKIs for more than 5 years, minimal residual disease (MRD) is often detected by a highly sensitive PCR method despite the absence of TKI-resistant ABL mutations. Recently, several groups have shown that BCR-ABL-expressing cells persist in the $CD34^{+}CD38^{-}$ human HSC fraction even after achievement of complete cytogenetic and molecular responses [35, 20, 27]. Of note, these cells retain a long-term repopulating capacity after xenotransplant into immunodeficient mice [20]. Based on these data, it is considered that TKIs are incapable of eradicating chronic-phase CML stem cells.

Recently, by using an inducible BCR-ABL transgenic mouse model, it has been demonstrated that CML stem cells can survive independent of BCR-ABL kinase activity [36]. In this model, p210 BCR-ABL expression is targeted to murine stem and progenitor cells via a tetracycline-off system. Upon tetracycline withdrawal, BCR-ABL expression is initiated at the HSC stage and a CML-like disease develops within a few weeks. Reintroduction of tetracycline completely blocked the BCR-ABL signaling and induced complete remission. However, CML-like disease was reconstituted from the remission marrow when tetracycline was stopped. This new mouse model formally proves that genetically induced CML stem cells can survive even if the expression of BCR-ABL oncogene was completely silenced for a certain period [36]. Thus, there might exist specific signaling pathways that support the survival of CML stem cells beyond the BCR-ABL kinase activity.

In clinics, in patients with complete molecular response (CMR) for more than 2 years, around 60 % of patients relapsed within 6 months after discontinuation of imatinib treatment [34]. The persistence of CML stem cells was observed even in patients treated with nilotinib, a second-generation strong TKI. At this moment, at most 50 % of chronic-phase CML patients achieve CMR and 40–50 % of these good responders successfully quit TKIs; thus, it is estimated that 75–80 % of chronic-phase CML patients need to continue TKI therapy throughout life. In order to "cure" CML, it is necessary to understand how CML stem cells survive under TKI treatment.

It is important to note that after the TKI discontinuation, a very low level of BCR-ABL transcripts remained detectable in a considerable fraction of patients who do not relapse. It is possible that these patients returned to the "pre-CML" phase in which CML stem cells are not addicted to BCR-ABL (Fig. 1.1). Another possibility is that some anti-leukemia immune responses inhibit CML stem cells to grow. Several groups have reported that treatment prior to TKI with interferon (IFN)-α is predictive of relapse-free survival upon the TKI discontinuation [37]. In this case, IFN-α is considered to target CML stem/progenitor cells as well as to facilitate an anti-leukemia immunity. These data suggest that combination of TKI and immune checkpoint therapies, such as anti-PD-1 or anti-PD-L1 antibody therapies, may be useful to eradicate CML stem cells.

## 1.6 Pathways That May Be Used for the Maintenance of CML Stem Cells

CML stem cells are likely to utilize key survival pathways that are inherent in normal HSCs. These pathways might also be good targets to eradicate CML stem cells. Previous studies have shown that Wnt/β-catenin [38] and Hedgehog [39] signaling pathways that are critical for normal HSC development and maintenance are also important for the maintenance of CML stem cells. Because inhibition of these pathways potentially influences the survival of normal HSCs, there is serious concern about whether the therapeutic window can be established appropriately in clinical trials. In addition, transcription factors such as Foxo family [40] and Hif1α [41] play critical roles in CML stem cell maintenance. BCL6 proto-oncogene was shown to be a key effector downstream of Foxo in self-renewal of CML stem cells [42]. Details are discussed in the following chapters.

It has been demonstrated that CSCs utilize the specific metabolic pathways. CML stem cells augment the expression of arachidonate 5-lipoxygenase (Alox5) which is responsible for producing leukotrienes, inflammatory substances [43]. The upregulation of Alox5 in CML stem cells occurs independent of BCR-ABL kinase activity. In the absence of Alox5, BCR-ABL transduction fails to induce a CML-like disease, and treatment with a 5-lipoxygenase inhibitor prolongs the survival of CML mice [43]. Importantly, normal HSCs are not affected by the inhibition of Alox5. Stearoyl-CoA desaturase 1 (Scd1), an endoplasmic reticulum enzyme that regulates fatty acid metabolism, is shown to be downregulated in CML stem cells [43]. Deletion of Scd1 gene accelerates the disease development in mouse CML model. Conversely, overexpression of Scd1 delays CML development, indicating that Scd1 might play a tumor-suppressive role [43]. Thus, the modulation of LSC-specific metabolism could also be useful to eradicate CML stem cells.

## 1.7 Conclusion

It has been considered that CML is a perfect model of oncogene addiction. Although proliferating CML progenitors are addictive to BCR-ABL kinase activity for their survival, most CML stem cells are resistant to TKI. To completely cure CML, it is necessary to fully understand the molecular events during development of CML stem cells from a single HSC that first acquires BCR-ABL fusion. In addition, elucidation of molecular events how CML stem cells survive during TKI therapy is critical. These studies are ongoing, and we are awaiting new drugs targeting such critical mechanisms.

## References


1. Reya T, Morrison SJ, Clarke MF, Weissman IL. Stem cells, cancer, and cancer stem cells. Nature. 2001;414(6859):105–11. doi:10.1038/35102167.
2. Bonnet D, Dick JE. Human acute myeloid leukemia is organized as a hierarchy that originates from a primitive hematopoietic cell. Nat Med. 1997;3(7):730–7.
3. Al-Hajj M, Wicha MS, Benito-Hernandez A, Morrison SJ, Clarke MF. Prospective identification of tumorigenic breast cancer cells. Proc Natl Acad Sci U S A. 2003;100(7):3983–8. doi:10.1073/pnas.0530291100.
4. Singh SK, Clarke ID, Terasaki M, Bonn VE, Hawkins C, Squire J, et al. Identification of a cancer stem cell in human brain tumors. Cancer Res. 2003;63(18):5821–8.
5. Li C, Heidt DG, Dalerba P, Burant CF, Zhang L, Adsay V, et al. Identification of pancreatic cancer stem cells. Cancer Res. 2007;67(3):1030–7. doi:10.1158/0008-5472.can-06-2030.
6. Ricci-Vitiani L, Lombardi DG, Pilozzi E, Biffoni M, Todaro M, Peschle C, et al. Identification and expansion of human colon-cancer-initiating cells. Nature. 2007;445(7123):111–5. doi:10.1038/nature05384.
7. Kim CF, Jackson EL, Woolfenden AE, Lawrence S, Babar I, Vogel S, et al. Identification of bronchioalveolar stem cells in normal lung and lung cancer. Cell. 2005;121(6):823–35. doi:10.1016/j.cell.2005.03.032.
8. Goldstein AS, Huang J, Guo C, Garraway IP, Witte ON. Identification of a cell of origin for human prostate cancer. Science. 2010;329(5991):568–71. doi:10.1126/science.1189992.
9. Ben-Neriah Y, Daley GQ, Mes-Masson AM, Witte ON, Baltimore D. The chronic myelogenous leukemia-specific P210 protein is the product of the bcr/abl hybrid gene. Science. 1986;233(4760):212–4.
10. Nowell PC, Hungerford DA. Chromosome studies in human leukemia. II. Chronic granulocytic leukemia. J Natl Cancer Inst. 1961;27:1013–35.
11. Rowley JD. Letter: a new consistent chromosomal abnormality in chronic myelogenous leukaemia identified by quinacrine fluorescence and Giemsa staining. Nature. 1973;243(5405):290–3.
12. Fialkow PJ, Gartler SM, Yoshida A. Clonal origin of chronic myelocytic leukemia in man. Proc Natl Acad Sci U S A. 1967;58(4):1468–71.
13. Fialkow PJ, Jacobson RJ, Papayannopoulou T. Chronic myelocytic leukemia: clonal origin in a stem cell common to the granulocyte, erythrocyte, platelet and monocyte/macrophage. Am J Med. 1977;63(1):125–30.
14. Mustjoki S, Richter J, Barbany G, Ehrencrona H, Fioretos T, Gedde-Dahl T, et al. Impact of malignant stem cell burden on therapy outcome in newly diagnosed chronic myeloid leukemia patients. Leukemia. 2013;27(7):1520–6. doi:10.1038/leu.2013.19.

15. Huntly BJ, Shigematsu H, Deguchi K, Lee BH, Mizuno S, Duclos N, et al. MOZ-TIF2, but not BCR-ABL, confers properties of leukemic stem cells to committed murine hematopoietic progenitors. Cancer Cell. 2004;6(6):587–96. doi:10.1016/j.ccr.2004.10.015.
16. Koschmieder S, Gottgens B, Zhang P, Iwasaki-Arai J, Akashi K, Kutok JL, et al. Inducible chronic phase of myeloid leukemia with expansion of hematopoietic stem cells in a transgenic model of BCR-ABL leukemogenesis. Blood. 2005;105(1):324–34. doi:10.1182/blood-2003-12-4369.
17. Reynaud D, Pietras E, Barry-Holson K, Mir A, Binnewies M, Jeanne M, et al. IL-6 controls leukemic multipotent progenitor cell fate and contributes to chronic myelogenous leukemia development. Cancer Cell. 2011;20(5):661–73. doi:10.1016/j.ccr.2011.10.012.
18. Cozzio A, Passegue E, Ayton PM, Karsunky H, Cleary ML, Weissman IL. Similar MLL-associated leukemias arising from self-renewing stem cells and short-lived myeloid progenitors. Genes Dev. 2003;17(24):3029–35. doi:10.1101/gad.1143403.
19. Krivtsov AV, Twomey D, Feng Z, Stubbs MC, Wang Y, Faber J, et al. Transformation from committed progenitor to leukaemia stem cell initiated by MLL-AF9. Nature. 2006;442 (7104):818–22. doi:10.1038/nature04980.
20. Chu S, McDonald T, Lin A, Chakraborty S, Huang Q, Snyder DS, et al. Persistence of leukemia stem cells in chronic myelogenous leukemia patients in prolonged remission with imatinib treatment. Blood. 2011;118(20):5565–72. doi:10.1182/blood-2010-12-327437.
21. Rongvaux A, Takizawa H, Strowig T, Willinger T, Eynon EE, Flavell RA, et al. Human hemato-lymphoid system mice: current use and future potential for medicine. Annu Rev Immunol. 2013;31:635–74. doi:10.1146/annurev-immunol-032712-095921.
22. Takenaka K, Prasolava TK, Wang JC, Mortin-Toth SM, Khalouei S, Gan OI, et al. Polymorphism in Sirpa modulates engraftment of human hematopoietic stem cells. Nat Immunol. 2007;8(12):1313–23. doi:10.1038/ni1527.
23. Yamauchi T, Takenaka K, Urata S, Shima T, Kikushige Y, Tokuyama T, et al. Polymorphic Sirpa is the genetic determinant for NOD-based mouse lines to achieve efficient human cell engraftment. Blood. 2013;121(8):1316–25. doi:10.1182/blood-2012-06-440354.
24. Foley SB, Hildenbrand ZL, Soyombo AA, Magee JA, Wu Y, Oravecz-Wilson KI, et al. Expression of BCR/ABL p210 from a knockin allele enhances bone marrow engraftment without inducing neoplasia. Cell Rep. 2013;5(1):51–60. doi:10.1016/j.celrep.2013.08.037.
25. Biernaux C, Loos M, Sels A, Huez G, Stryckmans P. Detection of major bcr-abl gene expression at a very low level in blood cells of some healthy individuals. Blood. 1995;86 (8):3118–22.
26. Bose S, Deininger M, Gora-Tybor J, Goldman JM, Melo JV. The presence of typical and atypical BCR-ABL fusion genes in leukocytes of normal individuals: biologic significance and implications for the assessment of minimal residual disease. Blood. 1998;92(9):3362–7.
27. Kumari A, Brendel C, Hochhaus A, Neubauer A, Burchert A. Low BCR-ABL expression levels in hematopoietic precursor cells enable persistence of chronic myeloid leukemia under imatinib. Blood. 2012;119(2):530–9. doi:10.1182/blood-2010-08-303495.
28. Miyamoto T, Nagafuji K, Akashi K, Harada M, Kyo T, Akashi T, et al. Persistence of multipotent progenitors expressing AML1/ETO transcripts in long-term remission patients with t(8;21) acute myelogenous leukemia. Blood. 1996;87(11):4789–96.
29. Miyamoto T, Weissman IL, Akashi K. AML1/ETO-expressing nonleukemic stem cells in acute myelogenous leukemia with 8;21 chromosomal translocation. Proc Natl Acad Sci U S A. 2000;97(13):7521–6.
30. Shima T, Miyamoto T, Kikushige Y, Yuda J, Tochigi T, Yoshimoto G, et al. The ordered acquisition of Class II and Class I mutations directs formation of human t(8;21) acute myelogenous leukemia stem cell. Exp Hematol. 2014;42(11):955–65. e1–5. doi:10.1016/j.exphem.2014.07.267.
31. Hochhaus A, O'Brien SG, Guilhot F, Druker BJ, Branford S, Foroni L, et al. Six-year follow-up of patients receiving imatinib for the first-line treatment of chronic myeloid leukemia. Leukemia. 2009;23(6):1054–61. doi:10.1038/leu.2009.38.

32. Jabbour E, Kantarjian HM, Saglio G, Steegmann JL, Shah NP, Boque C, et al. Early response with dasatinib or imatinib in chronic myeloid leukemia: 3-year follow-up from a randomized phase 3 trial (DASISION). Blood. 2014;123(4):494–500. doi:10.1182/blood-2013-06-511592.
33. Larson RA, Hochhaus A, Hughes TP, Clark RE, Etienne G, Kim DW, et al. Nilotinib vs imatinib in patients with newly diagnosed Philadelphia chromosome-positive chronic myeloid leukemia in chronic phase: ENESTnd 3-year follow-up. Leukemia. 2012;26(10):2197–203. doi:10.1038/leu.2012.134.
34. Mahon FX, Rea D, Guilhot J, Guilhot F, Huguet F, Nicolini F, et al. Discontinuation of imatinib in patients with chronic myeloid leukaemia who have maintained complete molecular remission for at least 2 years: the prospective, multicentre Stop Imatinib (STIM) trial. Lancet Oncol. 2010;11(11):1029–35. doi:10.1016/s1470-2045(10)70233-3.
35. Chomel JC, Bonnet ML, Sorel N, Bertrand A, Meunier MC, Fichelson S, et al. Leukemic stem cell persistence in chronic myeloid leukemia patients with sustained undetectable molecular residual disease. Blood. 2011;118(13):3657–60. doi:10.1182/blood-2011-02-335497.
36. Hamilton A, Helgason GV, Schemionek M, Zhang B, Myssina S, Allan EK, et al. Chronic myeloid leukemia stem cells are not dependent on Bcr-Abl kinase activity for their survival. Blood. 2012;119(6):1501–10. doi:10.1182/blood-2010-12-326843.
37. Takahashi N, Kyo T, Maeda Y, Sugihara T, Usuki K, Kawaguchi T, et al. Discontinuation of imatinib in Japanese patients with chronic myeloid leukemia. Haematologica. 2012;97(6):903–6. doi:10.3324/haematol.2011.056853.
38. Zhao C, Blum J, Chen A, Kwon HY, Jung SH, Cook JM, et al. Loss of beta-catenin impairs the renewal of normal and CML stem cells in vivo. Cancer Cell. 2007;12(6):528–41. doi:10.1016/j.ccr.2007.11.003.
39. Zhao C, Chen A, Jamieson CH, Fereshteh M, Abrahamsson A, Blum J, et al. Hedgehog signalling is essential for maintenance of cancer stem cells in myeloid leukaemia. Nature. 2009;458(7239):776–9. doi:10.1038/nature07737.
40. Naka K, Hoshii T, Muraguchi T, Tadokoro Y, Ooshio T, Kondo Y, et al. TGF-beta-FOXO signalling maintains leukaemia-initiating cells in chronic myeloid leukaemia. Nature. 2010;463(7281):676–80. doi:10.1038/nature08734.
41. Wang Y, Liu Y, Malek SN, Zheng P, Liu Y. Targeting HIF1alpha eliminates cancer stem cells in hematological malignancies. Cell Stem Cell. 2011;8(4):399–411. doi:10.1016/j.stem.2011.02.006.
42. Hurtz C, Hatzi K, Cerchietti L, Braig M, Park E, Kim YM, et al. BCL6-mediated repression of p53 is critical for leukemia stem cell survival in chronic myeloid leukemia. J Exp Med. 2011;208(11):2163–74. doi:10.1084/jem.20110304.
43. Chen Y, Hu Y, Zhang H, Peng C, Li S. Loss of the Alox5 gene impairs leukemia stem cells and prevents chronic myeloid leukemia. Nat Genet. 2009;41(7):783–92. doi:10.1038/ng.389.

# Chapter 2
# Molecular Mechanisms of CML Stem Cell Maintenance

**Atsushi Hirao, Yuko Tadokoro, and Masaya Ueno**

**Abstract** The molecular mechanisms regulating hematopoietic stem cell (HSC) behavior have been assumed to also control chronic myelogenous leukemia (CML) stem cells in vivo. For example, signals that are involved in stemness, the cell cycle, cellular metabolism, microenvironments, and epigenetic modification appear to control both HSC and CML stem cells. Therefore, CML stem cells have been believed to be able to survive and self-renew when exposed to inhibitors of BCR–ABL. However, detailed analyses have revealed that there are critical differences in how the self-renewal of these two types of stem cells depends on various signaling pathways, indicating that the regulation of CML stem cell self-renewal is not identical to that of HSCs. Such differences between HSC and CML stem cells could provide a therapeutic window for the total eradication of CML disease. Further dissection of these molecular mechanisms will lead to the development of successful therapeutics for CML patients.

**Keywords** CML stem cell • Stemness • Cell cycle • Metabolism • Microenvironments • Epigenetics

## 2.1 Introduction

Hematopoietic stem cells (HSCs) are able to reproduce themselves, a property known as self-renewal, and to give rise to mature hematopoietic cells. Most HSCs in bone marrow (BM) are in a quiescent state until a signal is received that the generation of additional mature blood cells is required. HSCs then proliferate, with some daughter cells differentiating and others undergoing self-renewal.

Several studies indicate that chronic myelogenous leukemia (CML) originates from HSCs that have sustained a chromosomal translocation, known as the Philadelphia chromosome (Ph), that results in the formation of a BCR–ABL fusion gene [1, 2]. The $Ph^+$ blood of CML patients contains stem cell-like populations that are

A. Hirao, MD, PhD (✉) • Y. Tadokoro • M. Ueno
Division of Molecular Genetics, Cancer and Stem Cell Research Program, Cancer Research Institute, Kanazawa University, Kakuma-machi, Kanazawa 920-1192, Japan
e-mail: ahirao@staff.akanazawa-u.ac.jp



M. Kizaki (ed.), *Molecular Pathogenesis and Treatment of Chronic Myelogenous Leukemia*, DOI 10.1007/978-4-431-55714-2_2

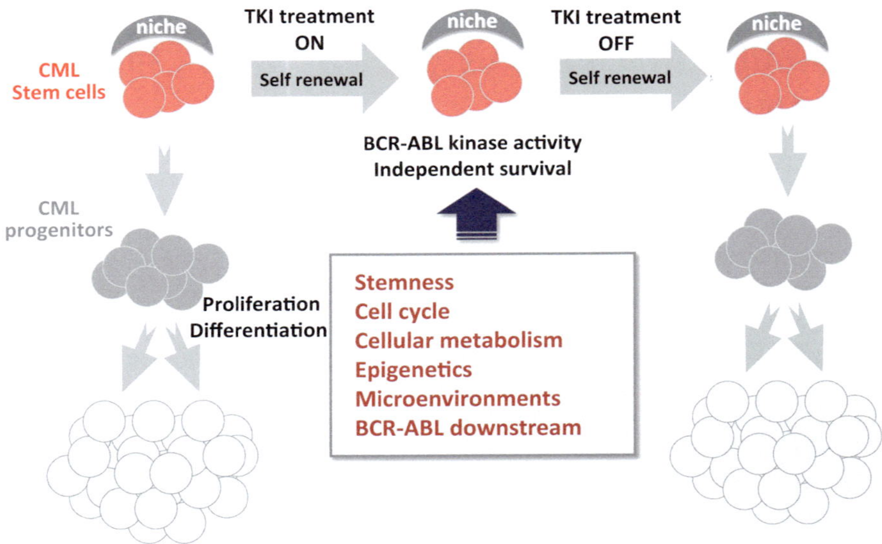


**Fig. 2.1** CML stem cell maintenance. CML stem cells self-renew as HSCs do when BCR–ABL kinase activity is inhibited by tyrosine kinase inhibitors (TKIs). Therefore, survival of CML stem cells causes recurrence of CML disease when TKI therapy is discontinued. Survival and self-renewal of CML stem cells despite TKI treatment are supported by several signals that are involved in stemness, the cell cycle, metabolism, epigenetics, or the microenvironment. In addition, molecules downstream of BCR–ABL that function independently of its kinase activity also support the TKI resistance of CML stem cells

phenotypically similar to normal HSCs. Like HSCs, CML stem cells generate both new stem cells and progenitors, because BCR–ABL does not affect the differentiation program in hematopoiesis. Tyrosine kinase inhibitors (TKIs), such as imatinib, nilotinib, and dasatinib, are effective for removing most CML cells; however, CML stem cells survive TKI therapy, causing relapse of CML disease when TKI therapy is discontinued [3, 4]. Therefore, it has been assumed that CML stem cells self-renew as HSCs do when BCR–ABL kinase activity is inhibited (Fig. 2.1).

Although the molecular mechanisms of CML disease development and progression in patients has been well investigated, it has not been clear whether these mechanisms maintain CML stem cells after the establishment of CML disease or whether CML stem cells are maintained by distinct molecular mechanisms. Because the disruption of signals required for the maintenance of CML stem cells will contribute to the eradication of CML disease, many researchers investigating CML disease have been interested in how CML stem cells are maintained. The maintenance of normal hematopoiesis provides some insight. HSCs are tightly regulated by both intrinsic and extrinsic factors in vivo. Therefore, numerous signals may also be involved in CML stem cell maintenance. For example, accumulating evidence has revealed the presence of "stemness" signals, that is, molecules and signaling pathways that play critical roles in maintaining the undifferentiated properties of various types of stem cells, including embryonic stem cells [5]. Such stemness signals are involved in control of CML stem cell function. Cell cycle regulation may be important, because CML stem cells cycle slowly, like HSCs in vivo, and there is evidence that loss of key cell cycle regulators leads to defective phenotypes in quiescence that are associated with reduced HSC function [6]. Cellular metabolism is also important for the maintenance of HSC function [7]. Furthermore, several microenvironmental components in BM, including the vasculature, endosteal osteolineage cells, and mature hematopoietic cells [8], may affect CML stem cells, although it is unclear whether the CML stem cell niche is identical to that of HSCs. In addition, modulation of metabolism is critical for HSC behaviors [9–12]. Epigenetic modifications are also important for controlling the undifferentiated status of HSCs [13].

Despite the similarities in the regulation of undifferentiated status between CML stem cells and HSCs, there are also critical differences between them. Even if a CML stem cell is derived from a HSC, additional characteristics associated with BCR–ABL are likely acquired during leukemogenesis. Therefore, dissection of BCR–ABL signals, whether or not they depend on its kinase activity, is needed to understand the mechanisms of CML stem cell maintenance. This chapter will introduce recent advances in the understanding of the molecular mechanisms regulating the maintenance of stem cell populations in CML.

## 2.2 Stemness

Increasing evidence points to shared core molecular stemness mechanisms between normal tissue stem cells and CML stem cells, which creates emerging possibilities for developing new therapeutics for CML. The Wnt and Hedgehog signals are most representative of stemness regulatory pathways. The Wnt proteins are secreted signaling molecules that regulate diverse processes, including embryogenesis, cell polarity, and cell fate modulation of stem/progenitor cells, and their deregulation is observed in many types of cancer [5, 14]. To date, 19 members of the Wnt family have been identified in primate, and these proteins activate two main Wnt signaling pathways, the canonical and noncanonical Wnt cascades. A hallmark of the canonical Wnt pathway is the nuclear localization of β-catenin. When the canonical Wnt signaling pathway is inactivated, β-catenin forms a complex with Axin, adenomatous polyposis coli, and glycogen synthase kinase-3β, and β-catenin is then phosphorylated and targeted for ubiquitinylation and subsequent degradation by proteasomes. Signaling is initiated when Wnt binds to Frizzled receptors and a member of the LDL receptor family, Lrp5/6. In the presence of Wnt signaling, β-catenin is uncoupled from the complex and translocates to the nucleus, where it binds Lef/Tcf transcription factors, thus activating transcription of target genes. The Wnt signaling pathway is critical for many types of tissue stem cells, including epidermal, intestinal, neural, and hematopoietic stem cells [5]. In a mouse model,

Wnt3A can induce self-renewal of HSCs and enhance their ability to reconstitute recipient hematopoiesis when transplanted into an irradiated recipient [15, 16]. Furthermore, treatment of undifferentiated human hematopoietic progenitors with Wnt5A leads to their expansion in vitro [17]. In the BM, Wnt proteins are produced by HSCs themselves as well as by the microenvironment, suggesting that Wnt proteins regulate HSCs in both an autocrine manner and paracrine manner [18]. Overexpression of Axin suppresses HSC growth [15], also supporting a pivotal role for the Wnt signaling pathway in the maintenance of HSC stemness. Paradoxically, conditional gene-targeting studies revealed that β-catenin, an essential downstream molecule in the canonical Wnt signaling pathway, is dispensable for normal hematopoiesis and lymphopoiesis [19]. Although the role of β-catenin signaling in the regulation of normal HSCs remains under debate, it is widely accepted that Wnt/β-catenin signaling is necessary for leukemogenesis and development of leukemia initiating cells (LICs) [20–23]. Granulocyte–macrophage progenitors (GMPs) from CML patients with blast crisis show the activation of Wnt/β-catenin signaling, as determined by Wnt reporter activity and accumulation of nuclear β-catenin [24]. Overactivation of Wnt signaling endows GMPs with the stem cell-like property of long-term renewal, which normal GMPs do not possess [24]. Interestingly, after CML was established in a mouse model of BCR–ABL-induced CML, deletion of β-catenin did not increase survival; however, deletion of β-catenin and cotreatment with imatinib synergized to eliminate CML stem cells [25]. This effect was also seen with pharmacological inhibition of β-catenin with indomethacin. These studies suggest that the Wnt/β-catenin signaling pathway is important for the establishment of stemness in progenitors, and it could become a therapeutic target in CML patients.

The Hedgehog (Hh) pathway is another important regulator of embryogenesis that has also been implicated in the development of multiple types of cancer [26]; it is essential for regulating the proliferation, migration, and differentiation of stem/progenitor cells. Genetic mutations of the Hh pathway are found in familial (Gorlin's syndrome) and sporadic basal cell carcinoma, as well as medulloblastoma, indicating a clear relationship between Hh pathway activity and oncogenesis [26]. In mammals, three Hh proteins, Desert Hedgehog (DHh), Indian Hedgehog (IHh), and Sonic Hedgehog (SHh), function as ligands for Patched (Ptch1). In the absence of an Hh ligand, the Ptch1 receptor inhibits the action of Smoothened (Smo), a G protein-coupled receptor. Binding of Hh ligands to Ptch1 causes internalization and degradation of Ptch1, releasing its suppression of Smo. Smo then interacts with Suppressor of fused (SUFU), which in turn activates glioma-associated oncogene homologue 1 (GLI1) and GLI2 and degrades GLI3, leading to the transcription of tumor-promoting genes.

The role of Hh signaling in normal hematopoiesis is controversial [27]. Evidence from genetic knockouts suggests that the Hh signaling pathway regulates definitive hematopoiesis during development, rather than early primitive hematopoiesis. Loss of Ihh causes hypoplasia of fetal liver, which is a major fetal hematopoietic organ [28]. In addition, overactivation of Hh signaling by single Ptch1 gene deletion ($Ptch1^{+/-}$) induces expansion but exhaustion of regenerating HSCs [29]. In contrast, studies using conditional *Smo* KO mice revealed that Hh signaling is dispensable for adult HSC function [30, 31]. The role of Hh signaling may be highly context dependent, changing with developmental stage, cell type, and even physiologic condition [27]. However, experimental CML models have suggested that the Hh signaling pathway is essential for the maintenance of CML stemness, and this pathway is therefore a therapeutic target. In the *Smo* KO CML mice, the CML stem cell population was significantly decreased, and the development of re-transplantable BCR–ABL-positive CML stem cells was abolished by the deletion of Smo genes [32]. In addition, treatment with both cyclopamine (Hh inhibitor) and nilotinib produces an additive effect over nilotinib alone in reducing the total number of progenitors and extending the time to relapse after discontinuation of therapy [33]. Therefore, a clinical strategy incorporating both Hh and BCR–ABL inhibition may have value in preventing the drug resistance and disease recurrence associated with TKI treatment alone.

## 2.3 Cell Cycle

Several studies have shown that CML stem cells cycle more slowly than progenitor CML cells [6]. The similarity in cell cycle status between normal HSCs and CML stem cells provides important clues about understanding the features of CML. One of the master regulators of the cell cycle in normal HSCs and CML stem cells is Fbxw7 (F-box and WD40 repeat domain-containing 7). Fbxw7 is an F-box protein component of an SCF (Skip-Cul1-F-box protein)-type ubiquitin ligase [34]. Fbxw7 has several substrates for ubiquitination, including c-Myc, cyclin E, and Notch1, and regulates both the cell cycle and cellular differentiation. Fbxw7 has three isoforms (α, β, and γ), and Fbxw7α is exclusively expressed in undifferentiated hematopoietic cells and T cell-committed progenitors. Ablation of Fbxw7 in hematopoietic cells has shown the importance of the Fbxw7/c-Myc axis in HSC maintenance [35, 36]. c-Myc is maintained in HSCs at a low level in the steady state and plays a critical role in the self-renewal and differentiation of HSCs [37]. Elimination of c-Myc increases the number of HSCs that can self-renew but fail to differentiate. Overexpression of c-Myc in HSCs enhances differentiation, resulting in HSC exhaustion. In mice with an Fbxw7 deletion, c-Myc protein accumulates in the HSC population, leading to cell cycle entry and premature loss by p53-dependent apoptosis of HSCs [35, 36]. This defective phenotype of *Fbxw7*-deficient HSCs is rescued by decreasing c-Myc protein expression [38]. Furthermore, the gene expression profile in *Fbxw7*-deficient HSCs/progenitor cells showed that differentiation-related genes were activated and genes enriched in HSCs were downregulated. Among genes regulating the cell cycle, loss of Fbxw7 in HSCs induced the upregulation of E2F2 and Ccnd1 and the downregulation of p57kip2. These affected genes have been suggested to be targets of c-Myc [39–41]. Conversely, forced expression of Fbxw7 in HSCs/progenitor cells suppresses the accumulation of c-Myc, resulting in the repression of cell cycle progression and maintenance of the high reconstitution activity of HSCs [42]. Fbxw7-overexpressing HSCs show increased expression levels of p21cip1 and p27kip1. Thus, the Fbxw7/c-Myc axis plays an important role in cell cycle regulation and the maintenance of HSCs [43]. In mouse CML models and human patients, Fbxw7 is highly expressed in the stem cell compartment compared to its expression in progenitor and differentiated cells. Genetic ablation of *Fbxw7* in CML cells suppresses the initiation and progression of CML disease [44, 45]. Loss of Fbxw7 induces the accumulation of c-Myc, cell cycle entry, and p53-dependent apoptosis, leading to exhaustion of CML stem cells. These functions in Fbxw7-deficient CML stem cells are rescued by a decrease in the c-Myc protein level or silencing of p53. Furthermore, the Fbxw7-deficient CML stem cells are sensitive to anticancer drug treatments. Importantly, the activation of BCR–ABL induces the upregulation of Fbxw7 expression, and the expression levels of Fbxw7 and c-Myc in CML stem cells are higher than those in normal HSCs. The expression pattern shows that Fbxw7 deficiency creates more dramatic defects in CML stem cells than in HSCs. The difference in cycle phenotypes between CML stem cells and HSCs may explain why Fbxw7-deficient CML stem cells show higher sensitivity to imatinib or Ara-C treatment than Fbxw7-deficient HSCs. Thus, Fbxw7 itself or related signals may be a therapeutic target for CML stem cells in combination with TKI.

FOXO transcription factors belong to the forkhead family of transcriptional regulators [46, 47]. In mammals, the FOXO group contains four members: FOXO1, FOXO3a, FOXO4, and FOXO6. FOXO proteins are normally present in an active state in a cell's nucleus. In response to growth factors or insulin, phosphatidylinositol 3-kinase (PI3K) is activated. PI3K in turn activates several serine/threonine kinases, including protein kinase B (PKB/Akt) and the related SGK family enzymes. Activated Akt phosphorylates FOXO proteins at three Akt phosphorylation sites, resulting in their export from the nucleus into the cytoplasm and subsequently their inactivation. FOXO activity is regulated by several environmental stimuli through posttranslational modifications, including phosphorylation, acetylation, ubiquitination, and methylation. The FOXO family has numerous target molecules that are involved in variety of cellular responses, including cell cycle arrest, DNA damage response, detoxification of reactive oxygen species (ROS), glucose metabolism, and mitochondrial activity. In normal quiescent HSCs, FOXO3a is localized in nuclei, whereas it is predominantly located in the cytoplasm of cycling progenitor cells [48, 49]. Deficiency of FOXO3a protein leads to impaired quiescence of HSCs and elevated ROS, resulting in defective capacity for hematopoietic regeneration after transplantation of HSCs [49–51]. The inhibition of ROS by N-acetyl cysteine reverses the defective phenotype of HSCs, indicating that FOXO proteins contribute to the maintenance of HSCs by suppressing ROS. In a mouse CML model, FOXO proteins were localized in the nuclei of CML stem cells and were associated with the inactivation of Akt, suggesting that the FOXO family may be activated in the these cells, as they are in normal HSCs [52]. FOXO3a is localized in both the cytoplasm and nuclei of $CD34^+$ cells from human CML patients (CML stem cells/progenitor cells), whereas it is localized mainly in the nuclei of normal $CD34^+$ cells [53]. The inactivation of

BCR–ABL by TKIs also activates FOXO by inactivating Akt. TKI treatment causes cell cycle arrest and apoptosis of CML cells that are associated with nuclear localization of FOXO1 and FOXO3a. TKI treatment induces several genes that are mediated by the FOXO family, including ATM, p57, and BCL6. Overexpression of FOXO3a in CML cell lines produces G1 arrest and apoptosis; however, CML stem cells derived from patients show an only slight increase in apoptosis when FOXO3a is activated, whereas remarkable cell cycle arrest occurs. Thus, FOXO family proteins are critical cell cycle regulators in CML stem cells, whereas apoptosis induced by FOXO activation may depend on cell context, and only cells with levels of FOXO activity over an "apoptosis threshold" may die. In human CML cell lines, knockdown of FOXO3a inhibits the cell cycle arrest induced by TKI treatment, followed by the induction of cell death. Importantly, FOXO3a deficiency increases the sensitivity of CML stem cells to TKI therapy in vivo. Thus, FOXO proteins play critical roles in the resistance of CML stem cells to TKI therapy [53, 52].

One molecule downstream of FOXO that is critical for the maintenance of CML stem cells is the transcription factor B cell lymphoma 6 (BCL6) [54, 55]. BCL6, which has a BTB domain, was originally identified as a proto-oncogene in diffuse large B cell lymphoma. Homodimerization of the BCL6 BTB domain forms a lateral groove motif, which is required to bind to the silencing mediator for retinoid and thyroid hormone receptor (SMRT) and N-CoR corepressors, thereby controlling expression of target genes [56]. BCL6 contributes to the maturation of mature B cells that is mediated by transcriptional repression of p53 and survival of pre-B cells. In addition, in BCR–ABL-transformed pre-B cell acute lymphoblastic leukemia ($Ph^+$ ALL), BCL6 is induced by TKI treatment, preventing cell death by suppressing p53 [54]. In human CML, the upregulation of BCL6 by TKI is restricted to $CD34^+$ cells. BCL6 deficiency sensitizes CML cell lines to TKI therapy in vitro [55]. Pharmacological inhibition of BCL6 transcription activity by a recombinant peptide leads to cell cycle arrest and apoptosis in CML stem cells. Thus, the FOXO–BCL6 axis contributes to the maintenance of CML stem cells.

The promyelocytic leukemia protein (PML), an essential component of PML bodies [57], is also involved in cell cycle regulation of CML stem cells [58]. PML is highly expressed in immature CML cells, whereas its expression is barely detected in differentiated neutrophils in CML patients. PML-deficient CML stem cells undergo the cell cycle in vivo and in vitro, associated with the impairment of CML stem cell function. Although it has been reported that PML suppresses mTOR activity via the inhibition of the Rheb–mTOR association [59], the defective phenotypes of CML stem cells are mediated by mTOR activation. Pharmacological PML downregulation by arsenic forces CML stem cells to enter the cell cycle, enhancing their sensitivity to chemotherapy.

## 2.4 Metabolism

HSCs utilize glycolysis rather than mitochondrial oxidative phosphorylation, whereas oxidative phosphorylation becomes dominant in hematopoietic progenitors; enhanced glycolysis results in the generation of a low level of ATP energy that is associated with low ROS [7]. Dysregulation of mitochondrial activity and ROS generation in HSCs causes loss of stem cell function. The glycolytic metabolism in HSCs may be supported by a mechanism of aerobic glycolysis similar to that observed in cancer. One of the key factors for aerobic glycolysis is a protein complex containing hypoxia-inducible factor (HIF) 1, which plays a critical role in the cellular metabolic response to hypoxia [60]. HIF1-α, whose protein stability is regulated by oxygen-dependent prolyl hydroxylases, forms a protein complex with a stable partner, HIF1-β. In hypoxic conditions, the upregulation of HIF1-α enhances glycolytic flow by inducing several key enzymes that enhance glycolysis. HIF1-α also inactivates pyruvate dehydrogenase kinases, which inhibit the conversion of pyruvate to acetyl-CoA, resulting in the suppression of the influx of glycolytic metabolites into the mitochondrial TCA cycle. Several studies using genetically engineered mouse models have indicated that the Meis1–HIF1 axis is essential for glycolytic metabolism in HSCs and therefore for maintaining HSC function [61–63], although there are controversies [64, 65]. The functions of the HIF2 complex, which consists of HIF2-α and HIF1-β, appear to overlap with those of HIF1, because HIF2-α is also induced by hypoxia. Gene knockdown experiments in human HSCs showed that HIF2-α, but not HIF1-α, is essential for HSC maintenance [66]. Thus, although the precise roles of these HIF complexes in HSC maintenance in vivo are complicated, appropriate regulation of metabolic conditions appears to be important for HSC maintenance. In a mouse CML model, HIF1-α is dispensable for the generation of CML-like disease [67]. However, when the leukemia cells lacking HIF1-α are transplanted into recipient mice, the development of CML in the mice is inhibited, indicating that HIF1 is essential for the maintenance of CML stem cells. Comparison of phenotypes of HIF1-α deficiency between CML and normal hematopoiesis shows that CML stem cell maintenance depends more on HIF1-α than does the maintenance of normal HSCs. These data may be consistent with the fact that the expression of HIF1-α is induced by BCR–ABL1. Thus, HIF1 may be a therapeutic target for CML therapy.

The regulation of lipid metabolism is also important for the maintenance of CML stem cells. The plasma concentration of leukotriene B4 (LTB4), a dihydroxy fatty acid derived from arachidonic acid through the 5-lipoxygenase (5-LO) pathway [68, 69], is increased in a mouse CML model [70]. In CML stem cells, Alox5, an enzyme that synthesizes LTB4 in the 5-LO pathway, is upregulated. Interestingly, the upregulation of *Alox5* in CML stem cells is dependent on BCR–ABL, but not on its enzymatic activity. Experiments with *Alox5*-deficient mice show that Alox5 is essential for the maintenance of CML stem cells, whereas it is dispensable for that of normal HSCs. The pharmacological inhibition of Alox5 by a selective 5-LO inhibitor, zileuton, also reduces CML stem cell number and prolongs survival of CML mice. Another molecule active in lipid metabolism, stearoyl-CoA desaturase-1 (SCD-1), is also involved in CML stem cell maintenance [71]. SCD-1, a key enzyme in fatty acid metabolism, is downregulated in CML stem cells, and its deficiency causes progression of CML disease. Because SCD-1 expression is induced by peroxisome proliferator-activated receptor γ (PPARγ), PPARγ agonists induce SCD-1, resulting in the suppression of CML stem cells.

## 2.5 Microenvironments

The presence of BCR–ABL-expressing cells changes the cytokine and chemokine levels in the BM microenvironment. Cytokines, including IL-1α, IL-1β, IL-6, G-CSF, and TNF-α, and chemokines, including MIP-1α, MIP-1β, and MIP-2, are upregulated in the BM in CML mouse models, and the CXCL12 level is reduced [72]. Some of these altered cytokines and chemokines have an impact on the fate or behavior of stem/progenitor cells in normal hematopoiesis and CML.

The level of IL-6, a proinflammatory cytokine, is elevated in the serum of CML patients [73, 74]. Myeloid-lineage cells in CML secrete IL-6, and the secreted IL-6 acts directly on both leukemic and normal multipotent progenitor cells (MPPs) by a paracrine loop. This biases the lymphoid differentiation of MPPs toward myeloid differentiation, resulting in the expansion of myeloid CML cells. The production of IL-6 by myeloid CML cells is controlled by BCR–ABL, because inhibition of BCR–ABL activity with TKI treatment downregulates the IL-6 expression level. In a study using IL-6 knockout mice, the decrease of IL-6 expression level delayed CML disease onset and restored the lymphoid differentiation, which showed aberrant pro-B cell features.

CXC motif chemokine ligand 12 (CXCL12/stromal cell-derived factor-1 [SDF-1]) and its receptor CXCR4 are important for the maintenance and retention of normal HSCs in BM [75]. During embryogenesis, CXCL12/CXCR4 signaling is essential for homing of HSCs and progenitor cells to BM and for the production of B-lymphoid cells [76, 77]. In adult hematopoiesis, CXCL12/CXCR4 signaling is essential for the maintenance and retention of HSCs in BM and for the production of B-lymphoid cells [78–81]. Whereas CXCR4 is expressed in several hematopoietic cell types, CXCL12 is expressed in stromal cells, osteoblasts, endothelial cells, nestin-expressing cells, and CXCL12 abundant reticular (CAR) cells. Studies of CXCL12 deletion in these CXCL12-expressing cells have demonstrated that CAR cells and endothelial cells function as a niche component. A study of conditional CXCL12 knockout mice showed that CXCL12 regulates the cell cycle status and number of HSCs in BM. Furthermore, treatment of mice with G-CSF reduces the CXCL12 level in BM. This downregulation of CXCL12 decreases HSC retention in BM and induces the mobilization of HSCs into peripheral blood [82]. In BM of both CML model mice and CML patients, increased production of G-CSF by CML cells downregulates CXCL12 [72]. This decrease of CXCL12 level results in the reduced homing of CML stem cells to BM and reduced retention there, leading to enhanced mobilization of CML stem cells into peripheral tissues. Another study reported that imatinib treatment upregulates the CXCR4 expression level in CML cells, suggesting that this signal may contribute to the resistance of CML stem cells to TKI therapy [83]. Thus, although the pathophysiological effects of the CXCR4/CXCL12 pathways on CML stem cells are still unknown, microenvironmental factors mediated by this signal critically affect CML stem cell behavior.

Recently, it was reported that the α-chain of the IL-2 receptor, also known as CD25, is expressed on some CML LICs in a CML mouse model [84]. Furthermore, expression of CD25 was also confirmed in the CML stem cell fraction, but not in the CML progenitor fraction, in patients. Importantly, CD25 is not expressed in healthy HSC and progenitor cells in mouse or human. In human CML patients, CD25 expression is elevated in the accelerated phase and in the blast crisis phase compared with the chronic phase, suggesting that CD25 signaling may contribute to CML progression. Studies using a mouse CML model showed that CML stem cells (FcεRIα$^-$lineage marker$^-$Sca-1$^+$c-Kit$^+$ cells; F$^-$LSK) consisted of two populations of cells, CD25 positive and CD25 negative. Although these cells can interconvert, CD25$^+$F$^-$LSK cells actively proliferate and have higher leukemia initiating capacity than CD25$^-$F$^-$LSK cells. Furthermore, CD25$^+$F$^-$LSK cells secrete higher levels of IL-4, IL-6, IL-13, and TGF-β, supporting the maintenance of CML disease. Although the serum IL-2 level is not elevated in CML mice, CML CD25$^+$F$^-$Lin$^-$ cells colocalize with IL-2$^+$Lin$^+$ cells in BM, suggesting that mature cells may function as niche cells for CML stem cells with the support of the IL-2/CD25 pathway. Administration of IL-2 to CML mice accelerates their death, and human IL-2 increases the colony-forming capacity of human CML samples. In contrast, genetic ablation of *IL2ra* or administration of a monoclonal antibody against CD25 or IL-2 increases the survival of CML mice. Thus, the IL-2/CD25 axis contributes to the maintenance of CML stem cells and progression. Moreover, the combination of TKI and anti-CD25 antibody treatments reduces the numbers of CML cells, including CML stem cells, in BM and spleen. Therefore, the IL-2/CD25 axis is expected to be a direct therapeutic target for the eradication of CML stem cells.

TGF-β signals are involved in the quiescence of HSCs [48, 85]. Glial cells play a critical role in the activation of latent TGF-β, supporting the quiescent status of HSCs in BM. Although HSCs lose their stem cell properties when FOXO proteins are inactivated during in vitro culture with cytokines, TGF-β can keep HSCs quiescent without a loss of biologic potential; this is associated with the nuclear localization of FOXO3a, indicating that TGF-β may regulate HSC function through FOXO activity. CML stem cells also exhibit activated Smad-2/Smad-3 in vivo [52]. Treatment with a TGF-β inhibitor in vivo induces relocation of FOXO3a into the cytoplasm and sensitizes CML stem cells to TKI therapy in CML-bearing mice. However, another study reported that the overexpression of TGF-β observed in transgenic mice that express the receptor for parathyroid hormone in osteoblastic cells also results in the suppression of CML stem cells [86]. These data suggest that the roles of TGF-β are complicated and that fine-tuning of the TGF-β signal may be important for supporting CML stem cell maintenance. Although it is unclear whether TGF-β affects CML stem cells directly or indirectly, manipulation of this signal may contribute to the development of a therapeutic approach for CML patients.

## 2.6 Epigenetic Modification

Multistep process of cell differentiation is controlled by epigenetic mechanisms [13]. Epigenetics is a regulatory mechanism by which gene expression is increased or decreased by DNA methylation or posttranslational modification of histone core proteins. Histone modifications of acetylation, methylation, and phosphorylation are involved in changes in the ability of regulatory transcription machinery proteins to access the chromatin of genomic DNA, thereby controlling gene expression. Histone deacetylation is involved in the maintenance of CML stem cells, and histone deacetylase (HDAC) inhibitors have been developed and are recognized as promising medications for CML disease. Treatment of CML stem cells with HDAC inhibitors increases the acetylation levels of H3 and H4 [87]. Treatment of CML stem cells with HDAC inhibitors or imatinib decreases phosphorylation of BCR–ABL, and the combination further suppresses the phosphorylation, leading to apoptosis. Interestingly, the combination induces more apoptosis in CML stem cells than in normal HSC and progenitor cells. HDAC inhibitors efficiently reduce the number of CML stem cells in vivo in mouse CML models or mouse models using xenografts of human CML cells. Gene expression profile analyses show that HDAC inhibitor treatment reduces sets of genes regulating the undifferentiated state (e.g., the Hox–Myc and Wnt-related pathways), cell cycle regulation, protein translation, and the cellular stress response. E2F, Ying Yang 1, and NRF1/2 are reduced, whereas G protein-coupled receptors are increased. Thus, modifications of histone acetylation are critical for the expression of a variety of genes that are involved in CML stem cell maintenance.

SIRT1 is a mammalian homologue of yeast silent information regulator 2 (Sir2), and both are NAD-dependent histone deacetylases. SIRT1 functions as a histone deacetylase of histones H4K16 and H1K26 and thus regulates chromatin modification. However, it also deacetylates numerous nonhistone proteins that are involved in transcription, cell cycle, and DNA repair. SIRT1 is upregulated by BCR–ABL via the activation of STAT5; therefore, SIRT1 expression in CML stem cells is higher than in HSCs [88, 89]. Consistent with this, SIRT1 plays critical roles in the generation and maintenance of CML stem cells, although the precise role of SIRT1 in normal HSCs is controversial. In a mouse model in which the BCR–ABL gene is introduced into hematopoietic cells, SIRT1 deficiency suppresses CML. Whereas mice receiving BCR–ABL-transformed wild-type BM cells develop CML disease within 3–4 weeks, disease development is significantly delayed in mice receiving cells derived from SIRT1-deficient BM cells. In human CML stem cells, knockdown of SIRT1 induces apoptosis and inhibits proliferation. Pharmacological inhibition of SIRT1 enhances sensitivity of CML stem cells to imatinib-induced apoptosis, but it does not remarkably affect normal HSC/progenitor cells. SIRT1 inhibition enhances acetylation of p53, which induces its transcriptional activity, leading to fewer CML stem cells. Interestingly, SIRT1 is also involved in the acquisition of genetic mutations in the BCR–ABL gene induced by imatinib treatment [90]. When KCL22 cells, a human CML cell line, were treated with imatinib, the cells initially died from apoptosis, followed by regrowth after 2 weeks in vitro subsequent to the acquisition of a BCR–ABL mutation. However, inhibition of SIRT1 inhibited the imatinib resistance. In contrast, inhibitors of class I and II HDAC, such as trichostatin A, did not show such inhibitory effects on imatinib resistance. SIRT1 inhibitors, but not class I/II HDAC inhibitors, also suppress γH2AX focus formation induced by DNA damage-inducing reagents. Furthermore, DNA damage repair pathways are affected by SIRT1 through the acetylation of Ku70, which is involved in nonhomologous end joining, and NBS1, which mediates homologous recombination, generating gene mutations. Thus, although it is unknown whether histone modification by SIRT1 is involved in regulating CML stem cell behavior, this molecule is essential for the maintenance of CML stem cells.

## 2.7 Kinase Activity-Independent BCR–ABL Signals

CML stem cells are able to survive TKI treatment, despite expressing higher levels of BCR–ABL than other subpopulations [24]. For example, when the TKI inhibition of BCR–ABL activity was evaluated by analyzing the inhibition of Crk-like protein (CrkL) phosphorylation, CrkL phosphorylation was inhibited in CML stem cells and progenitors to a similar degree, and CML stem cells treated with imatinib showed cell growth and survival comparable to those of HSCs; however, imatinib had remarkable effects on cell cycle arrest and apoptosis in CML progenitors [91]. These data indicate that CML stem cells are insensitive to TKI. One of the explanations is the presence of signaling pathways that are activated by BCR–ABL in a manner independent of its kinase activity. Although, as described above, Alox5 is upregulated by BCR–ABL, this upregulation is not prevented by TKI treatment, indicating that BCR–ABL controls CML stem cells via Alox5 independently of its kinase activity [70]. BCR–ABL also suppresses protein phosphatase 2A (PP2A), which activates β-catenin independently of its kinase activity [92]. The phosphatase activity of PPA2 in CML stem cells is lower than that in normal HSCs, due to higher expression of an endogenous PP2A inhibitor, SET. A chemical compound, FTY720, inhibits the association of SET with the catalytic subunit of PP2A, causing the activation of PP2A. The activation of PP2A by FTY720 or PP2A overexpression induces apoptosis in CML stem cells, whereas it does not affect normal HSCs, because the effect requires BCR–ABL. Therefore, PP2A-activating drugs are expected to be effective for targeting TKI-refractory CML stem cells.

## 2.8 Conclusion

Accumulating evidence indicates that CML stem cells are maintained by multiple signals. Some of the signals are involved in normal HSCs, indicating that CML stem cells and HSCs have similar properties. Therefore, we believe that increased knowledge of stem cell biology will accelerate progress in leukemia research. At the same time, detailed analyses have revealed the presence of molecules or signals that contribute to the maintenance of CML stem cells but not HSCs, providing an ideal therapeutic window. Future studies on CML stem cells are sure to give rise to new concepts in CML therapy.

## References

1. Ren R. Mechanisms of BCR-ABL in the pathogenesis of chronic myelogenous leukaemia. Nat Rev Cancer. 2005;5(3):172–83. doi:10.1038/nrc1567. nrc1567 [pii].
2. Quintas-Cardama A, Cortes J. Molecular biology of bcr-abl1-positive chronic myeloid leukemia. Blood. 2009;113(8):1619–30. doi:10.1182/blood-2008-03-144790.
3. Naka K, Hoshii T, Tadokoro Y, Hirao A. Molecular pathology of tumor-initiating cells: lessons from Philadelphia chromosome-positive leukemia. Pathol Int. 2011;61(9):501–8. doi:10.1111/j.1440-1827.2011.02688.x.
4. O'Hare T, Deininger MW, Eide CA, Clackson T, Druker BJ. Targeting the BCR-ABL signaling pathway in therapy-resistant Philadelphia chromosome-positive leukemia. Clin Cancer Res Off J Am Assoc Cancer Res. 2011;17(2):212–21. doi:10.1158/1078-0432.CCR-09-3314.
5. Reya T, Clevers H. Wnt signalling in stem cells and cancer. Nature. 2005;434(7035):843–50. doi:10.1038/nature03319.
6. Matsumoto A, Nakayama KI. Role of key regulators of the cell cycle in maintenance of hematopoietic stem cells. Biochim Biophys Acta. 2013;1830(2):2335–44. doi:10.1016/j.bbagen.2012.07.004.
7. Shyh-Chang N, Daley GQ, Cantley LC. Stem cell metabolism in tissue development and aging. Development. 2013;140(12):2535–47. doi:10.1242/dev.091777.
8. Kfoury Y, Mercier F, Scadden DT. SnapShot: the hematopoietic stem cell niche. Cell. 2014;158(1):228–228.e1. doi:10.1016/j.cell.2014.06.019.
9. Oh J, Lee YD, Wagers AJ. Stem cell aging: mechanisms, regulators and therapeutic opportunities. Nat Med. 2014;20(8):870–80. doi:10.1038/nm.3651. nm.3651 [pii].
10. Cheng CW, Adams GB, Perin L, Wei M, Zhou X, Lam BS, et al. Prolonged fasting reduces IGF-1/PKA to promote hematopoietic-stem-cell-based regeneration and reverse immunosuppression. Cell Stem Cell. 2014;14(6):810–23. doi:10.1016/j.stem.2014.04.014. S1934-5909(14)00151-9 [pii].
11. Mihaylova MM, Sabatini DM, Yilmaz OH. Dietary and metabolic control of stem cell function in physiology and cancer. Cell Stem Cell. 2014;14(3):292–305. doi:10.1016/j.stem.2014.02.008. S1934-5909(14)00059-9 [pii].
12. Nakada D, Levi BP, Morrison SJ. Integrating physiological regulation with stem cell and tissue homeostasis. Neuron. 2011;70(4):703–18. doi:10.1016/j.neuron.2011.05.011. S0896-6273(11)00392-8 [pii].
13. Cedar H, Bergman Y. Epigenetics of haematopoietic cell development. Nat Rev Immunol. 2011;11(7):478–88. doi:10.1038/nri2991.

14. Logan CY, Nusse R. The Wnt signaling pathway in development and disease. Annu Rev Cell Dev Biol. 2004;20:781–810. doi:10.1146/annurev.cellbio.20.010403.113126.
15. Reya T, Duncan AW, Ailles L, Domen J, Scherer DC, Willert K, et al. A role for Wnt signalling in self-renewal of haematopoietic stem cells. Nature. 2003;423(6938):409–14. doi:10.1038/nature01593.
16. Willert K, Brown JD, Danenberg E, Duncan AW, Weissman IL, Reya T, et al. Wnt proteins are lipid-modified and can act as stem cell growth factors. Nature. 2003;423(6938):448–52. doi:10.1038/nature01611.
17. Van Den Berg DJ, Sharma AK, Bruno E, Hoffman R. Role of members of the Wnt gene family in human hematopoiesis. Blood. 1998;92(9):3189–202.
18. Rattis FM, Voermans C, Reya T. Wnt signaling in the stem cell niche. Curr Opin Hematol. 2004;11(2):88–94.
19. Cobas M, Wilson A, Ernst B, Mancini SJ, MacDonald HR, Kemler R, et al. Beta-catenin is dispensable for hematopoiesis and lymphopoiesis. J Exp Med. 2004;199(2):221–9. doi:10.1084/jem.20031615.
20. Malhotra S, Kincade PW. Wnt-related molecules and signaling pathway equilibrium in hematopoiesis. Cell Stem Cell. 2009;4(1):27–36. doi:10.1016/j.stem.2008.12.004.
21. Muller-Tidow C, Steffen B, Cauvet T, Tickenbrock L, Ji P, Diederichs S, et al. Translocation products in acute myeloid leukemia activate the Wnt signaling pathway in hematopoietic cells. Mol Cell Biol. 2004;24(7):2890–904.
22. Wang Y, Krivtsov AV, Sinha AU, North TE, Goessling W, Feng Z, et al. The Wnt/beta-catenin pathway is required for the development of leukemia stem cells in AML. Science. 2010;327(5973):1650–3. doi:10.1126/science.1186624.
23. Yeung J, Esposito MT, Gandillet A, Zeisig BB, Griessinger E, Bonnet D, et al. Beta-Catenin mediates the establishment and drug resistance of MLL leukemic stem cells. Cancer Cell. 2010;18(6):606–18. doi:10.1016/j.ccr.2010.10.032.
24. Jamieson CH, Ailles LE, Dylla SJ, Muijtjens M, Jones C, Zehnder JL, et al. Granulocyte-macrophage progenitors as candidate leukemic stem cells in blast-crisis CML. N Engl J Med. 2004;351(7):657–67.
25. Heidel FH, Bullinger L, Feng Z, Wang Z, Neff TA, Stein L, et al. Genetic and pharmacologic inhibition of beta-catenin targets imatinib-resistant leukemia stem cells in CML. Cell Stem Cell. 2012;10(4):412–24. doi:10.1016/j.stem.2012.02.017.
26. Ng JM, Curran T. The Hedgehog's tale: developing strategies for targeting cancer. Nat Rev Cancer. 2011;11(7):493–501. doi:10.1038/nrc3079.
27. Mar BG, Amakye D, Aifantis I, Buonamici S. The controversial role of the Hedgehog pathway in normal and malignant hematopoiesis. Leukemia. 2011;25(11):1665–73. doi:10.1038/leu.2011.143.
28. Cridland SO, Keys JR, Papathanasiou P, Perkins AC. Indian hedgehog supports definitive erythropoiesis. Blood Cells Mol Dis. 2009;43(2):149–55. doi:10.1016/j.bcmd.2009.04.004.
29. Trowbridge JJ, Scott MP, Bhatia M. Hedgehog modulates cell cycle regulators in stem cells to control hematopoietic regeneration. Proc Natl Acad Sci U S A. 2006;103(38):14134–9. doi:10.1073/pnas.0604568103.
30. Hofmann I, Stover EH, Cullen DE, Mao J, Morgan KJ, Lee BH, et al. Hedgehog signaling is dispensable for adult murine hematopoietic stem cell function and hematopoiesis. Cell Stem Cell. 2009;4(6):559–67. doi:10.1016/j.stem.2009.03.016.
31. Gao J, Graves S, Koch U, Liu S, Jankovic V, Buonamici S, et al. Hedgehog signaling is dispensable for adult hematopoietic stem cell function. Cell Stem Cell. 2009;4(6):548–58. doi:10.1016/j.stem.2009.03.015.
32. Zhao C, Chen A, Jamieson CH, Fereshteh M, Abrahamsson A, Blum J, et al. Hedgehog signalling is essential for maintenance of cancer stem cells in myeloid leukaemia. Nature. 2009;458(7239):776–9. doi:10.1038/nature07737.

33. Dierks C, Beigi R, Guo GR, Zirlik K, Stegert MR, Manley P, et al. Expansion of Bcr-Abl-positive leukemic stem cells is dependent on Hedgehog pathway activation. Cancer Cell. 2008;14(3):238–49. doi:10.1016/j.ccr.2008.08.003.
34. Nakayama KI, Nakayama K. Ubiquitin ligases: cell-cycle control and cancer. Nat Rev Cancer. 2006;6(5):369–81. doi:10.1038/nrc1881. nrc1881 [pii].
35. Matsuoka S, Oike Y, Onoyama I, Iwama A, Arai F, Takubo K, et al. Fbxw7 acts as a critical fail-safe against premature loss of hematopoietic stem cells and development of T-ALL. Genes Dev. 2008;22(8):986–91. doi:10.1101/gad.1621808. gad.1621808 [pii].
36. Thompson BJ, Jankovic V, Gao J, Buonamici S, Vest A, Lee JM, et al. Control of hematopoietic stem cell quiescence by the E3 ubiquitin ligase Fbw7. J Exp Med. 2008;205 (6):1395–408. doi:10.1084/jem.20080277. jem.20080277 [pii].
37. Wilson A, Murphy MJ, Oskarsson T, Kaloulis K, Bettess MD, Oser GM, et al. c-Myc controls the balance between hematopoietic stem cell self-renewal and differentiation. Genes Dev. 2004;18(22):2747–63. doi:10.1101/gad.313104. 18/22/2747 [pii].
38. Reavie L, Della Gatta G, Crusio K, Aranda-Orgilles B, Buckley SM, Thompson B, et al. Regulation of hematopoietic stem cell differentiation by a single ubiquitin ligase-substrate complex. Nat Immunol. 2010;11(3):207–15. doi:10.1038/ni.1839. ni.1839 [pii].
39. Daksis JI, Lu RY, Facchini LM, Marhin WW, Penn LJ. Myc induces cyclin D1 expression in the absence of de novo protein synthesis and links mitogen-stimulated signal transduction to the cell cycle. Oncogene. 1994;9(12):3635–45.
40. Dauphinot L, De Oliveira C, Melot T, Sevenet N, Thomas V, Weissman BE, et al. Analysis of the expression of cell cycle regulators in Ewing cell lines: EWS-FLI-1 modulates p57KIP2 and c-Myc expression. Oncogene. 2001;20(25):3258–65. doi:10.1038/sj.onc.1204437.
41. Leone G, Sears R, Huang E, Rempel R, Nuckolls F, Park CH, et al. Myc requires distinct E2F activities to induce S phase and apoptosis. Mol Cell. 2001;8(1):105–13. S1097-2765(01) 00275-1 [pii].
42. Iriuchishima H, Takubo K, Matsuoka S, Onoyama I, Nakayama KI, Nojima Y, et al. Ex vivo maintenance of hematopoietic stem cells by quiescence induction through Fbxw7α overexpression. Blood. 2011;117(8):2373–7. doi:10.1182/blood-2010-07-294801. blood-2010-07-294801 [pii].
43. Takeishi S, Nakayama KI. Role of Fbxw7 in the maintenance of normal stem cells and cancer-initiating cells. Br J Cancer. 2014;111(6):1054–9. doi:10.1038/bjc.2014.259. bjc2014259 [pii].
44. Reavie L, Buckley SM, Loizou E, Takeishi S, Aranda-Orgilles B, Ndiaye-Lobry D, et al. Regulation of c-Myc ubiquitination controls chronic myelogenous leukemia initiation and progression. Cancer Cell. 2013;23(3):362–75. doi:10.1016/j.ccr.2013.01.025. S1535-6108 (13)00044-5 [pii].
45. Takeishi S, Matsumoto A, Onoyama I, Naka K, Hirao A, Nakayama KI. Ablation of Fbxw7 eliminates leukemia-initiating cells by preventing quiescence. Cancer Cell. 2013;23 (3):347–61. doi:10.1016/j.ccr.2013.01.026. S1535-6108(13)00045-7 [pii].
46. Lam EW, Brosens JJ, Gomes AR, Koo CY. Forkhead box proteins: tuning forks for transcriptional harmony. Nat Rev Cancer. 2013;13(7):482–95. doi:10.1038/nrc3539.
47. Greer EL, Brunet A. FOXO transcription factors at the interface between longevity and tumor suppression. Oncogene. 2005;24(50):7410–25.
48. Yamazaki S, Iwama A, Takayanagi SI, Eto K, Ema H, Nakauchi H. TGF-beta as a candidate bone marrow niche signal to induce hematopoietic stem cell hibernation. Blood. 2009;113 (6):1250–6. doi:10.1182/blood-2008-04-146480. blood-2008-04-146480 [pii].
49. Miyamoto K, Araki KY, Naka K, Arai F, Takubo K, Yamazaki S, et al. Foxo3a is essential for maintenance of the hematopoietic stem cell pool. Cell Stem Cell. 2007;1(1):101–12.
50. Yalcin S, Zhang X, Luciano JP, Mungamuri SK, Marinkovic D, Vercherat C, et al. Foxo3 is essential for the regulation of ataxia telangiectasia mutated and oxidative stress-mediated homeostasis of hematopoietic stem cells. J Biol Chem. 2008;283(37):25692–705. doi:10.1074/jbc.M800517200. M800517200 [pii].

51. Tothova Z, Kollipara R, Huntly BJ, Lee BH, Castrillon DH, Cullen DE, et al. FoxOs are critical mediators of hematopoietic stem cell resistance to physiologic oxidative stress. Cell. 2007;128(2):325–39.
52. Naka K, Hoshii T, Muraguchi T, Tadokoro Y, Ooshio T, Kondo Y, et al. TGF-β-FOXO signalling maintains leukaemia-initiating cells in chronic myeloid leukaemia. Nature. 2010;463(7281):676–80.
53. Pellicano F, Scott MT, Helgason GV, Hopcroft LE, Allan EK, Aspinall-O'Dea M, et al. The antiproliferative activity of kinase inhibitors in chronic myeloid leukemia cells is mediated by FOXO transcription factors. Stem Cells. 2014;32(9):2324–37. doi:10.1002/stem.1748.
54. Duy C, Hurtz C, Shojaee S, Cerchietti L, Geng H, Swaminathan S, et al. BCL6 enables Ph + acute lymphoblastic leukaemia cells to survive BCR-ABL1 kinase inhibition. Nature. 2011;473(7347):384–8. doi:10.1038/nature09883.
55. Hurtz C, Hatzi K, Cerchietti L, Braig M, Park E, Kim YM, et al. BCL6-mediated repression of p53 is critical for leukemia stem cell survival in chronic myeloid leukemia. J Exp Med. 2011;208(11):2163–74. doi:10.1084/jem.20110304.
56. Ahmad KF, Melnick A, Lax S, Bouchard D, Liu J, Kiang CL, et al. Mechanism of SMRT corepressor recruitment by the BCL6 BTB domain. Mol Cell. 2003;12(6):1551–64.
57. Bernardi R, Pandolfi PP. Structure, dynamics and functions of promyelocytic leukaemia nuclear bodies. Nat Rev Mol Cell Biol. 2007;8(12):1006–16. doi:10.1038/nrm2277. nrm2277 [pii].
58. Ito K, Bernardi R, Morotti A, Matsuoka S, Saglio G, Ikeda Y, et al. PML targeting eradicates quiescent leukaemia-initiating cells. Nature. 2008;453(7198):1072–8. doi:10.1038/nature07016. nature07016 [pii].
59. Bernardi R, Guernah I, Jin D, Grisendi S, Alimonti A, Teruya-Feldstein J, et al. PML inhibits HIF-1alpha translation and neoangiogenesis through repression of mTOR. Nature. 2006;442(7104):779–85. doi:10.1038/nature05029.
60. Semenza GL. Hypoxia-inducible factors in physiology and medicine. Cell. 2012;148(3):399–408. doi:10.1016/j.cell.2012.01.021.
61. Simsek T, Kocabas F, Zheng J, Deberardinis RJ, Mahmoud AI, Olson EN, et al. The distinct metabolic profile of hematopoietic stem cells reflects their location in a hypoxic niche. Cell Stem Cell. 2010;7(3):380–90. doi:10.1016/j.stem.2010.07.011.
62. Kocabas F, Zheng J, Thet S, Copeland NG, Jenkins NA, DeBerardinis RJ, et al. Meis1 regulates the metabolic phenotype and oxidant defense of hematopoietic stem cells. Blood. 2012;120(25):4963–72. doi:10.1182/blood-2012-05-432260.
63. Takubo K, Goda N, Yamada W, Iriuchishima H, Ikeda E, Kubota Y, et al. Regulation of the HIF-1alpha level is essential for hematopoietic stem cells. Cell Stem Cell. 2010;7(3):391–402. doi:10.1016/j.stem.2010.06.020.
64. Imanirad P, Solaimani Kartalaei P, Crisan M, Vink C, Yamada-Inagawa T, de Pater E, et al. HIF1alpha is a regulator of hematopoietic progenitor and stem cell development in hypoxic sites of the mouse embryo. Stem Cell Res. 2014;12(1):24–35. doi:10.1016/j.scr.2013.09.006.
65. Guitart AV, Subramani C, Armesilla-Diaz A, Smith G, Sepulveda C, Gezer D, et al. Hif-2alpha is not essential for cell-autonomous hematopoietic stem cell maintenance. Blood. 2013;122(10):1741–5. doi:10.1182/blood-2013-02-484923.
66. Rouault-Pierre K, Lopez-Onieva L, Foster K, Anjos-Afonso F, Lamrissi-Garcia I, Serrano-Sanchez M, et al. HIF-2alpha protects human hematopoietic stem/progenitors and acute myeloid leukemic cells from apoptosis induced by endoplasmic reticulum stress. Cell Stem Cell. 2013;13(5):549–63. doi:10.1016/j.stem.2013.08.011.
67. Zhang H, Li H, Xi HS, Li S. HIF1alpha is required for survival maintenance of chronic myeloid leukemia stem cells. Blood. 2012;119(11):2595–607. doi:10.1182/blood-2011-10-387381.

68. Radmark O, Werz O, Steinhilber D, Samuelsson B. 5-Lipoxygenase: regulation of expression and enzyme activity. Trends Biochem Sci. 2007;32(7):332–41. doi:10.1016/j.tibs.2007.06.002. S0968-0004(07)00144-2 [pii].
69. Wymann MP, Schneiter R. Lipid signalling in disease. Nat Rev Mol Cell Biol. 2008;9(2):162–76. doi:10.1038/nrm2335. nrm2335 [pii].
70. Chen Y, Hu Y, Zhang H, Peng C, Li S. Loss of the Alox5 gene impairs leukemia stem cells and prevents chronic myeloid leukemia. Nat Genet. 2009;41(7):783–92. doi:10.1038/ng.389. ng.389 [pii].
71. Zhang H, Li H, Ho N, Li D, Li S. Scd1 plays a tumor-suppressive role in survival of leukemia stem cells and the development of chronic myeloid leukemia. Mol Cell Biol. 2012;32(10):1776–87. doi:10.1128/MCB.05672-11.
72. Zhang B, Ho YW, Huang Q, Maeda T, Lin A, Lee SU, et al. Altered microenvironmental regulation of leukemic and normal stem cells in chronic myelogenous leukemia. Cancer Cell. 2012;21(4):577–92. doi:10.1016/j.ccr.2012.02.018. S1535-6108(12)00080-3 [pii].
73. Anand M, Chodda SK, Parikh PM, Nadkarni JS. Abnormal levels of proinflammatory cytokines in serum and monocyte cultures from patients with chronic myeloid leukemia in different stages, and their role in prognosis. Hematol Oncol. 1998;16(4):143–54. doi:10.1002/(SICI)1099-1069(199812). 16:4<143::AID-HON628>3.0.CO;2-U [pii].
74. Reynaud D, Pietras E, Barry-Holson K, Mir A, Binnewies M, Jeanne M, et al. IL-6 controls leukemic multipotent progenitor cell fate and contributes to chronic myelogenous leukemia development. Cancer Cell. 2011;20(5):661–73. doi:10.1016/j.ccr.2011.10.012. S1535-6108(11)00396-5 [pii].
75. Nagasawa T. CXC chemokine ligand 12 (CXCL12) and its receptor CXCR4. J Mol Med (Berl). 2014;92(5):433–9. doi:10.1007/s00109-014-1123-8.
76. Ara T, Nakamura Y, Egawa T, Sugiyama T, Abe K, Kishimoto T, et al. Impaired colonization of the gonads by primordial germ cells in mice lacking a chemokine, stromal cell-derived factor-1 (SDF-1). Proc Natl Acad Sci U S A. 2003;100(9):5319–23. doi:10.1073/pnas.0730719100. 0730719100 [pii].
77. Nagasawa T, Hirota S, Tachibana K, Takakura N, Nishikawa S, Kitamura Y, et al. Defects of B-cell lymphopoiesis and bone-marrow myelopoiesis in mice lacking the CXC chemokine PBSF/SDF-1. Nature. 1996;382(6592):635–8. doi:10.1038/382635a0.
78. Sugiyama T, Kohara H, Noda M, Nagasawa T. Maintenance of the hematopoietic stem cell pool by CXCL12-CXCR4 chemokine signaling in bone marrow stromal cell niches. Immunity. 2006;25(6):977–88. doi:10.1016/j.immuni.2006.10.016. S1074-7613(06)00515-2 [pii].
79. Tzeng YS, Li H, Kang YL, Chen WC, Cheng WC, Lai DM. Loss of Cxcl12/Sdf-1 in adult mice decreases the quiescent state of hematopoietic stem/progenitor cells and alters the pattern of hematopoietic regeneration after myelosuppression. Blood. 2011;117(2):429–39. doi:10.1182/blood-2010-01-266833. blood-2010-01-266833 [pii].
80. Greenbaum A, Hsu YM, Day RB, Schuettpelz LG, Christopher MJ, Borgerding JN, et al. CXCL12 in early mesenchymal progenitors is required for haematopoietic stem-cell maintenance. Nature. 2013;495(7440):227–30. doi:10.1038/nature11926. nature11926 [pii].
81. Ding L, Morrison SJ. Haematopoietic stem cells and early lymphoid progenitors occupy distinct bone marrow niches. Nature. 2013;495(7440):231–5. doi:10.1038/nature11885. nature11885 [pii].
82. Petit I, Szyper-Kravitz M, Nagler A, Lahav M, Peled A, Habler L, et al. G-CSF induces stem cell mobilization by decreasing bone marrow SDF-1 and up-regulating CXCR4. Nat Immunol. 2002;3(7):687–94. doi:10.1038/ni813.
83. Jin L, Tabe Y, Konoplev S, Xu Y, Leysath CE, Lu H, et al. CXCR4 up-regulation by imatinib induces chronic myelogenous leukemia (CML) cell migration to bone marrow stroma and promotes survival of quiescent CML cells. Mol Cancer Ther. 2008;7(1):48–58. doi:10.1158/1535-7163.MCT-07-0042. 7/1/48 [pii].

84. Kobayashi CI, Takubo K, Kobayashi H, Nakamura-Ishizu A, Honda H, Kataoka K, et al. The IL-2/CD25 axis maintains distinct subsets of chronic myeloid leukemia-initiating cells. Blood. 2014;123(16):2540–9. doi:10.1182/blood-2013-07-517847. blood-2013-07-517847 [pii].
85. Yamazaki S, Ema H, Karlsson G, Yamaguchi T, Miyoshi H, Shioda S, et al. Nonmyelinating Schwann cells maintain hematopoietic stem cell hibernation in the bone marrow niche. Cell. 2011;147(5):1146–58. doi:10.1016/j.cell.2011.09.053.
86. Krause DS, Fulzele K, Catic A, Sun CC, Dombkowski D, Hurley MP, et al. Differential regulation of myeloid leukemias by the bone marrow microenvironment. Nat Med. 2013;19 (11):1513–7. doi:10.1038/nm.3364.
87. Zhang B, Strauss AC, Chu S, Li M, Ho Y, Shiang KD, et al. Effective targeting of quiescent chronic myelogenous leukemia stem cells by histone deacetylase inhibitors in combination with imatinib mesylate. Cancer Cell. 2010;17(5):427–42. doi:10.1016/j.ccr.2010.03.011.
88. Li L, Wang L, Wang Z, Ho Y, McDonald T, Holyoake TL, et al. Activation of p53 by SIRT1 inhibition enhances elimination of CML leukemia stem cells in combination with imatinib. Cancer Cell. 2012;21(2):266–81. doi:10.1016/j.ccr.2011.12.020.
89. Yuan H, Wang Z, Li L, Zhang H, Modi H, Horne D, et al. Activation of stress response gene SIRT1 by BCR-ABL promotes leukemogenesis. Blood. 2012;119(8):1904–14. doi:10.1182/blood-2011-06-361691.
90. Wang Z, Yuan H, Roth M, Stark JM, Bhatia R, Chen WY. SIRT1 deacetylase promotes acquisition of genetic mutations for drug resistance in CML cells. Oncogene. 2013;32 (5):589–98. doi:10.1038/onc.2012.83.
91. Corbin AS, Agarwal A, Loriaux M, Cortes J, Deininger MW, Druker BJ. Human chronic myeloid leukemia stem cells are insensitive to imatinib despite inhibition of BCR-ABL activity. J Clin Invest. 2011;121(1):396–409. doi:10.1172/JCI35721.
92. Neviani P, Harb JG, Oaks JJ, Santhanam R, Walker CJ, Ellis JJ, et al. PP2A-activating drugs selectively eradicate TKI-resistant chronic myeloid leukemic stem cells. J Clin Invest. 2013;123(10):4144–57. doi:10.1172/JCI68951.

# Chapter 3
# Roles for Signaling Molecules in the Growth and Survival of CML Cells

**Itaru Matsumura**

**Abstract** Chronic myelogenous leukemia (CML) is caused by the reciprocal chromosomal translocation t(9:22)(q34;q11). This translocation yields *BCR-ABL* fusion gene on derivative chromosome 22 called as Philadelphia (Ph) chromosome. Although several forms of BCR-ABL are generated according to the breakpoints in the BCR gene, p210 BCR-ABL is observed in more than 95 % of CML patients. In contrast to the nuclear localization of c-ABL, BCR-ABL is localized in the cytoplasm and acts as a constitutively active tyrosine kinase as a tetramer. BCR-ABL has several functional domains, through which it interacts with downstream signaling molecules and transmits leukemogenic signals: a coiled-coil motif, SH2 domain, Y177, and Dbl homology domain from BCR and SH3, SH2, SH1(kinase), CRKL-binding, and actin-binding domains from c-ABL. Through these domains, BCR-ABL activates Ras/MAPK, PI3K/Akt, and STATs, each of which contributes to excessive cell growth, survival, and consequent leukemic transformation. In addition, SHP-2, c-Cbl, Gab2, and CRKL are involved in the leukemogenic activities of BCR-ABL. Although tyrosine kinase inhibitors (TKIs) have dramatically improved the prognosis of CML patients in chronic phase, a small proportion of patients show resistance to TKIs due to point mutations of the *BCR-ABL* gene and/or BCR-ABL-independent activation of Src family tyrosine kinases such as Lyn and HCK. In addition, CML stem cells are known to resistant to TKIs, in which JAK2, Wnt/β-catenin, and Sonic hedgehog pathways are activated in a BCR-ABL independent manner and contribute to TKI resistance.

**Keywords** BCR-ABL • Ras/MAPK • PI3K/Akt • Wnt/β-catenin • Sonic Hedgehog

---

I. Matsumura (✉)
Department of Hematology and Rheumatology, Kinki University, 377-2 Ohno-Higashi, Osaka-Sayama, Osaka 589-8511, Japan
e-mail: imatsumura@med.kindai.ac.jp



M. Kizaki (ed.), *Molecular Pathogenesis and Treatment of Chronic Myelogenous Leukemia*, DOI 10.1007/978-4-431-55714-2_3

## 3.1 Introduction

Chronic myelogenous leukemia (CML) is a malignant clonal disorder, which arises from hematopoietic stem cells (HSCs) harboring the reciprocal chromosomal translocation t(9:22)(q34;q11). The derivative chromosome 22 resulting from this translocation, which is called as Philadelphia (Ph) chromosome, is observed in more than 95 % of typical CML patients and utilized as a diagnostic hallmark of CML. This translocation joins c-*Abl* tyrosine kinase gene on chromosome 9 and breakpoint cluster region (*BCR*) gene on chromosome 22, leading to the generation of the fusion gene *BCR-ABL* on Ph chromosome. This fusion gene acts as a constitutively active tyrosine kinase and activates downstream pathways. A number of previous papers showed that overexpression of *BCR-ABL* in HSCs by retrovirus introduction or its transgenic mice causes CML-like disease in mouse models. In addition, the dramatic improvement of clinical outcomes of CML patients by the advent of tyrosine kinase inhibitors (TKIs) such as imatinib, nilotinib, and dasatinib provided clinical evidence that BCR-ABL is a main causative abnormality of CML. In this paper, I will review the functions of BCR-ABL and its downstream signaling molecules in the pathogenesis of CML.

## 3.2 Structure of BCR-ABL

As a result of the chromosomal translocation t(9:22)(q34;q11), three types of fusion genes, p210, p190, and p230 BCR-ABL, are generated according to the difference in the breakpoint in the *BCR* gene (Fig. 3.1). p210 BCR-ABL is generated from

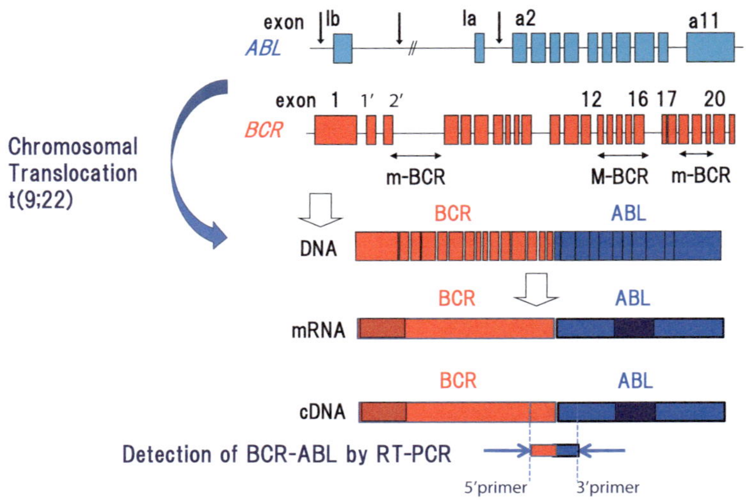


**Fig. 3.1** Formation of BCR-AB fusion gene by reciprocal chromosomal translocation t(9;22) and their breakpoints

translocations with the breakpoints ranging about 5.8 kb from exon 12 to exon 16 in the *BCR* gene, which is called as a major breakpoint cluster region (M-BCR). Meanwhile, the breakpoints in the minor BCR (m-BCR) yield p190 BCR-ABL and those in μ-BCR generate p230 BCR-ABL. p210 BCR-ABL is observed in more than 95 % of CML patients and in about 30–40 % of acute lymphoblastic leukemia (ALL) patients, while p190 BCR-ABL and p230 BCR-ABL are mainly observed in ALL and chronic neutrophilic leukemia (CNL), respectively. However, it still remains unknown how these three forms of BCR-ABL cause distinct disease types through their downstream signalings.

There are several functional domains in BCR-ABL, through which it interacts with downstream signaling molecules and transmits leukemogenic signals (Fig. 3.2). The N-terminal domain of BCR consisting from 63 amino acids with a coiled-coil motif induces tetramerization of BCR-ABL, which is essential for its biologic and leukemogenic activities [1–4]. In addition, Y177 was shown to be phosphorylated and interact with the SH2 domain of Grb2, leading to SHP-2 and Ras activation as described below. Because BCR-ABL harboring a point mutation at Y177 to phenylalanine (Y177F) can't transform fibroblasts [5], Y177 is supposed to be one of the key sites for transforming activity of BCR-ABL through SHP-2 and/or Ras/mitogen-activated protein kinase (MAPK; also called as an extracellular signal-regulated kinase, ERK) pathways. However, this mutant BCR-ABL still could confer factor-independent growth on hematopoietic cells [6]. So, the roles of Y177 would be somewhat different between fibroblasts and hematopoietic cells probably due to the difference in the cellular context. In addition, Src-homology-2 (SH2) domain is observed in the BCR-derived region. However, this domain seems to be dispensable for its tyrosine kinase and transforming activities. BCR also has an intrinsic serine-threonine kinase domain [7], while the role of this domain in the

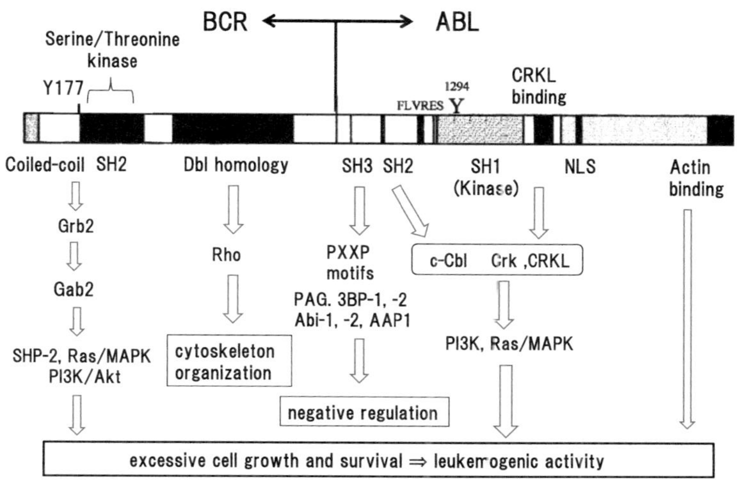


**Fig. 3.2** Functional domains of BCR-ABL and its downstream molecules

biologic function of BCR-ABL in CML is still unknown. In addition, BCR has a Dbl homology domain with a guanine nucleotide exchange activity [8], which can activate Rho, a member of small GTPases family involved in the cytoskeleton organization.

The N-terminal domain of ABL closely resembles to Src family kinases in that it possesses SH3, SH2, and SH1 (kinase) domains [9]. The SH3 domain usually functions as an adaptor domain, which mediates protein-protein interactions by binding to the conserved proline-rich motif, PXXP [10]. Deletion of domain confers oncogenic activity on c-Abl [11–14]. Furthermore, a mutant BCR-ABL lacking the oligomerization domain without transforming activity recovers transforming activity by the deletion of this domain [15]. These results suggest that this domain is a negative regulatory domain for transforming activity of BCR-ABL. As for the mechanism of this negative regulation, several proteins such as PAG. 3BP-1, 3BP-2, Abi-1, Abi-2, and AAP1 that interact with this domain and inhibit c-ABL activity have been identified [10, 15–21]. However, precise role of each molecule in the biologic function of c-ABL is not clear. In addition, it remains unknown whether these molecules inhibit kinase activity of BCR-ABL as well as of c-ABL. In contrast, it was also reported that the SH3 domain can act as a positive regulator of BCR-ABL activity. A previous paper showed that, although this domain is dispensable for the transforming activity of BCR-ABL in vitro, it is required for its full oncogenic activity in vivo [22]. In this report, proliferation of the cells expressing BCR-ABL without SH3 domain was apparently reduced compared with those expressing wild-type BCR-ABL in a transplantation model, which was accompanied by the decreased binding of these cells to the extracellular matrix and infiltration into bone marrow microenvironment in the recipient mice. As for the signal transduction from this domain, this domain was shown to play an important role as a docking site for phosphorylated tyrosine residues in their partner proteins [23]. This domain is necessary for the phosphatidylinositol 3-kinase (PI3K) signaling and essential for the induction of a critical cell-cycle regulator in G1/S transition, c-*myc* [24, 25]. Also, this domain activates Ras/MAPK pathway [5, 6]. If this domain is deleted or mutated, the formation of BCR-ABL will be totally different. So, this mutant BCR-ABL reveals tyrosine kinase activity different from wild-type BCR-ABL through the interaction with a distinct set of cellular proteins and unable to transform fibroblasts [14, 26]. However, this mutant BCR-ABL was still capable of transforming hematopoietic cell lines [27]. Thus, functional roles of this SH2 domain would be different between fibroblasts and hematopoietic cells as was the case with Y177F as described above.

In addition to the interaction with other cellular proteins, ABL kinase activity is regulated by intraprotein (intramolecule) interactions between the SH3 domain and the linker region between the SH2 and the kinase domain as observed in Src family kinases [28–30]. Especially, the intraprotein interaction between the SH2 domain and kinase domain is both necessary and sufficient for leukemogenic activity of BCR-ABL. Disruption of this interface abrogates downstream signals and completely abolishes in vivo leukemogenic activities of BCR-ABL [31]. In

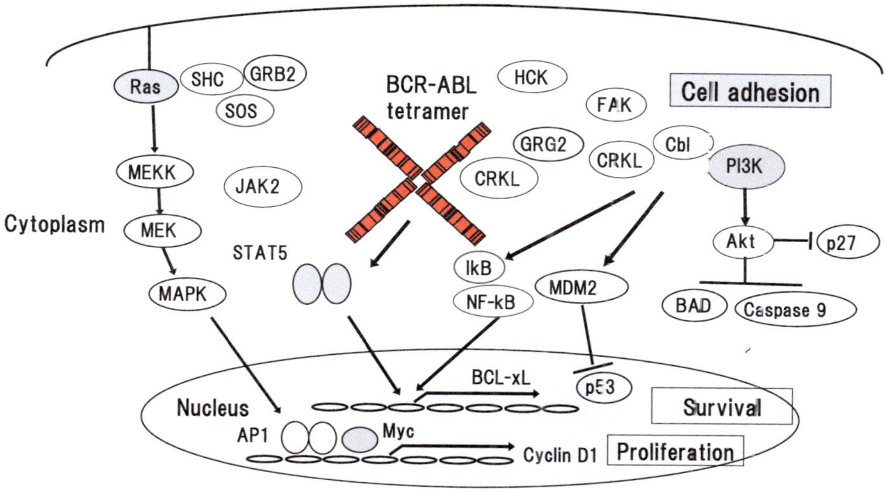


**Fig. 3.3** Signal transduction from BCR-ABL to downstream pathways

addition, disruption of this SH2-kinase interface sensitizes imatinib-resistant CML cells harboring *BCR-ABL* mutations to TKI. Furthermore, an engineered c-Abl SH2-binding fibronectin type III monobody HA4-7c12 was shown to inhibit BCR-ABL activity in primary CML cells (Fig. 3.3), suggesting that the SH2-kinase interface can be an allosteric target to construct a new therapeutic strategy.

The kinase domain is essential for BCR-ABL since mutants of BCR-ABL without kinase activity don't show transforming or leukemogenic activity in any experimental models. In addition, inhibition of BCR-ABL expression by anti-sense oligonucleotides reduced proliferation of BCR-ABL-positive cell lines and suppressed colony formation from primary CML progenitors in semisolid cultures [32]. Thus, this domain plays a central role in the biologic activity of BCR-ABL and is the most appropriate therapeutic target. Based on this concept, a number of TKIs that fit in the ATP-binding pocket and competitively inhibit ATP-binding of BCR-ABL have been developed [33–35]. Among them, the 1st generation of TKI, imatinib, initially showed dramatic clinical effects in patients with CML in chronic phase compared to the conventional therapy (cytarabine + interferon-$\alpha$), whereas it showed a limited degree of clinical efficacy for patients in the advanced (accelerated or blast crisis) phase [36–39]. However, about 15 % of CML patients in chronic phase still show resistance to imatinib. There are several mechanisms responsible for this resistance including amplification of the *BCR-ABL* gene, overexpression of *BCR-ABL* mRNA, point mutations of the *BCR-ABL* gene, and activation Src family tyrosine kinases [40–44]. Among them, point mutations of the *BCR-ABL* gene are most frequent and observed in 50–60 % of imatinib-resistant cases [45, 46]. At present, more than 60 point mutations of *BCR-ABL* have been identified, which are scattered throughout the kinase domain. To overcome these mutations, the 2nd generation of TKI (nilotinib, dasatinib, and bosutinib) have been developed and showed clinical efficacy for such cases. However, T315I mutation, which is called as a gatekeeper mutation, shows resistance to both 1st and 2nd generations of TKIs. For this mutation, the 3rd generation of TKI, ponatinib, which is effective for all types of point mutations of *BCR-ABL* including T315I, was developed [47, 48]. Ponatinib was approved and used in Europe and the USA, showing stable clinical efficacy for patient with CML with T315I mutation. In addition to these ATP-binding competitors, an allosteric inhibitor, GNF-2.5, which modifies the structure of the ATP-binding domain, was shown to inhibit BCR-ABL activity [49].

The kinase domain is linked to the C-terminal noncatalytic domain, which is important for biologic functions of c-Abl as well as of BCR-ABL. This domain contains the binding sites for adaptor proteins (Crk-like protein) [50, 51], a nuclear localization sequence (NLS), a DNA-binding domain [52], a p53 binding site [53], and a G- and F-actin-binding domains [1, 2, 54]. Among them, although NLS-, DNA-, and p53-binding domains are necessary for the physiological function of c-Abl, they are not required for leukemogenic activity of BCR-ABL [52, 53]. As to the role of CRKL-binding domain, a deletion mutant of BCR-ABL lacking this domain revealed reduce transformation activity by 50 % in fibroblasts [51], while it effectively conferred factor-independent growth on hematopoietic cell lines [50], suggesting the different role for this domain between hematopoetic cells and non-hematopoietic cells. The G- and F-actin-binding domain in the C-terminus is shared by another ABL family tyrosine kinase, Arg (also called as ABL2), and is indispensable for BCR-ABL to transform Rat1 fibroblasts and to confer anchorage-independent growth on NIH3T3 cells and factor-independent growth on hematopoietic cells [2, 55].

## 3.3 Original Function of c-ABL

c-*ABL* was first identified as a cellular homologue of the Abelson murine leukemia virus (v-*ABL*), which causes ALL/lymphoma in mice. In the v-*ABL* oncogene, viral gag sequences were fused to the truncated c-*ABL* gene lacking the NH2-terminal region that is implicated in its autoregulation. c-ABL forms a non-receptor tyrosine kinase family together with Arg, both of which have the common unique actin-binding domains in the C-terminus as describe above [56]. To examine the functional roles of c-ABL in vivo, its knockout mice were generated. However, c-*ABL*-deficient mice were embryonic lethal from unknown reason. Previous studies demonstrated that ABL mainly exists in the nucleus and induces apoptosis in response to DNA damage through the cooperation with the p53 homologue, p73. In addition, recent analyses showed that ABL kinases are activated by a variety of stimuli including growth factors and chemokines and the engagement of cadherin and integrin, thereby regulating cytoskeleton remodeling, cell adhesion, and migration [56]. In addition, ABL kinases are implicated in the regulation of endothelial barrier function [57, 58]. So, pharmacological inhibition of ABL kinase by imatinib reduces interstitial fluid pressure in lung and colon cancer models [8, 19, 59].

## 3.4 Biologic Activity of BCR-ABL

In contrast to the nuclear localization of c-ABL, BCR-ABL primarily localizes in cytoplasm. This cytoplasmic localization is necessary for its biologic activities because BCR-ABL entrapped into the nucleus by leptomycin B induces apoptosis through its tyrosine kinase activities [60]. In addition, tetramer formation is essential for BCR-ABL to reveal tyrosine kinase activity, because mutant BCR-ABL lacking the N-terminal tetramerization domain loses its transforming activities [1–4].

As for the biologic activities of BCR-ABL in leukemogenesis, a number of in vitro experiments have shown that BCR-ABL enables primitive hematopoietic cells as well as factor-dependent hematopoietic cell lines such as Ba/F3, 32D, and FDC-P1 to proliferate and survive continuously under factor-deprived conditions [61–64]. In addition, enforced expression of p210 or p190 BCR-ABL in Rat-1 fibroblasts causes a distinct morphologic change and confers both tumorigenicity and ability of anchorage-independent growth [65]. Furthermore, when bone marrow cells infected with retrovirus expressing p210 BCR-ABL are transplanted into lethally irradiated mice, recipient mice develop various types of hematologic malignancies including granulocytic hyperplasia resembling human CML, myelomonocytic leukemia, ALL, lymphomas, and erythroid leukemia [66–68]. Moreover, transgenic mice expressing p210 BCR-ABL develop pre-B or T-cell lymphomas, T-ALL, or myeloproliferative disorder like CML [69–71]. In addition, TKIs such as imatinib, nilotinib, and dasatinib are dramatically effective for CML. Together, these results indicate that BCR-ABL is a main causative gene of CML. In addition, it should be noted that BCR-ABL by itself can't immortalize hematopoietic progenitor cells without self-renewal activity because only HSCs but not hematopoietic progenitor cells that were transfected with BCR-ABL can cause leukemia in the recipient mice in a transplantation model.

## 3.5 Regulation of Signaling Molecules by BCR-ABL

Growth and survival of hematopoietic cells are regulated by a number of hematopoietic growth factors. Upon the stimulation with the ligand, receptors for hematopoietic growth factors transmit mitogenic and anti-apoptotic signals through activation of intracellular downstream molecules. To keep homeostasis of hematopoiesis, these cytokine signals are subsequently eliminated by negative feedback mechanisms including ubiquitin/proteasome-dependent protein degradation, activation of phosphatases, and induction of inhibitory molecules. In contrast, activated mutants of the upstream tyrosine kinases such as tandem duplication of FLT3 (FLT3-ITD), activating point mutations of KIT, and TEL-PDGFR cause sustained activation of downstream cascades. Similarly, BCR-ABL constitutively activates various signaling molecules including Ras/ MAPK pathway, PI3K/Akt pathway, and signal transducers and activators of transcription (STATs, STAT1 and STAT5), Src family tyrosine kinases, JAK2, and so on (Fig. 3.3), thereby causing excessive growth, survival, and consequent malignant transformation of HSCs.

## 3.6 Ras/MAPK

Ras family proteins belong to a superfamily of GTPases that is localized to the inner surface of the plasma membrane [72, 73]. Ras family proteins play a pivotal role in a number of signaling pathways mediated by growth factors, cytokines, and cell adhesion. Activated tyrosine kinases become to associate with adapter proteins such as Shc and Grb2, which in turn recruit guanine nucleotide exchange factors (GEFs), thereby activating Ras. Once induced, Ras activates a serine/threonine kinase, Raf, which then phosphorylates MAPK kinases (also called as MEKs). Activated MAPK moves into the nucleus and phosphorylates and activates nuclear transcription factors such as Elk-1. MAPK also activates downstream kinases such as RSKs (also known as MAPK-activated protein kinases), which regulate cell-cycle regulation and apoptosis. MAPK-activated RSK catalyzes a proapoptotic protein Bad, thereby inhibiting Bad-mediated apoptosis. Furthermore, the Ras-Raf-MEK-MAPK cascade modulates cell proliferation by regulating the expression and/or activity of several proteins, including cell-cycle regulators (e.g., cyclin D1, $p21^{WAF1}$, $p27^{KIP1}$, and cdc25A) and transcription factors (e.g., c-*fos*, c-*jun*, and c-*myc*). Aberrant activation of MEK and MAPK has been demonstrated in various types of leukemic cells including CML cells [72–75].

In a previous study, we showed that induced expression of a dominant negative (DN) form of Ras (N17) inhibited the growth of p210 BCR-ABL-positive K562 cells by 90 %, while DN STAT5 (694 F) and DN PI3K (Δp85) inhibited the growth by 55 and 40 %, respectively [76]. During these cultures, the expression of cyclin D2 and cyclin D3 was suppressed by N17, 694F, and Δp85, that of cyclin E by N17, and that of cyclin A by Δp85. In addition, we found that N17 induced apoptosis in a small proportion of K562 cells, whereas 694F and Δp85 were hardly effective. During these cultures, the expression of Bcl-2 was suppressed by N17, 694F, and Δp85 and that of Bcl-XL by N17. Furthermore, although K562 was resistant to interferon-α- and dexamethasone-induced apoptosis, disruption of one pathway by N17, 694F, or Δp85 sensitized K562 to these reagents. In addition, coexpression of two DN mutants in any combinations induced severe apoptosis. These results suggest that cooperation among Ras/MAPK, STAT5, and PI3K is required for full leukemogenic activities of BCR-ABL, whereas Ras/MAPK seemed to be most important for BCR-ABL-dependent cell growth and survival.

## 3.7 PI3K/Akt

PI3K is another important signaling pathway controlling serine/threonine phosphorylation [74, 75, 77]. PI3K consists of two subunits, the p85 regulatory subunit and the p110 catalytic subunit. The p85 subunit binds to the ligand-activated and autophosphorylated tyrosine kinases. As a result, the p110 subunit and their downstream substrate Akt (previously called as PKB) are recruited to the membrane. PI3K/Akt pathway activates several downstream targets including p70 RSK, forkhead transcription factors (FOXOs), and NF-κB. Akt is a serine/threonine kinase and an important component of the cell survival machinery. PI3K-activated Akt provokes a number of signaling events. For example, Akt phosphorylates an NF-κB inhibitor, IκB. Upon phosphorylation, IκB is degraded by 26S proteasome and releases NF-κB, which then moves into the nucleus and induces the transcription of a number of target genes involved in cell survival such as Bcl-XL and IAPs and cell adhesion such as E-selectin, VCAM-1, and ICAM-1. Akt also phosphorylates the proapoptotic protein Bad, which leads to higher levels of free anti-apoptotic Bcl-XL, thereby inhibiting the cell-death protease, caspase-9. A tumor suppressor, PTEN, is a phosphatase that removes a phosphate from the three position of the inositol ring of the PIP3,4,5 phospholipids. PTEN has been shown to act as a negative regulator for Akt through its phosphatase activity.

The mammalian target of rapamycin (mTOR) is a serine/threonine kinase and acts as another important downstream effector of the PI3K/Akt signaling pathway, which mediates cell survival and proliferation. mTOR exists in two different complexes. mTOR forms mTORC1 by binding to Raptor, mLST8, and PRAS40, which promotes cell growth with p70 S6K as one of the main substrate. The other complex, mTORC2, is formed by the binding of mTOR to Rictor, mSIN1, and mLST8, which acts as a crucial Akt regulator.

FoxO transcription factors are human homologues of the *C. elegans* transcription factor DAF-16, sharing a highly conserved DNA-binding domain, forkhead box or winged-helix domain. At present, four main members (FoxO1, FoxO3a, FoxO4, and FoxO6) have been identified in the subfamily of class O. Among them, FoxO3a is considered to function as a tumor suppressor by regulating the expression of genes involved in apoptosis, cell-cycle arrest, oxidative stresses, and autophagy such as proapoptotic BIM, $p27^{KIP1}$, p57, and Pdk1. Phosphorylation is the most important regulatory mechanism of FoxO3a, whereas its activity is also regulated by acetylation and ubiquitination. Although FoxO3a can be phosphorylated by several kinases, Akt is a pivotal kinase among them. When growth factors or insulin are deprived, FoxO3a translocates into the nucleus and induces the transcription of its target genes as described above, thereby inducing apoptosis and/or cell-cycle arrest (Fig. 3.4). In contrast, under the culture with growth factors or insulin, FoxO3a is phosphorylated by Akt and translocated into the cytoplasm through the interaction with 14-3-3 nuclear export protein, becoming an inactive form. Then, phosphorylated FoxO3a is trapped by an ubiquitin E3 ligase and subsequently degraded by the 26S proteasome, implying that Akt is a critical

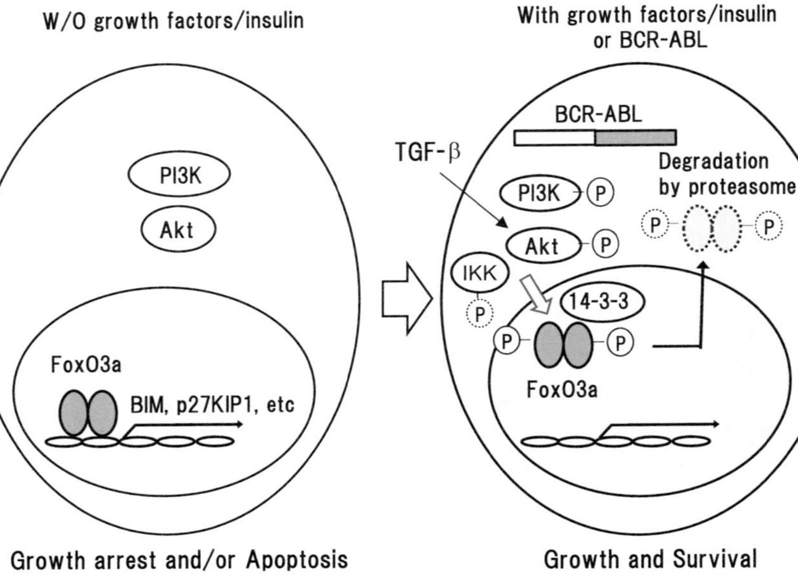


**Fig. 3.4** Regulation of FoxO3a by growth factors/insulin and BCR-ABL in CML cells

negative regulator of FoxO3a. However, a recent analysis showed that IκB kinase (IKK) also phosphorylates FoxO3a at serine 644, thereby keeping it in cytoplasm and inhibiting its transcriptional activity in an Akt-independent manner.

With regard to the biologic roles of PI3K/Akt in CML, a mutant BCR-ABL, which can't activate PI3K, doesn't reveal leukemogenic activity in vitro and in vivo, indicating that PI3K/Akt pathway is essential for the leukemogenic activity of BCR-ABL [22, 78]. In addition, DN PI3K inhibits the growth and survival of BCR-ABL-positive K562 cells together with DN Ras/MAPK and DN STAT5 as described above [76]. Also, imatinib and an mTORC1 inhibitor, rapamycin, synergistically induce apoptosis in CML cells [79]. Moreover, simultaneous inhibition of mTORC1 and mTORC2 effectively induces apoptosis in CML cells with T315I mutation, for which both 1st and 2nd generations of TKIs are ineffective [80]. Furthermore, it is of clinical importance that inhibitors of PI3K/mTOR pathway sensitize CML stem cells to nilotinib, suggesting that PI3K/Akt pathway is also involved in the survival of CML stem cells [81, 82].

However, to our surprise, Akt phosphorylation was found to be reduced in CML stem cells, which resulted in the nuclear translocation (activation) of FoxO3a [83]. In this paper, serial transplantation of BCR-ABL-transformed cells originating from *Foxo3a*$^{-/-}$ mice showed decreased leukemogenic activity compared to those from *Foxo3a*$^{+/+}$ mice, indicating that FoxO3a is essential for the maintenance of CML stem cells. Furthermore, TGF-β was shown to be a pivotal activator of Akt in CML stem cells and controls FoxO3a localization, suggesting a critical role for the TGF-β–Akt-FoxO pathway in the maintenance of CML stem cells. In contrast, it was recently reported that FoxO1 and Fox3a are inactivated and relocalized to the cytoplasm by BCR-ABL activity in CD34$^+$ CML cells [84]. TKI treatment reduced phosphorylation of FoxOs, leading to their relocalization from cytoplasm (inactive) to nucleus (active), where they induced the expression of target genes, such as Cyclin D1, ATM, CDKN1C, and BCL6, and thereby induced G1 arrest. In addition, overexpression of FoxO3a inhibited the growth of CML cells in combination with TKI with similar results seen for inhibitors of PI3K/Akt/mTOR signaling. These data demonstrate that TKI induces G1 arrest through inhibition of the PI3K/Akt pathway and reactivation of FoxOs in CML cells. Thus, the roles for PI3KAkt/FoxO3a are rather complicated in CML cells and their stem cells. Further studies are required to clarify their precise functions, especially with attention on their crosstalk with other signaling pathways.

## 3.8 STATs

STATs are coded by six known mammalian genes including 10 different proteins including different isomers of STAT1, STAT3, STAT4, STAT5A, STAT5B, and STAT6 [85, 86]. Like other transcription factors, STATs have a well-defined structure including a DNA-binding domain, a conserved NH2-terminal domain, a COOH-terminal transactivation domain, and SH2 and SH3 domains. STATs mediate signals from various cytokines such as erythropoietin (EPO), thrombopoietin (TPO), granulocyte-colony stimulating factor (G-CSF), granulocyte macrophage-colony stimulating factor (GM-CSF), interleukin-2 (IL-2), IL-3, IL-5, IL-7, and IL-15. Upon tyrosine phosphorylation by upstream tyrosine kinases such as JAKs, activated STATs dimerize and translocate into the nucleus, where they activate specific target genes. A number of previous studies have shown that STATs mediate cytokine-dependent cell growth and survival by regulating the expression of cyclins, c-*myc*, and Bcl-XL. Among STAT family members, STAT5 is essential for the development of hematopoietic cells, because STAT5A$^{-/-}$STAT5B$^{-/-}$ mice suffer from severe anemia and are embryonic lethal due to the disruption of EPO signaling [87]. In addition, STAT5 activity was shown to be necessary for the maintenance of HSCs [88].

STAT5 is directly activated by BCR-ABL in CML cells. Also, it can be activated by JAK2 through the mediation of AHI-1 (Fig. 3.5). Regarding the roles of STAT5 in BCR-ABL-dependent growth and survival, previous studies showed that DN STAT5 suppressed apoptosis resistance, factor-independent proliferation, and leukemogenic potential of a CML-derived cell line, K562 and BCR-ABL-transformed 32D and Ba/F3 [89–91]. In addition, a recent paper showed that STAT5B is more involved in BCR-ABL-dependent growth and survival than STAT5A, while IL-3 activates STAT5A and STAT5B equivalently [92].

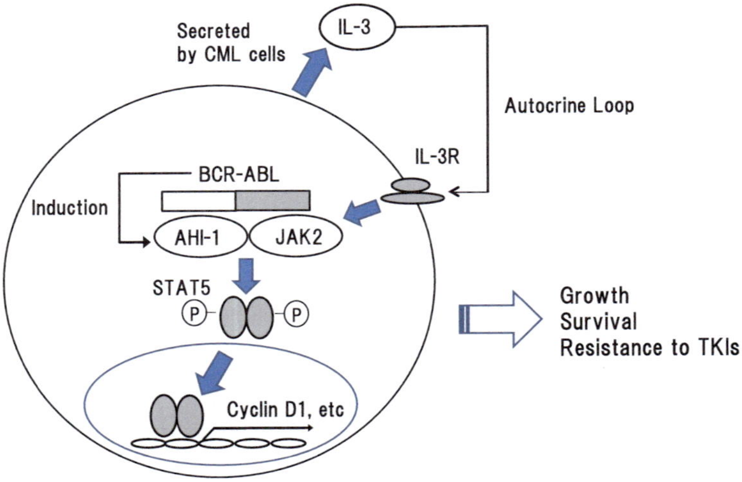


**Fig. 3.5** Roles for AHI-1, JAK2, and STAT5 in CML cells

## 3.9 SHP-2

A tyrosine phosphatase, SHP-2, is ubiquitously expressed but highly expressed in hematopoietic cells, which has two N-terminal SH2 (N-SH2 and C-SH2) domains, a central protein tyrosine phosphatase domain, and C-terminal tyrosine phosphorylation sites. SHP-2 is involved in various signaling pathways from growth factors, cytokines, and extracellular matrix. Especially, it augments intracellular signaling from receptor tyrosine kinases. In addition, SHP-2 is known to form a stable complex with BCR-ABL, c-cbl, and Grb2-associated binder 2 (GAB2) through its SH2 domains [93, 94]. In this complex, SHP-2 is heavily tyrosine phosphorylated and plays an essential role in transforming activity of BCR-ABL for hematopoietic cells because leukemogenic activity of BCR-ABL was severely reduced in SHP-2-deficient hematopoietic cells in vitro and in vivo [95]. These results suggest that SHP-2 would be a promising therapeutic target in CML cells. To confirm this hypothesis, Sha F. et al. generated monobodies binding to the N- and C-SH2 domains of SHP-2, respectively, both of which work as competitors of SH2-phosphotyrosine interactions [96]. The monobody targeting the N-SH2 domain impaired the interaction between SHP-2 and its upstream activator, GAB2, probably by sequestering SHP-2 from the BCR-ABL protein complex. In addition, they found that inhibition of either N-SH2 or C-SH2 was sufficient to inhibit BCR-ABL-induced SHP-2 activity and to block MAPK activation, suggesting a new potent and specific therapeutic strategy for CML using the antagonists of protein-protein interactions.

## 3.10 Gab2

Gab2 is a member of Gab family docking proteins, which bind to receptor tyrosine kinases and other tyrosine-phosphorylated proteins via Grab2, thereby transmitting the signals to downstream molecules such as SHP-2, Ras/MAPK, PI3K/Akt, and JAK/STAT pathways. In CML cells, Grb2 binds to Y177 of BCR-ABL and bridges BCR-ABL and the C-terminal SH3 domain of Gab2. When this interaction was disrupted by Y177F mutation, BCR-ABL-dependent growth of Ba/F3 cells was severely impaired, where tyrosine phosphorylation of Gab2 and PI3K/Akt and Ras/MAPK activation were severely reduced [97]. In addition, BCR-ABL is not capable of activating PI3K/Akt and Ras/MAPK pathways effectively in Gab2-deficient hematopoietic cells [98]. Furthermore, Gab2 signaling is involved in TKI resistance in CML cells. These results indicate that Gab2 is essential for signal transductions of BCR-ABL and its leukemogenic activities [99].

## 3.11 c-Cbl, CRKL, and Cas (Crk-Associated Substrate)

v-Cbl was originally identified as an oncogene that causes murine leukemias. Then, later studies demonstrated that its cellular homologue, c-Cbl, regulates a number of signals from receptors for IL-2, IL-3, GM-CSF, EPO, stem cell factor, and so on through the interaction with CRKL, p85 PI3K, and Grb2 [100–103]. c-Cbl interacts with the SH2 domain of BCR-ABL [104] and phosphorylated c-Cbl binds to the SH2 domain of CRKL [105], of which complex formation is specifically observed in CML cells but not in normal hematopoietic cells. CRKL included in complex is supposed to mediate BCR-ABL signals to downstream PI3K/Akt and Ras/MAPK pathways (Fig. 3.2) [106]. In addition, a previous paper showed that inhibition of CRKL expression by antisense oligonucleotides severely reduced the growth of Ph-positive cells but not of BCR-ABL-negative hematopoietic cells [107], suggesting a key role of CRKL in the biologic activity of CML.

Cas is primarily localized at the cytoskeleton and one of the most heavily phosphorylated Crk-binding protein in v-Crk-transformed cells [108]. Cas has an SH3 domain in the N-terminus and a number of following tyrosine residues, most of which can act as potential binding sites for the SH2 domains in the partner proteins. In normal cells, Cas regulates integrin signals in combination with focal adhesion kinase (FAK) and the Src family kinases [109, 110], both of which are implicated in BCR-ABL signals. In CML cells, Cas is tyrosine phosphorylated and associates with the SH2 domain of CRKL [111]. Thus, it is supposed that Cas would transmit BCR-ABL signals to downstream molecules like c-Cbl and critically regulate the effects of BCR-ABL on cytoskeleton.

## 3.12 Src Family Tyrosine Kinases

Src family tyrosine kinases are first identified non-receptor tyrosine kinases including Src, Lyn, Lck, and Hck, which play crucial roles in cell growth, survival, and adhesion by mediating signals from growth factors and cytokines [112]. In addition, Src family kinases are key regulators of immune reactions in T and B lymphocytes by mediating the antigen engagement. c-*Src* was originally identified as a cellular homologue of the transforming oncogene Rous sarcoma virus (v-*Src*). v-*Src* activates a number of signaling proteins such as Ras/MAPK, STATs, and PI3K/Akt, thereby transforming NIH3T3 cells and conferring factor-independent growth on IL-3-dependent murine cell lines 32Dcl3 and Ba/F3 [108, 113–119]. Src family kinases are also activated in CML cells at the early stage of chronic phase in a BCR-ABL-dependent manner. However, Hck and Lyn are often overexpressed in imatinib-resistant CML cells without BCR-ABL mutations [120]. In addition, Lyn was constitutively phosphorylated and activated in imatinib-resistant CML cells without BCR-ABL mutations in a BCR-ABL-independent manner [121]. In these cells, Lyn forms a complex with the Gab2 and c-Cbl at its phosphorylation sites (Y193 and Y459), thereby inducing sustained tyrosine phosphorylation of Gab2 and BCR-ABL even in the presence of imatinib [122]. However, because no mutation was found in the kinase domain or C-terminal regulatory domain, it remains unknown how Lyn is activated in these cells [121]. In addition, suppression of Lyn expression by siRNA or pharmacological inhibition of its activity by dasatinib effectively induced cell death in imatinib-resistant CML cells, validating the use of TKIs with Src inhibitory activity such as dasatinib, bosutinib, and ponatinib for imatinib-resistant CML cases without BCR-ABL mutations.

## 3.13 JAK2

JAK2 is a family member of Janus family tyrosine kinases including JAK1, JAK2, and JAK3 and Tyk1 and Tyk2. This family of tyrosine kinases has tandem pseudokinase and tyrosine kinase domains in common. JAK family tyrosine kinases transmit signals from the receptor for cytokines, interferons, and hormones. Among them, JAK2 is known to mainly transmit signals from the receptors for EPO, TPO, and G-CSF [123]. In agreement with these findings, definitive hematopoiesis was severely impaired in the fetal liver of JAK2 knockout mice and these mice are embryonic lethal around day 12.5 due to severe anemia [124]. In addition, selective deletion of Jak2 in adult mouse hematopoietic cells leads to lethal anemia and thrombocytopenia [125, 126]. These results indicate that JAK2 plays a key role in the development of hematopoietic cells. Upon activation, JAK2 activates Ras/MAPK, STATs, and PI3K/Akt. In addition, JAK2 is activated in BCR-ABL-transformed cells. However, even if BCR-ABL activity is inhibited by TKI, JAK2 activity is kept in residual CML stem cells by IL-3 and G-CSF produced by themselves in the bone marrow microenvironment, thereby contributing to their resistance to TKI (Fig. 3.5) [127].

Abelson helper integration site 1 (AHI-1) is an oncogene that was identified by provirus insertional mutagenesis in v-*ABL*-transformed murine pre-B-cell lymphoma. Overexpression of AHI-1 augments the growth of hematopoietic cells in vitro and causes leukemia in vivo [128]. AHI-1 is highly expressed in CML stem/progenitor cells, where it forms a complex with BCR-ABL and JAK2 (Fig. 3.5) [128]. Suppression of AHI-1 expression by SiRNA reduces the growth of in CML stem/progenitor cells in vitro. In addition, it was shown that AHI-1 regulates phosphorylation status of BCR-ABL, JAK2, and STAT5 in CML cells. So, it is supposed to enhance the function of BCR-ABL. Furthermore, AHI-1-BCR-ABL-JAK2-AHI-1 complex is responsible for TKI resistance in CML stem/progenitor cells [129, 130]. These results suggest that JAK2-AHI-1 will be a potential therapeutic target in CML as well as BCR-ABL. Based on this hypothesis, Lin H et al. recently reported that dual inhibition of Jak2 and BCR-ABL by BMS-911543 in combination with TKIs effectively eliminates TKI-resistant CML stem/progenitor cells [131].

## 3.14 Wnt/β-Catenin

Wnt (wingless-type) ligands activate three different pathways: canonical Wnt/β-catenin, noncanonical planar cell polarity, and noncanonical Wnt/calcium pathways. The canonical Wnt/β-catenin pathway is the most studied pathway, where Wnt ligands form a complex with Frizzled (FZD) receptor and the coreceptor, low-density lipoprotein receptor-related protein 5 (LRP5) or LRP6. Without the Wnt ligand activation, β-catenin is phosphorylated by glycogen synthase kinase-3β (GSK-3β) and/or casein kinase Iα (CKIα) and subjected to degradation by ubiquitin/proteasome system (Fig. 3.6). Upon the receptor activation, phosphorylation of β-catenin is reduced and the function of "destruction complex" consisting of adenomatous polyposis coli (APC) protein and Axin is inhibited, resulting in cytoplasmic β-catenin stabilization and accumulation. Then, β-catenin translocates into the nucleus. Nuclear β-catenin acts as a transcriptional coactivator and interacts with transcriptions factors including T-cell factor (TCF) and lymphoid enhancer factor (LEF), thereby inducing the transcription of target genes such as c-Myc, cyclin D1, MMP7, and c-Jun and c-Fos family members. In addition, Wnt signaling also activates Rac, Rho, JNK, and protein kinase C (PKC) pathways through the other nonconononical pathways independently of β-catenin, thereby regulating cell polarity, movement, and survival. WNT/β-catenin pathway is supposed to play an important role in self-renewal of HSCs, since enforced expression of mutant β-catenin with S33 mutation resistance to degradation is sufficient to maintain HSC population and effectively reconstitutes hematopoiesis in vivo [132]. Also, lack of WNT signals result in multilineage differentiation of

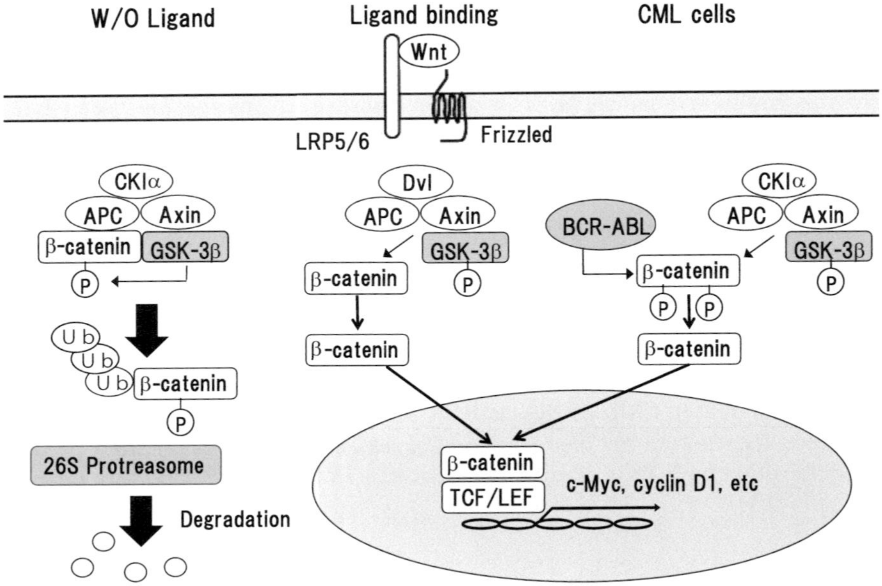


**Fig. 3.6** Regulation of canonical Wnt/β-catenin pathway by its ligand and in CML cells

HSCs [133]. These results suggest that WNT/β-catenin signaling is implicated in the maintenance of normal HSCs.

As for the relationship between BCR-ABL and β-catenin, BCR-ABL was shown to phosphorylate β-catenin at tyrosine residues at 86 and 654 through the direct interaction (Fig. 3.6) [134]. Phosphorylated β-catenin binds to the transcription factor TCF4 and promotes target gene transcription. GSK3β is constitutively activated by the phosphorylation at tyrosine 216 and predominantly located to the cytoplasm in primary CML stem/progenitor cells compared with that in normal cells. Although BCR-ABL by itself does not influence GSK3-β-autophosphorylation, it inhibits the binding of β-catenin to Axin/GSK3β and its subsequent serine/threonine phosphorylation through these tyrosine phosphorylations. In this context, imatinib inhibits tyrosine phosphorylation of β-catenin and restores its binding to the Axin/GSK3β-complex, thereby inhibiting β-catenin/TCF-mediated transcription. These findings indicate that BCR-ABL-induced tyrosine phosphorylation of β-catenin contributes to its protein stabilization and subsequent gene transcription in CML cells. Also, missplicing of GSK3β was shown to contribute to the development of CML stem cells [135]. In addition, a recent study demonstrated that CML stem cells are protected from TKI by N-cadherin and Wnt/β-catenin signaling in the bone marrow microenvironment [136].

A previous study showed that silencing of β-catenin expression by SiRNA inhibits growth and colony-forming activity of CML cells [137]. Also, CML stem cells but not normal HSCs can be eliminated by inhibition of GSK3β-activity [138]. These results suggest that CML stem cells are more dependent on

WNT/β-catenin signaling for their maintenance than normal hematopoietic stem cells. Moreover, CML stem cells lacking β-catenin have decreased activity of infiltrating into the lung and liver in the injected mice, suggesting that β-catenin is also required for full biologic activity of BCR-ABL [137].

Furthermore, Jamieson et al. showed that, although CML stem cells originate from most immature HSCs but not from progenitor cells lacking self-renewal activity in chronic phase of CML, granulocyte/macrophage progenitor (GMP)-like cells acquiring self-renewal activity act as CML stem cells in the advanced stages (accelerated phase and blastic transformation) of CML patients due to the aberrant activation of WNT/β-catenin signaling [139]. In addition, they demonstrated that a GSK3β-inhibitor effectively inhibited the growth of CML cells in the recipient mice in transplantation model.

## 3.15 Sonic Hedgehog (Shh)

*Shh* is one of the three vertebrate hedgehog genes (*Indian*, *Desert*, and *Sonic*) homologous to the *Drosophila* hedgehog. Shh signaling is regulated by the interaction of three key molecules including the Shh ligand, its receptor patched 1 (Ptch1), and the pathway activator smoothened (Smo). Although Smo is trapped by ligand-unbound Ptch1, the binding of Shh ligand to Ptch1 results in the release of Smo, leading to activation of a transcription factor Gli and subsequent activation of the Shh/Gli-mediated gene transcription (Fig. 3.7). Shh acts as a morphogen and governs and precisely regulates development of multicellular organisms. So, deregulated Shh signaling is implicated in birth defects. In addition, Shh signaling plays an important role in the development and/or maintenance of many human cancers and cancer stem cells [140].

A previous study showed that SMO levels were higher and Ptch1 levels were lower in CML cells from patients with high Sokal risk compared to those in the other risk groups, indicating that Shh signaling is more active in this risk group

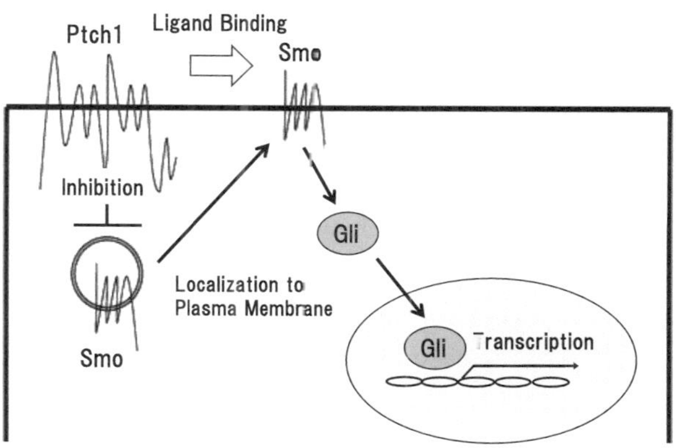


**Fig. 3.7** Regulation of Shh pathway by its ligand

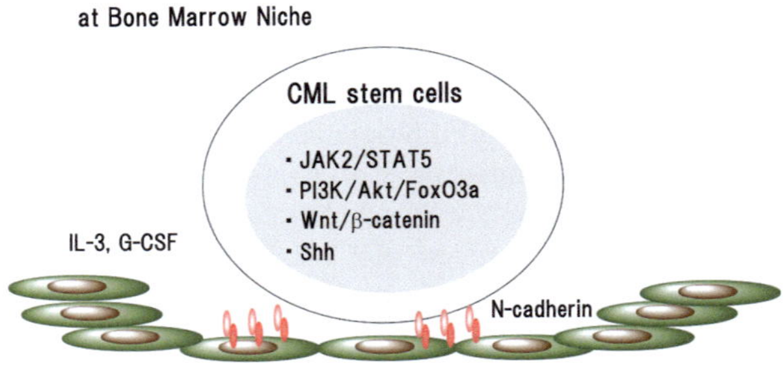


**Fig. 3.8** Signaling molecules involved in BCR-ABL-independent survival of residual CML stem cells during TKI treatment

[141]. Furthermore, Shh signaling activity was correlated with *BCR-ABL* mRNA level and upcoming molecular relapse during TKI treatment. Also, activation of Shh signaling precedes molecular relapse by several months in most patients carrying T315 mutation [141]. Moreover, activation of Shh signaling is observed in about 50 % of CML cases in chronic phase, about 70 % of CML cases in accelerated phase, and more than 80 % of CML cases in blast crisis. In addition, deregulation of signaling network among Shh, Wnt, Notch, and Hox in $CD34^+$ CML cells was shown to be involved in blastic transformation from chronic phase, which is accompanied by upregulated expression of Patched1, Frizzled2, Lef1, $p21^{WAF1}$, and cyclin D1 [142]. Together, these results indicate that Shh activity is correlated with disease activity and influences disease status. In addition to matured CML cells, aberrant activation of Shh signaling is observed in $CD34^+$c-$kit^+$ CML progenitor cells [143]. Furthermore, constitutively active Smo augments the number of CML stem cells and accelerates disease progression. Also, $Smo^{-/-}$ HSCs transformed by BCR-ABL have decreased leukemogenic activity in the transplantation model and these cells are consequently exhausted due to the impaired self-renewal activity [144]. In agreement with these findings, a Smo inhibitor, cyclopamine, impairs CML development by CML stem cells in a mouse transplantation model [140]. These results indicate that Shh signal is required for the development of CML and maintenance of CML stem cells (Fig. 3.8), validating the use of Shh inhibitor such as LDE225 as a therapeutic drug for CML alone or in combination with TKI.

## References

1. McWhirter JR, et al. Activation of tyrosine kinase and microfilament-binding functions of c-abl by bcr sequences in bcr/abl fusion proteins. Mol Cell Biol. 1991;11(3):1553–65.
2. McWhirter JR, et al. An actin-binding function contributes to transformation by the Bcr-Abl oncoprotein of Philadelphia chromosome-positive human leukemias. EMBO J. 1993;12 (4):1533–46.
3. McWhirter JR, et al. A coiled-coil oligomerization domain of Bcr is essential for the transforming function of Bcr-Abl oncoproteins. Mol Cell Biol. 1993;13(12):7587–95.

4. Tauchi T, et al. A coiled-coil tetramerization domain of BCR-ABL is essential for the interactions of SH2-containing signal transduction molecules. J Biol Chem. 1997;272(2):1389–94.
5. Cortez D, et al. Structural and signaling requirements for BCR-ABL-mediated transformation and inhibition of apoptosis. Mol Cell Biol. 1995;15(10):5531–41.
6. Goga A, et al. Alternative signals to RAS for hematopoietic transformation by the BCR-ABL oncogene. Cell. 1995;82(6):981–8.
7. Maru Y, et al. The BCR gene encodes a novel serine/threonine kinase activity within a single exon. Cell. 1991;67(3):459–68.
8. Chuang TH, et al. Abl and Bcr are multifunctional regulators of the Rho GTP-binding protein family. Proc Natl Acad Sci U S A. 1995;92(22):10282–6.
9. Ramakrishnan L, et al. Abl genes. Biochim Biophys Acta. 1989;989(2):209–24.
10. Ren R, et al. Identification of a ten-amino acid proline-rich SH3 binding site. Science. 1993;259(5098):1157–61.
11. Franz WM, et al. Deletion of an Nterminal regulatory domain of the c-abl tyrosine kinase activates its oncogenic potential. EMBO J. 1989;8(1):137–47.
12. Jackson P, et al. N-terminal mutations activate the leukemogenic potential of the myristoylated form of c-abl. EMBO J. 1989;8(2):449–56.
13. Jackson PK, et al. Mutation of a phenylalanine conserved in SH3-containing tyrosine kinases activates the transforming ability of c-Abl. Oncogene. 1993;8(7):1943–56.
14. Mayer BJ, et al. Mutagenic analysis of the roles of SH2 and SH3 domains in regulation of the Abl tyrosine kinase. Mol Cell Biol. 1994;14(5):2883–94.
15. Maru Y, et al. Deletion of the ABL SH3 domain reactivates de-oligomerized BCR-ABL for growth factor independence. FEBS Lett. 1996;379(3):244–6.
16. Pendergast AM, et al. Evidence for regulation of the human ABL tyrosine kinase by a cellular inhibitor. Proc Natl Acad Sci U S A. 1991;88(13):5927–31.
17. Walkenhorst J, et al. Analysis of human c-Abl tyrosine kinase activity and regulation in S. pombe. Oncogene. 1996;12(7):1513–20.
18. Wen ST, et al. The PAG gene product, a stress-induced protein with antioxidant properties, is an Abl SH3-binding protein and a physiological inhibitor of c-Abl tyrosine kinase activity. Genes Dev. 1997;11(19):2456–67.
19. Cicchetti P, et al. Identification of a protein that binds to the SH3 region of Abl and is similar to Bcr and GAP-rho. Science. 1992;257(5071):803–6.
20. Dai Z, et al. Abi-2, a novel SH3-containing protein interacts with the c-Abl tyrosine kinase and modulates c-Abl transforming activity. Genes Dev. 1995;9(21):2569–82.
21. Zhu J, et al. c-ABL tyrosine kinase activity is regulated by association with a novel SH3-domain-binding protein. Mol Cell Biol. 1996;16(12):7054–62.
22. Skorski T, et al. The SH3 domain contributes to BCR/ABL-dependent leukemogenesis in vivo: role in adhesion, invasion, and homing. Blood. 1998;91(2):406–18.
23. Songyang Z, et al. SH2 domains recognize specific phosphopeptide sequences. Cell. 1993;72(5):767–78.
24. Skorski T, et al. Transformation of hematopoietic cells by BCR/ABL requires activation of a PI-3k/Akt-dependent pathway. EMBO J. 1997;16(20):6151–61.
25. Afar DE, et al. Differential complementation of Bcr-Abl point mutants with c-Myc. Science. 1994;264(5157):424–6.
26. Mayer BJ, et al. Point mutations in the abl SH2 domain coordinately impair phosphotyrosine binding in vitro and transforming activity in vivo. Mol Cell Biol. 1992;12(2):609–18.
27. Ilaria RL, et al. The SH2 domain of p210bcr/abl is not required for the transformation of hematopoetic factor-dependent cells. Blood. 1995;86(10):3897–904.
28. Barila D, et al. An intramolecular SH3-domain interaction regulates c-Abl activity. Nat Genet. 1998;18(3):280–2.
29. Moarefi I, et al. Activation of the Src-family tyrosine kinase Hck by SH3 domain displacement. Nature. 1997;385(6617):650–3.

30. Sicheri F, et al. Crystal structure of the Src family tyrosine kinase Hck. Nature. 1997;385 (6617):602–9.
31. Grebien F, et al. Targeting the SH2-kinase interface in Bcr-Abl inhibits leukemogenesis. Cell. 2011;147(2):306–19.
32. Rowley PT, et al. The effect of bcr-abl antisense oligonucleotide on DNA synthesis and apoptosis in K562 chronic myeloid leukemia cells. Leuk Res. 1996;20(6):473–80.
33. Druker BJ, et al. Effects of a selective inhibitor of the Abl tyrosine kinase on the growth of Bcr-Abl positive cells. Nat Med. 1996;2(5):561–6.
34. Deininger MW, et al. The tyrosine kinase inhibitor CGP57148B selectively inhibits the growth of BCR-ABL-positive cells. Blood. 1997;90(9):3691–8.
35. Carroll M, et al. CGP 57148, a tyrosine kinase inhibitor, inhibits the growth of cells expressing BCR-ABL, TEL-ABL and TEL-PDGFR fusion proteins. Blood. 1997;90 (12):4947–52.
36. O'Brien SG, et al. Imatinib compared with interferon and low-dose cytarabine for newly diagnosed chronic-phase chronic myeloid leukemia. N Engl J Med. 2003;348(11):994–1004.
37. Kantarjian H, et al. Hematologic and cytogenetic responses to imatinib mesylate in chronic myelogenous leukemia. N Engl J Med. 2002;346(24):645–52.
38. Druker BJ, et al. Five-year follow-up of patients receiving imatinib for chronic myeloid leukemia. N Engl J Med. 2006;355(23):2408–17.
39. Druker BJ, et al. Activity of a specific inhibitor of the BCR-ABL tyrosine kinase in the blast crisis of chronic myeloid leukemia and acute lymphoblastic leukemia with the Philadelphia chromosome. N Engl J Med. 2001;344(14):1038–42.
40. le Coutre P, et al. Induction of resistance to the Abelson inhibitor STI571 in human leukemic cells through gene amplification. Blood. 2000;95(5):1758–66.
41. Mahon FX, et al. Selection and characterization of BCR-ABL positive cell lines with differential sensitivity to the tyrosine kinase inhibitor STI571: diverse mechanisms of resistance. Blood. 2000;96(3):1070–9.
42. Gorre ME, et al. Clinical resistance to STI-571 cancer therapy caused by BCR-ABL gene mutation or amplification. Science. 2001;293(5531):876–80.
43. Hochhaus A, et al. Molecular and chromosomal mechanisms of resistance to imatinib (STI571) therapy. Leukemia. 2002;16(11):2190–6.
44. Apperley JF. Part II: management of resistance to imatinib in chronic myeloid leukaemia. Lancet Oncol. 2007;8(12):1116–28.
45. Branford S, et al. Detection of BCR-ABL mutations in patients with CML treated with imatinib is virtually always accompanied by clinical resistance, and mutations in the ATP phosphate-binding loop (P-loop) are associated with a poor prognosis. Blood. 2003;102 (1):276–83.
46. Quintás-Cardama A, et al. Molecular biology of *bcr-abl1*–positive chronic myeloid leukemia. Blood. 2009;113(8):1619–30.
47. Cortes JE, et al. Ponatinib in refractory Philadelphia chromosome-positive leukemias. N Engl J Med. 2012;367(22):2075–88.
48. Cortes JE, et al. A phase 2 trial of ponatinib in Philadelphia chromosome-positive leukemias. N Engl J Med. 2013;369(19):1783–96.
49. Zhang J, et al. Targeting Bcr-Abl by combining allosteric with ATP-binding-site inhibitors. Nature. 2010;463(7280):501–6.
50. Heaney C, et al. Direct binding of CRKL to BCR-ABL is not required for BCR-ABL transformation. Blood. 1997;89(1):297–306.
51. Senechal K, et al. The CRKL adaptor protein transforms fibroblasts and functions in transformation by the BCR-ABL oncogene. J Biol Chem. 1996;271(38):23255–61.
52. Kipreos ET, et al. Cell cycle-regulated binding of c-Abl tyrosine kinase to DNA. Science. 1992;256(5055):382–5.
53. Goga A, et al. p53 dependent growth suppression by the c-Abl nuclear tyrosine kinase. Oncogene. 1995;11(4):791–9.

54. Van Etten RA, et al. The COOH terminus of the c-Abl tyrosine kinase contains distinct F- and G-actin binding domains with bundling activity. J Cell Biol. 1994;124(3):325–40.
55. Renshaw MW, et al. The human leukemia oncogene bcr-abl abrogates the anchorage requirement but not the growth factor requirement for proliferation. Mol Cell Biol. 1995;15(3):1286–93.
56. Greuber EK, et al. Role of ABL family kinases in cancer: from leukaemia to solid tumours. Nat Rev Cancer. 2013;13(8):559–71.
57. Aman J, et al. Effective treatment of edema and endothelial barrier dysfunction with imatinib. Circulation. 2012;126(23):2728–38.
58. Dudek SM, et al. Abl tyrosine kinase phosphorylates nonmuscle Myosin light chain kinase to regulate endothelial barrier function. Mol Biol Cell. 2010;21(22):4042–56.
59. Clark BR, et al. Cell adhesion in the stromal regulation of haemopoiesis. Baillieres Clin Haematol. 1992;5(3):619–52.
60. Vigneri P, et al. Induction of apoptosis in chronic myelogenous leukemia cells through nuclear entrapment of BCR-ABL tyrosine kinase. Nat Med. 2001;7(2):228–34.
61. Gishizky ML, et al. Initiation of deregulated growth of multipotent progenitor cells by bcr-abl in vitro. Science. 1992;256(5058):836–9.
62. Daley GQ, et al. Transformation of an interleukin 3-dependent hematopoietic cell line by the chronic myelogenous leukemia-specific P210bcr/abl protein. Proc Natl Acad Sci U S A. 1988;85(23):9312–6.
63. Hariharan IK, et al. bcr-abl oncogene renders myeloid cell line factor independent: potential autocrine mechanism in chronic myeloid leukemia. Oncogene Res. 1988;3(4):387–99.
64. Laneuville P, et al. Expression of the chronic myelogenous leukemia-associated p210bcr/abl oncoprotein in a murine IL-3 dependent myeloid cell line. Oncogene. 1991;6(2):275–82.
65. Lugo TG, et al. The BCR-ABL oncogene transforms Rat-1 cells and cooperates with v-myc. Mol Cell Biol. 1989;9(3):1263–70.
66. Daley GQ, et al. Induction of chronic myelogenous leukemia in mice by the P210bcr/abl gene of the Philadelphia chromosome. Science. 1990;247(4944) 824–30.
67. Elefanty AG, et al. bcr-abl, the hallmark of chronic myeloid leukaemia in man, induces multiple haemopoietic neoplasms in mice. EMBO J. 1990;9(4):1069–78.
68. Kelliher MA, et al. Induction of a chronic myelogenous leukemia-like syndrome in mice with v-abl and BCR/ABL. Proc Natl Acad Sci U S A. 1990;87(17)):6649–53.
69. Hariharan IK. A bcr-v-abl oncogene induces lymphomas in transgenic mice. Mol Cell Biol. 1989;9(7):2798–805.
70. Honda H, et al. Expression of p210bcr/abl by metallothionein promoter induced T-cell leukemia in transgenic mice. Blood. 1995;85(10):2853–61.
71. Honda H, et al. Development of acute lymphoblastic leukemia and myeloproliferative disorder in transgenic mice expressing p210bcr/abl: a novel transgenic model for human Ph1-positive leukemias. Blood. 1998;91(6):2067–75.
72. Lancet JE, et al. Farnesyltransferase inhibitors in hematologic malignancies: new horizons in therapy. Blood. 2003;102(12):3880–9.
73. Morgan MA, et al. Therapeutic efficacy of prenylation inhibitors in the treatment of myeloid leukemia. Leukemia. 2003;17(8):1482–98.
74. Ravandi F, et al. Modulation of cellular signaling pathways: prospects for targeted therapy in hematological malignancies. Clin Cancer Res. 2003;9(2):535–50.
75. Mizuki M, et al. Oncogenic receptor tyrosine kinase in leukemia. Cell Mol Biol. 2003;49(6):907–22.
76. Sonoyama J, et al. Functional cooperation among Ras, STAT5, and phosphatidylinositol 3-kinase is required for full oncogenic activities of BCR/ABL in K562 cells. J Biol Chem. 2002;277(10):8076–82.
77. Matsumura I, et al. Roles for deregulated receptor tyrosine kinases and their downstream signaling molecules in hematologic malignancies. Cancer Sci. 2008;99(3):479–85.

78. Skorski T, et al. Phosphatidylinositol-3 kinase activity is regulated by BCR/ABL and is required for the growth of Philadelphia chromosome-positive cells. Blood. 1995;86 (2):726–36.
79. Sillaber C, et al. Evaluation of antileukaemic effects of rapamycin in patients with imatinib-resistant chronic myeloid leukaemia. Eur J Clin Invest. 2008;38(1):43–52.
80. Carayol N, et al. Critical roles for mTORC2- and rapamycin-insensitive mTORC1-complexes in growth and survival of BCR-ABL-expressing leukemic cells. Proc Natl Acad Sci U S A. 2010;107(28):12469–74.
81. Airiau K, et al. PI3K/mTOR pathway inhibitors sensitize chronic myeloid leukemia stem cells to nilotinib and restore the response of progenitors to nilotinib in the presence of stem cell factor. Cell Death Dis. 2013;4, e827.
82. Ding J, et al. Inhibition of PI3K/mTOR overcomes nilotinib resistance in BCR-ABL1 positive leukemia cells through translational down-regulation of MDM2. PLoS One. 2013;8(12), e83510.
83. Naka K, et al. TGF-beta-FOXO signalling maintains leukaemia-initiating cells in chronic myeloid leukaemia. Nature. 2010;463(7281):676–80.
84. Pellicano F, et al. The antiproliferative activity of kinase inhibitors in chronic myeloid leukemia cells is mediated by FOXO transcription factors. Stem Cells. 2014;32(9):2324–37.
85. Rane SG, Reddy EP. JAKs, STATs and Src kinases in hematopoiesis. Oncogene. 2002;21 (21):3334–58.
86. Darnell Jr JE. STATs and gene regulation. Science. 1997;277(5532):1630–5.
87. Teglund S, et al. Stat5a and Stat5b proteins have essential and nonessential, or redundant, roles in cytokine responses. Cell. 1998;93(5):841–50.
88. Schepers H, et al. STAT5 is required for long-term maintenance of normal and leukemic human stem/progenitor cells. Blood. 2007;110(8):2880–8.
89. Nieborowska-Skorska M, et al. Signal transducer and activator of transcription (STAT)5 activation by BCR/ABL is dependent on intact Src homology (SH)3 and SH2 domains of BCR/ABL and is required for leukemogenesis. J Exp Med. 1999;189(8):1229–42.
90. de Groot RP, et al. STAT5 activation by BCR-Abl contributes to transformation of K562 leukemia cells. Blood. 1999;94(3):1108–12.
91. Sillaber C, et al. STAT5 activation contributes to growth and viability in Bcr/Abl-transformed cells. Blood. 2000;95(6):2118–25.
92. Schaller-Schönitz M, et al. BCR-ABL affects STAT5A and STAT5B differentially. PLoS One. 2014;9(5), e97243.
93. Sattler M, et al. The phosphatidylinositol polyphosphate 5-phosphatase SHIP and the protein tyrosine phosphatase SHP-2 form a complex in hematopoietic cells which can be regulated by BCR/ABL and growth factors. Oncogene. 1997;15(19):2379–84.
94. Scherr M, et al. Enhanced sensitivity to inhibition of SHP2, STAT5, and Gab2 expression in chronic myeloid leukemia (CML). Blood. 2006;107(8):3279–87.
95. Chen J, et al. SHP-2 phosphatase is required for hematopoietic cell transformation by Bcr-Abl. Blood. 2007;109(2):778–85.
96. Sha F, et al. Dissection of the BCR-ABL signaling network using highly specific monobody inhibitors to the SHP2 SH2 domains. Proc Natl Acad Sci U S A. 2013;110(37):14924–9.
97. Pendergast AM, et al. BCR-ABL-induced oncogenesis is mediated by direct interaction with the SH2 domain of the GRB-2 adaptor protein. Cell. 1993;75(1):175–85.
98. Sattler M, et al. Critical role for Gab2 in transformation by BCR/ABL. Cancer Cell. 2002;1 (5):479–92.
99. Wöhrle FU, et al. Gab2 signaling in chronic myeloid leukemia cells confers resistance to multiple Bcr-Abl inhibitors. Leukemia. 2013;27(1):118–29.
100. Barber DL, et al. Erythropoietin and interleukin-3 activate tyrosine phosphorylation of CBL and association with CRK adaptor proteins. Blood. 1997;89(9):3166–74.

101. Gesbert F, et al. Interleukin-2 stimulation induces tyrosine phosphorylation of p120-Cbl and CrkL and formation of multimolecular signaling complexes in T lymphocytes and natural killer cells. J Biol Chem. 1988;273(7):3986–93.
102. Odai H, et al. The proto-oncogene product c-Cbl becomes tyrosine phosphorylated by stimulation with GM-CSF or Epo and constitutively binds to the SH3 domain of Grb2/Ash in human hematopoietic cells. J Biol Chem. 1995;270(18):10800–5.
103. Wisniewski D, et al. c-kit ligand stimulates tyrosine phosphorylation of the c-Cbl protein in human hematopoietic cells. Leukemia. 1996;10(9):1436–42.
104. Bhat A, et al. Interactions of CBL with BCR-ABL and CRKL in BCR-ABL-transformed myeloid cells. J Biol Chem. 1997;272(26):16170–5.
105. de Jong R, et al. CRKL is complexed with tyrosine-phosphorylated Cbl in Ph-positive leukemia. J Biol Chem. 1995;270(37):21468–71.
106. Pisick E, Xu G, Li JL, Prasad KV, Griffin JD. The proto-oncogene product p120CBL and the adaptor proteins CRKL and c-CRK link c-ABL, p190BCR/ABL and p210BCR/ABL to the phosphatidylinositol-3' kinase pathway. Oncogene. 1996;12(4):839–46.
107. Tari AM, Arlinghaus R, Lopez-Berestein G. Inhibition of Grb2 and Crkl proteins results in growth inhibition of Philadelphia chromosome positive leukemic cells. Biochem Biophys Res Commun. 1997;235(2):383–8.
108. Sakai R, et al. A novel signaling molecule, p130, forms stable complexes in vivo with v-Crk and v-Src in a tyrosine phosphorylation-dependent manner. EMBO J. 1994;13(16):3748–56.
109. Nojima Y, et al. Integrin-mediated cell adhesion promotes tyrosine phosphorylation of p130Cas, a Src homology 3-containing molecule having multiple Src homology 2-binding motifs. J Biol Chem. 1995;270(25):15398–402.
110. Harte MT, et al. p130Cas, a substrate associated with v-Src and v-Crk, localizes to focal adhesions and binds to focal adhesion kinase. J Biol Chem. 1996;271(23):13649–55.
111. Salgia R, et al. p130CAS forms a signaling complex with the adaptor protein CRKL in hematopoietic cells. J Biol Chem. 1996;271(41):25198–203.
112. Erpel T, et al. Src family protein tyrosine kinases and cellular signal transduction pathways. Curr Opin Cell Biol. 1995;7(2):176–82.
113. Odajima J, et al. Full oncogenic activities of v-Src are mediated by multiple signaling pathways Ras as an essential mediator for cell survival. J Biol Chem. 2000;275 (31):24096–105.
114. Chaturvedi P, et al. Abrogation of interleukin-3 dependence of myeloid cells by the v-src oncogene requires SH2 and SH3 domains which specify activation of STATs. Mol Cell Biol. 1997;17(6):3295–304.
115. Guan JL, et al. Regulation of focal adhesion-associated protein tyrosine kinase by both cellular adhesion and oncogenic transformation. Nature. 1992;358(6388):690–2.
116. Nori M, et al. Inhibition of v-src-induced transformation by a GTPase-activating protein. Mol Cell Biol. 1991;11(5):2812–8.
117. Aftab DT, et al. Ras-independent transformation by v-Src. Proc Natl Acad Sci U S A. 1997;94 (7):3028–33.
118. DeClue JE, et al. Suppression of src transformation by overexpression of full-length GTPase-activating protein (GAP) or of the GAP C terminus. Mol Cell Biol. 1991;11(5):2819–25.
119. Oldham SM, et al. Ras, but not Src, transformation of RIE-1 epithelial cells is dependent on activation of the mitogen-activated protein kinase cascade. Oncogene. 1998;16(20):2565–73.
120. Wu J, et al. Association between imatinib-resistant BCR-ABL mutation-negative leukemia and persistent activation of LYN kinase. J Natl Cancer Inst. 2008;100(13):926–39.
121. Pene-Dumitrescu T, et al. Expression of a Src family kinase in chronic myelogenous leukemia cells induces resistance to imatinib in a kinase-dependent manner. J Biol Chem. 2010;285(28):21446–57.
122. Wu J, et al. Lyn regulates BCR-ABL and Gab2 tyrosine phosphorylation and c-Cbl protein stability in imatinib-resistant chronic myelogenous leukemia cells. Blood. 2008;111 (7):3821–9.

123. Parganas E, et al. Jak2 is essential for signaling through a variety of cytokine receptors. Cell. 1998;93(3):385–95.
124. Neubauer H, et al. Jak2 deficiency defines an essential developmental checkpoint in definitive hematopoiesis. Cell. 1998;93(3):397–409.
125. Park SO, et al. Conditional deletion of Jak2 reveals an essential role in hematopoiesis throughout mouse ontogeny: implications for Jak2 inhibition in humans. PLoS One. 2013;8 (3), e59675.
126. Grisouard J, et al. Selective deletion of Jak2 in adult mouse hematopoietic cells leads to lethal anemia and thrombocytopenia. Haematologica. 2014;99(4):e52–4.
127. Jiang X, et al. Chronic myeloid leukemia stem cells possess multiple unique features of resistance to BCR-ABL targeted therapies. Leukemia. 2007;21(5):926–35.
128. Zhou LL, et al. AHI-1 interacts with BCR-ABL and modulates BCR-ABL transforming activity and imatinib response of CML stem/progenitor cells. J Exp Med. 2008;205 (11):2657–71.
129. Liu X, et al. Molecular and structural characterization of the SH3 domain of AHI-1 in regulation of cellular resistance of BCR-ABL(+) chronic myeloid leukemia cells to tyrosine kinase inhibitors. Proteomics. 2012;12(13):2094–106.
130. Chen M, et al. Targeting primitive chronic myeloid leukemia cells by effective inhibition of a new AHI-1-BCR-ABL-JAK2 complex. J Natl Cancer Inst. 2013;105:405–23.
131. Lin H, et al. Selective JAK2/ABL dual inhibition therapy effectively eliminates TKI-insensitive CML stem/progenitor cells. Oncotarget. 2014;5(18):8637–50.
132. Reya T, et al. A role for Wnt signalling in self-renewal of haematopoietic stem cells. Nature. 2003;423:409–14.
133. Baba Y, et al. Constitutively active β-catenin confers multilineage differentiation potential on lymphoid and myeloid progenitors. Immunity. 2005;23:599–609.
134. Coluccia AM, et al. Bcr-Abl stabilizes β-catenin in chronic myeloid leukemia through its tyrosine phosphorylation. EMBO J. 2007;26:1456–66.
135. Abrahamsson AE, et al. Glycogen synthase kinase 3β missplicing contributes to leukemia stem cell generation. Proc Natl Acad Sci U S A. 2009;106(10):3925–9.
136. Zhang B, et al. Microenvironmental protection of CML stem and progenitor cells from tyrosine kinase inhibitors through N-cadherin and Wnt-β-catenin signaling. Blood. 2013;121(10):1824–38.
137. Zhao C, Blum J, Chen A, et al. Loss of β-catenin impairs the renewal of normal and CML stem cells in vivo. Cancer Cell. 2007;12(6):528–41.
138. Reddiconto G, et al. Targeting of GSK3β promotes imatinib-mediated apoptosis in quiescent CD34+ chronic myeloid leukemia progenitors, preserving normal stem cells. Blood. 2012;119(10):2335–45.
139. Jamieson CH, et al. Granulocyte-macrophage progenitors as candidate leukemic stem cells in blast-crisis CML. N Engl J Med. 2004;351(7):657–67.
140. Zhao C, Chen A, Jamieson CH, et al. Hedgehog signalling is essential for maintenance of cancer stem cells in myeloid leukaemia. Nature. 2009;458(7239):776–9.
141. Cea M, et al. Tracking molecular relapse of chronic myeloid leukemia by measuring Hedgehog signaling status. Leuk Lymphoma. 2013;54(2):342–52.
142. Sengupta A, et al. Deregulation and cross talk among Sonic hedgehog, Wnt, Hox and Notch signaling in chronic myeloid leukemia progression. Leukemia. 2007;21(5):949–55.
143. Su W, et al. Sonic hedgehog maintains survival and growth of chronic myeloid leukemia progenitor cells through b-catenin signaling. Exp Hematol. 2012;40(5):418–27.
144. Dierks C, Beigi R, Guo GR, et al. Expansion of Bcr-Abl-positive leukemic stem cells is dependent on Hedgehog pathway activation. Cancer Cell. 2008;14:238–49.

# Chapter 4
# Goals of CML Treatment in the Tyrosine Kinase Inhibitor Era

**Jerald Radich and Daniel Egan**

**Abstract** The widespread introduction of tyrosine kinase inhibitor (TKI) therapy has radically changed the treatment strategy and goals of treatment of chronic myeloid leukemia (CML). In the past, allogeneic transplantation offered the only alternative for "curative" therapy, and the use of this modality was limited by patient age and donor availability. In a mere decade of use, TKI therapy has pushed transplantation to a salvage therapy, and most chronic-phase patients can expect prolonged response, with a small risk of progression to advanced-phase disease. Indeed, we now can speak of a "functional cure" and can now even consider discontinuing therapy for those patients without molecular evidence of disease. Given the multiple tyrosine kinase inhibitors now available to clinicians, as well as sensitive and relatively noninvasive methods to monitor disease response, we are now at the enviable phase of being able to optimize response based on the individual treatment goals of the patient and physician.

**Keywords** Chronic myeloid leukemia • Chronic myelogenous leukemia • Tyrosine kinase inhibitor • Monitoring • BCR-ABL

## 4.1 Introduction

The widespread introduction of tyrosine kinase inhibitor (TKI) therapy has radically changed the treatment strategy and goals of treatment of chronic myeloid leukemia (CML). In the past, allogeneic transplantation offered the only alternative for "curative" therapy, and the use of this modality was limited by patient age and donor availability. In a mere decade of use, TKI therapy has pushed transplantation to a salvage therapy, and most chronic-phase patients can expect prolonged response, with a small risk of progression to advanced-phase disease. Indeed, we now can speak of a "functional cure" and can now even consider discontinuing therapy for those patients without molecular evidence of disease.

J. Radich, MD (✉) • D. Egan, MD
Clinical Research Division, Fred Hutchinson Cancer Research Center, Seattle, WA, USA
e-mail: jradich@fredhutch.org



M. Kizaki (ed.), *Molecular Pathogenesis and Treatment of Chronic Myelogenous Leukemia*, DOI 10.1007/978-4-431-55714-2_4

When considering treatment goals in the twenty-first century, it is important to consider a few "ground truths" in CML in the age of TKIs:

### 4.1.1 *The Majority of Chronic-Phase CML Case Do Remarkably Well*

For example, patients treated with imatinib in chronic phase have an excellent response to therapy, with nearly 70 and 90 % achieving a complete cytogenetic remission (CCyR) at 1 year and 5 years, respectively [1, #461]. At 8 years of follow-up, ~90 % of patients treated with imatinib on the IRIS trial were still alive [2]. Rates of CCyR are even higher with the "second-generation" TKIs nilotinib and dasatinib (though so far, these gains compared to imatinib have not translated into survival differences) [2–5].

### 4.1.2 *TKI Failures Are Not Unusual*

Approximately 60 % of patients treated with imatinib on the IRIS trial remained in CCyR after 6 years of therapy [6]. These patients whom IM failed (not the other way around, which is the conventional language) causes are divided into tertiles of primary resistance, toxicity, and resistance/progression. A point mutation in the Abelson (ABL) tyrosine kinase domain, which affects TKI binding and ABL inhibition, may be detected in roughly half of those with imatinib resistance [7–9]. For those patients who fail frontline imatinib, salvage therapy with the second-generation TKIs (dasatinib, nilotinib) can yield a CCyR in 40–50 % of cases [10, 11]. For cases in which initial therapy with a second generation fails, salvage with another second-generation TKI, or a "third-generation" bosutinib or ponatinib, can yield major and complete cytogenetic remission, but generally at a lower frequency [12, 13]. However, cases that initially respond to second-line therapy often relapse, sometimes with a new mutation. Patients in this category can either be treated with other TKIs (bosutinib, ponatinib), but if one is looking for cure, allogeneic transplant remains the best bet for highly resistant disease [14, 15].

### 4.1.3 *Advanced-Phase Disease Is Still Difficult to Treat*

Patients who become resistant to TKI therapy and progress to accelerated and blast phase continue to be a therapeutic challenge. In this context, second-generation TKIs can yield a response, but it is not generally long lived. For example, 27 % and 43 % of myeloid and lymphoid BC, respectively, achieved a CCyR on dasatinib.

Unfortunately, the response was rather short lived, as the median PFS was 5 and 3 months for myeloid and lymphoid BC, respectively [16, 17]. Transplantation may be effective, but survival rates are considerably less than those performed in chronic phase. This underlines the importance on adherence to therapy, as well as monitoring of disease response (see below).

In CML, we are in the enviable position of having many different treatment modalities and sensitive measures to monitor disease response. How do we best use these tools to optimize therapy in our patients?

## 4.2 Outcomes and the Tools to Measure Them

The diagnostic and monitoring toolbox includes the peripheral complete blood count (CBC), marrow metaphase cytogenetics to discover the Ph chromosome, in situ fluorescence hybridization (FISH) for the *BCR-ABL* DNA translocation, and peripheral blood quantitative RT-PCR (qPCR) for the chimeric BCR-ABL mRNA (Table 4.1). At diagnosis, all patients should undergo complete disease staging with a bone marrow aspiration and biopsy. Using the marrow aspirate sample, cytogenetic analysis is used to confirm the presence of the Ph and has the added ability to screen for additional chromosomal abnormalities, which would be indicative of accelerated-phase disease. In cases where a bone marrow is difficult, FISH can be used to diagnose CML, but will obviously not pick up other clonal abnormalities unless specific probes are added to the analysis. qPCR testing should also be performed to determine the baseline pretreatment BCR-ABL transcript level, and it is best to perform it on peripheral blood, as this will be the source of material as treatment progresses.

In general, treatment with TKIs can be viewed as a series of benchmarks that consider both the *degree* of reduction in disease markers, as well as the *rapidity* of response, both of which have clearly been shown to correlate with long-term outcomes in numerous clinical trials. Two nonprofit professional organizations, the US-based National Comprehensive Cancer Network (NCCN) and the European Leukemia Net (ELN), publish recommendations to guide clinicians in the best

**Table 4.1** Methods to detect minimal residual disease in CML

| Method | Target | Sensitivity | Advantages | Disadvantages |
|---|---|---|---|---|
| Metaphase Chromosome Cytogenetics | t(9;22) | 1–5 % | The gold standard and detection of other chromosomal changes | Needs dividing cells, so generally only successful form of bone marrow sample |
| FISH | *BCR-ABL* DNA | 0.1–5 % | Can use peripheral blood or bone marrow | Relatively insensitive compared to RT-PCR |
| Quantitative RT-PCR | *BCR-ABL* mRNA | 0.001–0.01 % | Very sensitive and uses peripheral blood | Not well standardized across labs |

**Table 4.2** Response criteria in CML

| Level of response | Definition |
|---|---|
| Complete hematological response | Normal CBC and differential |
| Minor cytogenetic response | 35–90 % Ph-positive metaphases |
| Partial cytogenetic response | 1–34 % Ph-positive metaphases |
| Complete cytogenetic response | 0 % Ph-positive metaphases |
| Major molecular response | ≥3-log reduction of *BCR-ABL* mRNA; 0.1 % IS |
| Complete molecular remission | Negativity by qPCR at a sensitivity of at least 4.5 logs (0.0032 % IS) |

therapeutic and monitoring strategies for CML, with guidelines based on the most recent medical evidence. As of the time of publication, the 2015 NCCN and 2013 ELN guidelines represent the most recent consensus recommendations, the content of which are remarkably similar between the two groups [18, 19].

Once TKI treatment has begun, the first measure of response is hematological remission, which is simply the normalization of peripheral complete blood counts and normalization in spleen size. The term "complete hematologic response" (CHR) is specifically defined as normalization in peripheral blood counts (total leukocyte count of less than $10 \times 10^9$/L, platelet count of less than $450 \times 10^9$/L, and absence of circulating immature myeloid cells) and absence of splenomegaly (Table 4.2). The achievement of a CHR within 3 months of initiating therapy is widely recognized as a critical objective of modern therapy and is incorporated as the first milestone in guidelines from both the ELN and NCCN. For chronic-phase patients, this occurs in >90 % of patients within the first 3 months of therapy (and for the majority, sooner than that) [20]. ELN guidelines suggest the additional criterion of basophils comprising less than 5 % of the peripheral blood differential. Failure to achieve hematological remission, if the patient has been adherent to prescribed therapy, is an indication to change to another TKI.

Reduction in the amount of detectable Ph, as measured by conventional metaphase cytogenetics, represents the next stratum of response assessment. Cytogenetic responses are based on sequential bone marrow cytogenetic analyses, with evaluation of at least 20 metaphases required for optimal interpretation. A minor cytogenetic response (mCyR) and major cytogenetic response (MCyR) are defined by the presence of t(9;22) in 35–65 % and 1–35 % of metaphases, respectively. The more stringent definition of "complete cytogenetic response" (CCyR) indicates the absence of detectable Ph in at least 20 metaphases. For consistency between clinical trials, the standard approach to determining CCyR has been through conventional metaphase cytogenetics, and thus patient outcomes have been historically based on this. There is evidence to suggest that if such evaluation is not available, FISH <1 % (considering at least 200 cells) appears to be equivalent to CCyR [21] (Table 4.3).

Cytogenetic response continues to be the standard indicator of therapeutic success with TKI therapy. In the landmark IRIS trial, where patients were treated

**Table 4.3** A comparison of "optimal" and "failure" criteria for NCCN and ELN guidelines

| | NCCN Guidelines®: version 1.2015 | | 2013 European LeukemiaNet guidelines[d] | | |
|---|---|---|---|---|---|
| | Optimal | Failure (change of therapy advised) | Optimal | Warning | Failure[e] (change of therapy advised) |
| 3 months | BCR-ABL ≤10 % (IS) or PCyR | BCR-ABL >10 % (IS) or lack of PCyR[a,b] | BCR-ABL ≤10 % (IS) or Ph+ ≤35 % | BCR-ABL >10 % (IS) and/or Ph+ 65–95 % | Lack CHR or Ph+ >95 % |
| 6 months | BCR-ABL ≤10 % (IS) or ≥ PCyR | BCR-ABL >10 % (IS) or lack of PCyR | BCR-ABL ≤1 % (IS) and/or CCyR | BCR-ABL 1–10 % (IS) and/or Ph+ 1–35 % | BCR-ABL >10 % (IS) and/or Ph+ >35 % |
| 12 months | CCyR or BCR-ABL ≤1 % (IS) | < PCyR[a,c] or BCR-ABL >10 % (IS) | BCR-ABL ≤0.1 % (IS) | BCR-ABL =0.1–1 % (IS) | BCR-ABL >1 % (IS) and/or Ph+ >0 % |
| 18 months | CCyR | Less than CCyR or cytogenetic relapse | | | |

Referenced with permission from the NCCN Clinical Practice Guidelines in Oncology (NCCN Guidelines®) for Chronic Myelogenous Leukemia V.1.2015.  Accessed [Month and Day, Year]. To view the most recent and complete version of the guideline, go online to NCCN.org. NATIONAL COMPREHENSIVE CANCER NETWORK®, NCCN®, NCCN GUIDELINES®, and all other NCCN Content are trademarks owned by the National Comprehensive Cancer Network, Inc.

*PCyR* partial cytogenetic response, *IS* international scale, *CHR* complete hematologic response, *Ph+* Philadelphia chromosome (by cytogenetic analysis), *TKI* tyrosine kinase inhibitor, *CCA* clonal cytogenetic abnormalities, *NCCN* National Comprehensive Cancer Network®, *ELN* European LeukemiaNet

[a]Consider dose escalation of imatinib to 800 mg, if not a candidate for alternate TKI or omacetaxine

[b]Continuation of same dose TKI may be considered if the primary treatment was dasatinib or nilotinib

[c]Continuation of same dose TKI may be considered with PCyR at 12 months

[d]ELN guidelines summarized are for response assessment of first-line TKI therapy only. See reference for response assessment of second-line therapy

[e]At any point in time, other indicators of treatment failure include: (1) any loss of CHR, CCyR, PCyR, or MMR; (2) new point mutations in BCR-ABL; or (3) CCA in Ph+ cells

with imatinib versus interferon plus cytarabine, achievement of a CCyR at 6 months (on either treatment arm) was associated with a decreased risk of disease progression to advanced phase at a median of 42 months of follow-up [1]. Impact of CCyR on survival has also remained in patients receiving high-dose imatinib or second-generation TKIs [22]. Both the ELN and NCCN recognize the achievement of CCyR within a year of therapy as an extremely important milestone [18, 19].

The most sensitive, and convenient, method of measuring disease response during therapy is by BCR-ABL qPCR. With current methods, laboratories are able to detect as low as a single CML cell in a background of up to at least 100,000 normal cells. This high level of sensitivity allows routine disease monitoring to be performed on peripheral blood. *BCR-ABL* transcript levels determined by qRT-PCR are highly correlated with disease burden as determined by cytogenetics or FISH (at least, in the range that all three can be comparatively measured), and many centers with expertise in qRT-PCR use *BCR-ABL* transcript monitoring to monitor patients instead of cytogenetics, once cytogenetics have been performed at diagnosis to establish the diagnosis and stage of disease [23, 24].

There is no "standard" BCR-ABL qPCR assay, as the labs have variations in the platform used, primers, and even housekeeping genes that are used as controls. Much of what has been established for molecular monitoring stems from the landmark IRIS study (the phase 3 trial that established imatinib as the new standard for CML). In IRIS, a baseline *BCR-ABL* transcript level (measured as *BCR-ABL/BCR*) was determined through PCR testing of peripheral blood samples from 30 untreated, chronic-phase CML patients in each of the three IRIS laboratories [25]. Median values for the 30 samples served as the baseline *BCR-ABL/BCR* level for each laboratory, to which subsequent patient samples would be compared. The *BCR-ABL* log reduction value for each patient was calculated by comparing a result to the median value of the diagnostic reference group. A 3-log reduction from the median baseline was deemed a "major molecular response" (MMR), and this correlated with an excellent progression-free survival. Amazingly, other studies confirmed the importance of the MMR (see below), and MMR quickly became an important response metric [3, 5, 26, 27].

Unfortunately, the original specimen pool that was used to determine the baseline BCR-ABL/BCR transcript levels in the IRIS study has since been depleted. However, prior to the consumption of these specimens, an equivalent measure of *BCR-ABL* transcript levels was engineered, and thus a standard for *BCR-ABL* has been established, known as the International Scale [28]. Through exchange of samples with an IS reference laboratory, an "IS conversion factor" can be established for a particular lab, which will then allow for standardization of results to the IS. The IS has been conveniently aligned with important milestones for treatment, with a value of 1 % IS correlating with a complete cytogenetic response (CCyR) and an IS of 0.1 % indicating the level of MMR.

## 4.3 What Is the Best Definition of Response to Therapy in CML?

Molecular responses are defined using qRT-PCR for detection of BCR-ABL mRNA transcript levels. Fortunately, peripheral blood may be used for such monitoring by qRT-PCR. A major molecular response (MMR), a milestone that correlates with long-term prognosis (see below), is defined by a transcript level less than 0.1 %, or a greater than 3-log scale reduction, on the International Scale (IS). More stringent responses, such as "MR$^{4}$" and "MR$^{4.5}$" suggest molecular remission with undetectable transcripts at 4-log and 4.5-log scale reductions, respectively, from the IRIS baseline.

## 4.4 Treatment Milestones

There are several sequential treatment landmarks which are clearly associated with clinical outcome.

### *4.4.1 Complete Hematologic Response (CHR)*

The complete normalization of counts generally occurs quickly, certainly within the first 3 months of therapy. Failure to reach a CHR obviously precludes a deeper cytogenetic and molecular response and triggers an immediate change of TKI therapy. In addition, failure to achieve a CHR should trigger suspicion about poor adherence to therapy.

### *4.4.2 Cytogenetic Response*

Cytogenetic monitoring of the level of Ph+ metaphases is the next prognostic factor for predicting long-term response to TKI therapy once patients have achieved a CHR. Achieving a CCyR is an independent prognostic factor for survival and should therefore be considered a goal of therapy [1, 29, 30]. Failure to achieve any reduction in the number of Ph+ cells after 6 months of imatinib therapy and failure to achieve an MCyR response after 12 months of imatinib therapy predict for <20 % chance of ever achieving a CCyR [31]. Additionally, studies have shown that achieving an MCyR at 3 months is associated with prolonged time to disease progression in patients with late chronic-phase and accelerated-phase CML [32, 33].

### *4.4.3 Major Molecular Response (MMR)*

While attaining a CCyR remains a major therapeutic milestone, the further achievement of MMR seems to be a "safe haven," as secondary resistance and progression is relatively unusual once MMR has been achieved. In the IRIS trial, considering only those patients with a CCyR, there was a 97 % progression-free survival at 54 months in the subset with more than 3-log reduction (MMR), at 12 months, as opposed to an 89 % progression-free survival in the subset with less than an MMR at 12 months [34]. Additional studies have confirmed that achievement of MMR at either 12 or 18 months is associated with a longer duration of CCyR and higher rates of progression-free survival [35, 36]. Furthermore, loss of MMR after initially achieving one is associated with an increased risk of disease relapse [37].

### 4.4.4 Complete Molecular Remission (CMR)

In vitro studies have demonstrated that the CML "stem cell" does not depend on BCR-ABL kinase activity for survival [38]. Given that finding, the prevailing assumption had been that patients would require TKI therapy forever. This is yet another example of popular assumptions being wrong. In fact, several studies have shown that for those (relatively rare) patients with persistently undetectable *BCR-ABL*, many patients may discontinue therapy without relapse of their disease, even by PCR criteria. The STIM trial and the Australasian Leukemia and Lymphoma Group's CML8 TWISTER trial represent two landmark clinical trials investigating the clinical course of patients with undetectable disease by PCR testing [39, 40]. Both trials required that patients have undetectable BCR-ABL mRNA for at least 2 years to be considered eligible for TKI discontinuation, and in both a remarkably similar proportion of enrolled patients, 40 % maintained long-term remission after discontinuation of imatinib. Happily, those patients who did relapse responded to subsequent TKI therapy, though not all reverted back to an undetectable *BCR-ABL* transcript level.

In reality, the term "undetectable *BCR-ABL*" is complicated, as *BCR-ABL* can become undetectable given (1) a very low *BCR-ABL* level despite employment of a sensitive test; (2) a higher level of disease burden, but an inadequate sample size; and (3) almost any *BCR-ABL* level with a poorly sensitive test. Obviously, only the first such scenario would satisfy clinical requirements to consider discontinuing therapy. Thus, the concept of a complete molecular remission (CMR) pertains to that degree of response in which BCR-ABL is undetectable by PCR methods, backed with the potentially depth that the assay is able to reach given the number of cells tested. The copy number of the control gene estimates the cell numbers. Thus, CMR 4.5 would refer to undetectable disease in a sample adequate to assess a 4.5-log reduction in BCR-ABL level. Ongoing discontinuation studies differ by the depth of response required to consider discontinuation, but generally require at least a 4-log read depth. For example, the PCR sensitivity criteria for the above-referenced CML8 and STIM trials were set at a 4.5-log and 5-log reduction, respectively, from the IRIS baseline [39, 40]. It reasons that earlier and deeper molecular responses attained with second-generation TKIs might allow more patients to successfully discontinue TKI therapy, and prospective trials to address this issue are ongoing (Fig. 4.1).

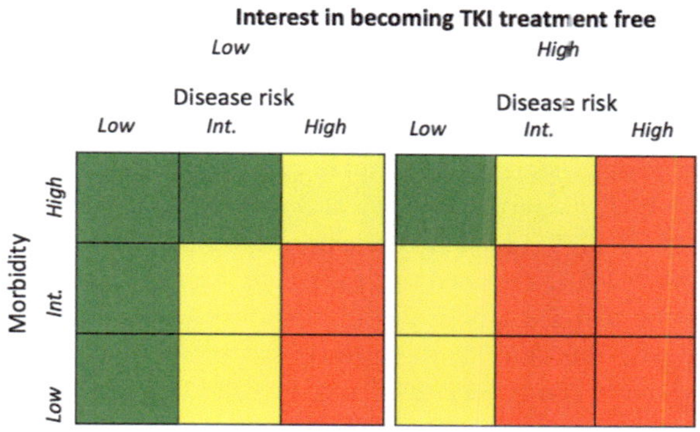


**Fig. 4.1** An imaginary treatment grid based on morbidity, disease risk (Sokal), and desire to obtain a sustained CMR and successfully discontinue therapy. The colors are a heat map, where *green* is a strong choice toward imatinib, *yellow* intermediate choice between imatinib and a second-generation TKI, and *red* a strong preference toward a second-generation TKI

## 4.5 The Significance of Early Molecular Response (EMR)

Previous guidelines identified the presence or absence of a complete hematologic response at 3 months after initiation of therapy as a suggested "early" metric to evaluate treatment response. More recently, it was shown that early cytogenetic responses by 3–6 months correlate with increased progression-free survival and overall survival [31, 41]. Both major guidelines have been updated to emphasize a partial cytogenetic response by 3 months as being optimal. In addition, there is increasingly convincing evidence that the degree of early molecular response by 3–6 months of therapy is favorably associated with long-term outcomes. For example, among patients receiving imatinib, Marin et al. showed that 97 % of patients with BCR-ABL/ABL <10 % at 3 months were alive at 7 years, compared to only 54 % of those with BCR-ABL/ABL >10 % at 3 months [41]. Jain et al. also showed that in patients taking imatinib or second-generation TKIs, the 3-year event-free survival was 95–98 % for those with a BCR-ABL level of <10 % IS at 3 months, versus an event-free survival of only 61 % for those with a transcript level of >10 % at 3 months [42].

The current 2015 NCCN guidelines now suggest *BCR-ABL* <10 % IS at 3 months as an important response criterion, with switching to a different TKI considered if *BCR-ABL* levels are greater than 10 %. ELN guidelines do not call for a change at 3 months, but do suggest a change at the 6-month mark. There are a few important considerations: (1) there is no published data that switching TKIs at 3 or 6 months will affect the natural history of the disease – bad biology may trump our clinical strategy; (2) most progressions to advanced-phase disease occur early, so waiting to 6 months may allow some patients to progress. However, again, there is no assurance that switching to another TKI would change the biology of the disease and prevent progression; and (3) a poor response early on, especially by 3 months, may be due to lack of drug exposure, given side effects or other problems with adherence. These patients may have responsive biology in the long run, once they are able to amply tolerate the drug.

Of course, making a somewhat arbitrary categorical variable (10 % IS at 3 or 6 months) out of a rich, continuous variable can be problematic. Is a patient that goes from 100 % IS at diagnosis to 11 % at 3 months really the same as a patient who goes from 15 to 11 %? Is someone who goes from 100 % IS to 11 % really different than 100–9 %? As opposed to an absolute response threshold of molecular response, it may be that the kinetics of treatment response is more predictive of long-term prognosis. Branford et al. showed that patients with more than 10 % *BCR-ABL* at 3 months could further be risk stratified by considering the rate of decline in *BCR-ABL* transcripts [43]. Those patients with a "halving time" of more than 76 days after commencing imatinib had a statistically significant poorer survival at 4 years (58 %), as opposed to 95 % for those with a halving time of less than 76 days. The survival curve for those with an early response of $<$10 % *BCR-ABL* at 3 months overlapped with the survival curve for those with $>$10 % *BCR-ABL* but a more rapid halving time. This would suggest that even patients starting out with a high disease burden may have similar long-term outcomes depending on the rate of response. Interestingly, the rate in which patients achieve a deep molecular response seems to be independently predictive of sustained remission after stopping imatinib, providing further evidence that the rate of molecular response is of prognostic value, and raises the intriguing question of whether second-generation agents may have a possible advantage in increasing a patient's chances of ultimately achieving future sustained molecular remissions off of therapy.

## 4.6 New Advances in Disease Monitoring

**Alternative PCR Methods** The fact that more than half of patients enrolled on TKI discontinuation trials demonstrate relapse, despite previously having undetectable BCR-ABL transcripts for a sustained period of time, illustrates the fact that in most patients, leukemic cells continue to survive below the limit of detection using standard qPCR methods. It reasons that increasingly sensitive methods of detection may better stratify patients in regard to risk of relapse, perhaps with a more stringent definition of a complete molecular response. Because the proportions of final (saturated) PCR products do not necessarily equal the relative quantities of initial template, simply increasing the number of amplification cycles will not increase sensitivity and may result in errors in replication. In addition, because of the high degree of technical variation that exists with qPCR, in that laboratory conditions and reagents contribute to poor reproducibility between different locations, or even separate runs in one location, there is interest in developing newer, more precise methods for monitoring of BCR-ABL.

**DNA PCR** While detection of BCR-ABL mRNA forms the primary basis for molecular monitoring in CML, amplification of DNA template that includes a particular patient's breakpoint region allows for the possibility of DNA qPCR. It should be noted that use of a housekeeping control gene is necessary. Using a nested approach, and using mixing to create dilute positive controls, an Australian group demonstrated a level of sensitivity down to 1:10$^6$ with DNA qPCR. Using patient samples, there was good correlation between RNA and DNA qPCR, and in addition, among the 16 samples with undetectable mRNA transcript, half were detectable by DNA qPCR. In a recent 2014 publication from the group, in which samples from 92 CML patients were monitored for MRD, DNA qPCR was shown to be more precise at the level of MRD [44].

**Digital PCR** This represents a newer, alternative method of quantitative detection of rare transcripts [45, 46]. The method involves partitioning the original specimen into hundreds, or thousands (or more) of tiny chambers, or droplets, so that the presence or absence of target template in each partition yields a binary, or "digital," result (positive or negative). Using the Poisson distribution, the presence or absence of PCR product allows for quantification of rare target sequences. It has been estimated that digital PCR increases the limit of detection by 1 or 2 logs. The method has the additional advantages of having low technical variation (greater similarity between repeat runs), and calibration curves are not required to yield an absolute numerical value. While not yet integrated into clinical trials for CML, recent work by Jennings et al. demonstrates the feasibility, precision, and sensitivity of digital PCR compared to qPCR in the detection of *BCR-ABL* [47]. Through the use of microfluidic platforms, digital PCR is poised to become increasingly feasible.

**"Duplex" Next-Generation Sequencing** *Most sequencing methods for ABL mutations use the* Sanger sequencing method, using a PCR-derived DNA template of the target sequence. This method can detect a mutation if it occurs in approximately 10–20 % of the total targets. This is fine for sequencing of patients in frank relapse, but is inadequate to understand the kinetics of mutation emergence. "Next-generation sequencing" (NGS) methods rely on creating libraries of DNA fragments and sequencing short stretches, then aligning and rebuilding the fragments of the genome into an assembled consensus sequence. This potentially adds another order of magnitude in sensitivity. Studies have used NGS to detect ABL mutations and have shown that in many cases there is a complicated kinetic structure of competing mutational clones, some becoming dominant and creating a relapse, while others emerging and then receding [48]. However, it is estimated that as many as 1 % of the mutation reads are erroneous during the technical issues in generating the DNA libraries, and this obviously impacts the understanding of the significance of rare frequency mutations. A new way to obviate this potential technical artifact is "duplex" NGS, in which DNA libraries are made from both the complementary DNA strands. In composing the aggregate sequence, mutations are only "called" if they appeared in both strands. The chance that such a complementary mutation will occur in both strands is exceeding unlikely, and thus the false positive error rate is remarkably reduced by several orders of magnitude [49].

## 4.7 Conclusion: Toward Patient-Specific Goals

The NCCN and ELN have promoted guidelines on CML care. These are quite useful, but are somewhat generic given the broad range of CML patients in regard to age, disease state, comorbidities, and expectations. Given the options in TKIs and the various disease endpoints (CCyR, survival, progression-free survival, treatment-free survival), what types of things should we consider when tailoring therapy to each patient?

Age has important implications both on treatment expectations, as well as potential comorbidities. For example, in a 70-year-old, a reasonable treatment expectation might be to obtain a CCyR, which could potentially extend survival, rather than the expectation of CMR and discontinuation, which is more appealing for younger patients who may want children, let alone hoping to be treatment-free for decades. Thus, in this hypothetical elderly patient, imatinib might be a fine choice, especially given the cardiovascular toxicity of many of the second-generation TKIs.

In addition, the disease state comes into play. Patients with a low Sokol/Hansford/Euro score may not need the extra activity of the second-generation medications, while those with a higher disease score, and thus with a higher chance of progression, would be prime candidates for stronger TKI activity. Thus, one can imagine a treatment grid, where youth and disease stage drive choices more toward second-generation TKIs, while advancing age and low disease score lean toward imatinib therapy.

Health economics will likely also influence treatment algorithms. With the option of generic imatinib and more costly, but more potent, second-generation TKIs, two interesting treatment strategies emerge: first, starting therapy with generic imatinib and aggressive switching to second-generation TKIs if milestones are not met, or starting with second-generation TKI and switching to generic imatinib as "maintenance" (much like therapy for acute leukemia).

Rarely has the basic fundamentals of treatment options and goals changed so dramatically in such a small time. CML is a sterling example of the power of having a drug target, a drug, and reliable markers of disease burden.

## References

1. Druker BJ, Guilhot F, O'Brien SG, Gathmann I, Kantarjian H, Gattermann N, et al. Five-year follow-up of patients receiving imatinib for chronic myeloid leukemia. N Engl J Med. 2006;355(23):2408–17.
2. Deininger M, O'Brien SG, Guilhot F, Goldman JM, Hochhaus A, Hughes TP, et al. International randomized study of interferon vs STI571 (IRIS) 8-year follow up: sustained survival and low risk for progression or events in patients with newly diagnosed chronic myeloid leukemia in chronic phase (CML-CP) treated with imatinib. Blood. 2009;114:462. ASH Abstract 1126.

3. Kantarjian H, Shah NP, Hochhaus A, Cortes J, Shah S, Ayala M, et al. Dasatinib versus imatinib in newly diagnosed chronic-phase chronic myeloid leukemia. N Engl J Med. 2010;362(24):2260–70.
4. Radich JP, Kopecky KJ, Appelbaum FR, Kamel-Reid S, Stock W, Malnassy G, et al. A randomized trial of dasatinib 100 mg versus imatinib 400 mg in newly diagnosed chronic-phase chronic myeloid leukemia. Blood. 2012;120(19):3898–905.
5. Saglio G, Kim DW, Issaragrisil S, le Coutre P, Etienne G, Lobo C, et al. Nilotinib versus imatinib for newly diagnosed chronic myeloid leukemia. N Engl J Med. 2010;362(24):2251–9.
6. Hochhaus A, O'Brien SG, Guilhot F, Druker BJ, Branford S, Foroni L, et al. Six-year follow-up of patients receiving imatinib for the first-line treatment of chronic myeloid leukemia. Leukemia. 2009;23(6):1054–61.
7. Branford S, Rudzki Z, Walsh S, Parkinson I, Grigg A, Szer J, et al. Detection of BCR-ABL mutations in patients with CML treated with imatinib is virtually always accompanied by clinical resistance, and mutations in the ATP phosphate-binding loop (P-loop) are associated with a poor prognosis. Blood. 2003;102(1):276–83.
8. Khorashad JS, de Lavallade H, Apperley JF, Milojkovic D, Reid AG, Bua M, et al. Finding of kinase domain mutations in patients with chronic phase chronic myeloid leukemia responding to imatinib may identify those at high risk of disease progression. J Clin Oncol. 2008;26 (29):4806–13.
9. Soverini S, Martinelli G, Rosti G, Bassi S, Amabile M, Poerio A, et al. ABL mutations in late chronic phase chronic myeloid leukemia patients with up-front cytogenetic resistance to imatinib are associated with a greater likelihood of progression to blast crisis and shorter survival: a study by the GIMEMA Working Party on Chronic Myeloid Leukemia. J Clin Oncol. 2005;23(18):4100–9.
10. Hughes T, Saglio G, Branford S, Soverini S, Kim DW, Muller MC, et al. Impact of baseline BCR-ABL mutations on response to nilotinib in patients with chronic myeloid leukemia in chronic phase. J Clin Oncol. 2009;27(25):4204–10.
11. Muller MC, Cortes JE, Kim DW, Druker BJ, Erben P, Pasquini R, et al. Dasatinib treatment of chronic-phase chronic myeloid leukemia: analysis of responses according to preexisting BCR-ABL mutations. Blood. 2009;114(24):4944–53.
12. Cortes JE, Kim DW, Pinilla-Ibarz J, le Coutre P, Paquette R, Chuah C, et al. A phase 2 trial of ponatinib in Philadelphia chromosome-positive leukemias. N Engl J Med. 2013;369 (19):1783–96.
13. Cortes JE, Kantarjian HM, Brummendorf TH, Kim DW, Turkina AG, Shen ZX, et al. Safety and efficacy of bosutinib (SKI-606) in chronic phase Philadelphia chromosome-positive chronic myeloid leukemia patients with resistance or intolerance to imatinib. Blood. 2011;118(17):4567–76.
14. Oehler VG, Gooley T, Snyder DS, Johnston L, Lin A, Cummings CC, et al. The effects of imatinib mesylate treatment before allogeneic transplantation for chronic myeloid leukemia. Blood. 2007;109(4):1782–9.
15. Radich JP, Gooley T, Bensinger W, Chauncey T, Clift R, Flowers M, et al. HLA-matched related hematopoietic cell transplantation for chronic-phase CML using a targeted busulfan and cyclophosphamide preparative regimen. Blood. 2003;102(1):31–5.
16. Cortes J, Rousselot P, Kim DW, Ritchie E, Hamerschlak N, Coutre S, et al. Dasatinib induces complete hematologic and cytogenetic responses in patients with imatinib-resistant or -intolerant chronic myeloid leukemia in blast crisis. Blood. 2007;109(8):3207–13.
17. Guilhot F, Apperley J, Kim DW, Bullorsky EO, Baccarani M, Roboz GJ, et al. Dasatinib induces significant hematologic and cytogenetic responses in patients with imatinib-resistant or -intolerant chronic myeloid leukemia in accelerated phase. Blood. 2007;109(10):4143–50.
18. O'Brien S, Radich JP, Abboud CN, et al. NCCN Clinical Practice Guidelines in Oncology (NCCN Guidelines®) chronic myelogenous leukemia version 1.2015. © 2015 National Comprehensive Cancer Network, Inc. Available at NCCN.org. Accessed 11 Apr 2015.
19. Baccarani M, Deininger MW, Rosti G, et al. European LeukemiaNet recommendations for the management of chronic myeloid leukemia: 2013. Blood. 2013;122:872–84.

20. O'Brien SG, Deininger MW. Imatinib in patients with newly diagnosed chronic-phase chronic myeloid leukemia. Semin Hematol. 2003;40(2 Suppl 2):26–30.
21. Testoni N, Marzocchi G, Luatti S, et al. Chronic myeloid leukemia: a prospective comparison of interphase fluorescence in situ hybridization and chromosome banding analysis for the definition of complete cytogenetic response: a study of the GIMEMA CML WP. Blood. 2009;114:4939–43.
22. Jabbour E, Kantarjian H, O'Brien S, et al. The achievement of an early complete cytogenetic response is a major determinant for outcome in patients with early chronic phase chronic myeloid leukemia treated with tyrosine kinase inhibitors. Blood. 2011;118:4541–6.
23. Hardling M, Wei Y, Palmqvist L, et al. Serial monitoring of BCR-ABL transcripts in chronic myelogenous leukemia (CML) treated with imatinib mesylate. Med Oncol. 2004;21:349–58.
24. Bao F, Munker R, Lowery C, et al. Comparison of FISH and quantitative RT-PCR for the diagnosis and follow-up of BCR-ABL-positive leukemias. Mol Diagn Ther. 2007;11:239–45.
25. Hughes TP, Kaeda J, Branford S, et al. Frequency of major molecular responses to imatinib or interferon alfa plus cytarabine in newly diagnosed chronic myeloid leukemia. N Engl J Med. 2003;349:1423–32.
26. Jabbour E, Kantarjian HM, Saglio G, et al. Early response with dasatinib or imatinib in chronic myeloid leukemia: 3-year follow-up from a randomized phase 3 trial (DASISION). Blood. 2014;123:494–500.
27. Larson RA, Hochhaus A, Hughes TP, et al. Nilotinib vs imatinib in patients with newly diagnosed Philadelphia chromosome-positive chronic myeloid leukemia in chronic phase: ENESTnd 3-year follow-up. Leukemia. 2012;26:2197–203.
28. Hughes T, Deininger M, Hochhaus A, et al. Monitoring CML patients responding to treatment with tyrosine kinase inhibitors: review and recommendations for harmonizing current methodology for detecting BCR-ABL transcripts and kinase domain mutations and for expressing results. Blood. 2006;108:28–37.
29. Cortes J, Quintas-Cardama A, Jabbour E, et al. The clinical significance of achieving different levels of cytogenetic response in patients with chronic phase chronic myeloid leukemia after failure to front-line therapy: is complete cytogenetic response the only desirable endpoint? Clin Lymphoma Myeloma Leuk. 2011;11(5):421–6.
30. Kantarjian HM, Talpaz M, O'Brien S, Smith TL, Giles FJ, Faderl S, et al. Imatinib mesylate for Philadelphia chromosome-positive, chronic-phase myeloid leukemia after failure of interferon-alpha: follow-up results. Clin Cancer Res. 2002;8(7):2177–87.
31. Marin D, Marktel S, Bua M, Szydlo RM, Franceschino A, Nathan I, et al. Prognostic factors for patients with chronic myeloid leukaemia in chronic phase treated with imatinib mesylate after failure of interferon alfa. Leukemia. 2003;17(8):1448–53.
32. Guilhot F, Larson RA, O'Brien SG, et al. Time to Complete Cytogenetic Response (CCyR) does not affect long-term outcomes for patients on imatinib therapy. Blood. 2007;110: abstract 27.
33. Tam CS, Kantarjian H, Garcia-Manero G, et al. Failure to achieve a major cytogenetic response by 12 months defines inadequate response in patients receiving nilotinb or dasatinib as second or subsequent line therapy for CML. Blood. 2008;112(3):516–8.
34. Paschka P, Muller MC, Merx K, et al. Molecular monitoring of response to imatinib (Glivec) in CML patients pretreated with interferon alpha. Low levels of residual disease are associated with continuous remission. Leukemia. 2003;17:1687–94.
35. Hughes TP, Hochhaus A, Branford S, et al. Long-term prognostic significance of early molecular response to imatinib in newly diagnosed chronic myeloid leukemia: an analysis from the International Randomized Study of Interferon and STI571 (IRIS). Blood. 2010;116:3758–65.
36. Kantarjian H, O'Brien S, Shan J, et al. Cytogenetic and molecular responses and outcome in chronic myelogenous leukemia: need for new response definitions? Cancer. 2008;112:837–45.
37. Press RD, Galderisi C, Yang R, et al. A half-log increase in BCR-ABL RNA predicts a higher risk of relapse in patients with chronic myeloid leukemia with an imatinib-induced complete cytogenetic response. Clin Cancer Res. 2007;13:6136–43.

38. Hamilton A, Helgason GV, Schemionek M, et al. Chronic myeloid leukemia stem cells are not dependent on Bcr-Abl kinase activity for their survival. Blood. 2012;119:1501–10.
39. Mahon FX, Rea D, Guilhot J. Intergroupe Francais des Leucemies Myeloides Chroniques. Discontinuation of imatinib in patients with chronic myeloid leukemia who have maintained complete molecular remission for at least 2 years: the prospective, multicenter Stop Imatinib (STIM) trial. Lancet Oncol. 2010;11:1029–35.
40. Ross DM, Branford S, Seymour JF, et al. Safety and efficacy of imatinib cessation for CML patients with stable undetectable minimal residual disease: results from the TWISTER study. Blood. 2013;122:515–22.
41. Marin D, Ibrahim AR, Lucas C, et al. Assessment of BCR-ABL1 transcript levels at 3 months is the only requirement for predicting outcome for patients with chronic myeloid leukemia treated with tyrosine kinase inhibitors. J Clin Oncol. 2012;30:232–8.
42. Jain P, Kantarjian H, Nazha A, et al. Early responses predict better outcomes in patients with newly diagnosed chronic myeloid leukemia: results with four tyrosine kinase inhibitor modalities. Blood. 2013;121:4867–74.
43. Branford S, Yeung DT, Parker WT, et al. Prognosis for patients with CML and >10% BCR-ABL1 after 3 months of imatinib depends on the rate of BCR-ABL1 decline. Blood. 2014;124:511–8.
44. Bartley PA, Latham S, Budgen B, et al. A DNA real-time quantitative PCR method suitable for routine monitoring of low levels of minimal residual disease in chronic myeloid leukemia. J Mol Diagn. 2015;17:185–92.
45. Goh H-G, Lin M, Fukushima F, et al. Sensitive quantitation of minimal residual disease in chronic myeloid leukemia using nanofluidic digital polymerase chain reaction assay. Leuk Lymphoma. 2011;52:896–904.
46. Huggett FJ, Cowen S, Foy CA. Considerations for digital PCR as an accurate molecular diagnostic tool. Clin Chem. 2015;61:1–10.
47. Jennings LJ, George D, Czech J, Yu M, Joseph L. Detection and quantification of BCR-ABL1 fusion transcripts by droplet digital PCR. J Mol Diagn. 2014;16(2):174–9.
48. Soverini S, De Benedittis C, Polakova KM, et al. Unraveling the complexity of tyrosine kinase inhibitor-resistant populations by ultra-deep sequencing of the BCR-ABL kinase domain. Blood. 2013;122:1634–48.
49. Schmitt MW, Kennedy SR, Salk JJ, Fox EJ, Hiatt JB, Loeb LA. Detection of ultra-rare mutations by next-generation sequencing. Proc Natl Acad Sci U S A. 2012;109:14508–13.

# Chapter 5
# Biomarkers for Determining the Prognosis of CML

**Naoto Takahashi**

**Abstract** Tyrosine kinase inhibitors (TKIs) have dramatically improved the clinical outcome and prognosis for chronic myelogenous leukemia (CML) patients. However, some patients develop acquired resistance to TKI treatment. Several mechanisms for imatinib resistance in CML have been proposed, and "biomarkers" are used at diagnosis and during TKI treatment to predict CML patient outcome. In this chapter, we discuss prognostic scoring systems used at diagnosis such as the Sokal score, Hasford score, European Treatment and Outcome Study score, early molecular response to TKI as a surrogate endpoint, pharmacokinetic factors such as plasma concentration of TKIs, polymorphisms of drug transporters, immunological biomarkers such as T-cell profiling, and a common intronic deletion polymorphism in the gene-encoding BCL2-like 11 (BIM) as candidates for biomarkers associated with clinical endpoints.

**Keywords** Chronic myelogenous leukemia • Tyrosine kinase inhibitor • Biomarker • Surrogate endpoint • Treatment-free remission

## 5.1 Introduction

Imatinib mesylate, a competitive tyrosine kinase inhibitor (TKI), is considered the first-line therapy drug for Ph+ chronic myelogenous leukemia (CML) and has dramatically improved the clinical outcome and prognosis for CML patients [1]. Despite the marked improvement in CML treatment, approximately 20 % of CML patients develop resistance to imatinib during the first 5 years of treatment [2]. Several mechanisms for imatinib resistance in CML have been proposed, including the baseline presence or later emergence of a BCR-ABL1 point mutation, BCR-ABL1 overexpression or other genetic variants [3, 4], a high Sokal risk score at baseline [5], and pharmacokinetic factors such as drug metabolism or drug transport [6, 7], drug-drug interactions [8, 9], and adherence [10]. Recently, a

N. Takahashi, MD, PhD (✉)
Department of Hematology, Nephrology and Rheumatology, Akita University, 1-1-1 Hondo, Akita 010-8543, Japan
e-mail: naotot@doc.med.akita-u.ac.jp



M. Kizaki (ed.), *Molecular Pathogenesis and Treatment of Chronic Myelogenous Leukemia*, DOI 10.1007/978-4-431-55714-2_5

common intronic deletion polymorphism in the gene-encoding BCL2-like 11 (BIM) was reported as an explanation for the heterogeneity of TKI responses between individuals [11]. Evaluating or analyzing such a biological marker, a so-called biomarker, may make it possible to predict TKI response and subsequently outcomes in CML patients. In this chapter, we discuss several candidate biomarkers for TKI treatment in CML.

## 5.2 What Is a Biomarker?

Biomarkers are clinical and diagnostic tools that can predict clinical endpoints in basic and clinical research as well as in general practice. Biomarkers are objectively measured and evaluated as an indicator of normal biological process, pathogenic processes, or pharmacologic responses to therapeutic intervention [12]. Example of biomarkers include everything from medical symptoms to basic chemistries to more complex laboratory tests of blood and other tissues [13], including DNA for analyzing mutations or polymorphisms and RNA for measuring expression of target genes.

A major goal of CML treatment in general practice is to improve morbidity and mortality. In other words, a primary endpoint for CML treatment is increased overall survival (OS). If OS of CML patients treated with TKI is the same as that of the general population, it indicates that we have achieved the major goal of CML treatment. Another endpoint is progression-free survival (PFS) either to the accelerated phase (AP) or the blast phase (BP). If progression to AP or BP is completely controlled, patients with CML in the chronic phase (CML-CP) will not die from disease-related causes. Thus, prevention of CML progression to AP or BP is another major goal of CML treatment.

A true biomarker would be associated with OS as the primary endpoint. When we evaluate the biomarker at diagnosis or during treatment, we should ideally be able to predict OS. In this review, we define "biomarker of CML" as an indicator that is objectively measured in blood or other tissues. Before a discussion of biomarkers in the narrow sense, we summarize the prognostic scoring systems at diagnosis and surrogate endpoints in treatment as biomarkers in the broad sense.

### *5.2.1 Prognostic Scoring Systems at Diagnosis*

Three prognostic scoring systems have been reported to predict the clinical response to TKI and outcome: Sokal score [14], Hasford score [15], and European Treatment and Outcome Study (EUTOS) score [16]. In general practice, these systems are a simple indicator based on clinical symptoms and hematologic data.

Although Sokal and Hasford scores were established during the pre-imatinib era, they worked well for predicting prognosis among patients with CML-CP who were treated with imatinib. On the other hand, the EUTOS score was established using data on patients treated with imatinib as an initial therapy in 2011 and was only based on spleen size and blood basophil percentage prior to any treatment. In the 2060 patients evaluated in the original report, the EUTOS score predicted both complete cytogenetic response (CCyR) and PFS better than that of the Sokal or Hasford score [16]. The EUTOS score discriminated between high-risk and low-risk groups of patients, and the 5-year PFS was significantly better in the low-risk than in the high-risk group (90 % vs. 82 %, $P = 0.006$) [16]. These results were confirmed in validation samples in the report, and independent studies have investigated its prognostic power [17–23]. However, several groups found that the EUTOS score did not predict the OS, PFS, and/or CCyR [24–26]. Studies at M.D. Anderson Cancer Center reported that the EUTOS score could predict CCyR, but not OS or PFS in 465 cases receiving standard doses of imatinib, high doses of imatinib, or second-generation TKIs [26]. Baccarani et al. have suggested that there is no evidence that any one of the three risk scores is superior or more convenient [27]. Two prospective randomized studies, the ENESTnd study [28–30] and the DASISION study [31, 32], reported a significantly higher rate of CCyR and major molecular response (MMR) in a group taking second-generation TKIs compared with a control group taking imatinib across all risk categories according to either the Sokal score or Hasford score. Second-generation TKIs might overcome a poor prognosis in these studies. However, event-free survival is excellent in patients with a low-risk score even when imatinib is used, suggesting that these patients may be managed safely with imatinib. It is necessary to establish a new prognostic scoring system for patients treated with second-generation TKIs as a first-line therapy.

### 5.2.2 *Surrogate Endpoint*

A primary endpoint, which is generally OS or PFS, requires a long period of observation. Surrogate endpoints without a long duration of observation act as substitutes for such a primary endpoint. During TKI treatment, response can be assessed with internationally standardized real-time quantitative polymerase chain reaction. According to European LeukemiaNet recommendation, BCR-ABL1 transcript level >10 % of the standardized baseline at 6 months and >1 % at 12 months defines "failure." The treatment for patients who are classified into the failure category should be changed [27]. BCR-ABL1 transcript levels ≤0.1 % at 12 months, which is considered a major molecular response (MMR), is defined as "optimal response." Optimal response is associated with the best long-term outcome [27]. Patients who achieved MMR by 18 months experienced remarkably durable responses, with no progression to AP/BC and 95 % OS at 7 years [33].

Recently, BCR-ABL1 transcript levels <10 % at 3 months or <1 % at 6 months were reported to be prognostically significant in several studies, corresponding to an early molecular response (EMR) [33–37]. Patients who do not achieve a BCR-ABL1 transcript level of <10 % at 3 months still may achieve a BCR-ABL1 transcript level <1 % at 6 months. The EMR to TKIs might be the best prognostic factor for use as a new surrogate endpoint in CML treatment.

A new clinical endpoint is treatment-free remission (TFR). Recently, some clinical trials showed that approximately 40 % of CML patients who developed a sustained, deep molecular response using imatinib could discontinue imatinib without experiencing molecular relapse [38–40], although only stem cell transplantation can render patients durably molecularly negative and "cured." TFR might be very close to a "cure" that can be obtained by TKIs. In several imatinib stop studies, molecular recurrences were observed within 6 months after cessation of imatinib [38–40]. Accordingly, TFR at 6 months might be another surrogate endpoint in CML treatment.

## 5.3 Candidate for Biomarkers Associated with Clinical Endpoints

### *5.3.1 Plasma Concentration of TKIs*

It was recently reported that variations in the imatinib plasma trough concentration correlated with the clinical response of patients (Table 5.1) [10, 41–43]. Picard et al. reported that a steady-state imatinib concentration, when measured at least 12 months after starting treatment with a standard imatinib dose, correlated with both cytogenetic and molecular responses [42]. The investigators suggested that the threshold for imatinib concentration should be set above 1000 ng/mL as a concentration significantly associated with an MMR. Thus, the efficacy of the threshold concentration of imatinib should be set above 1000 ng/mL for CML patients.

The relationship between plasma concentration of second-generation TKIs and clinical efficacy has been reported in only a few studies. Giles et al. evaluated the

**Table 5.1** Molecular response and plasma trough concentration of imatinib

| | | | $C_0$ (ng/mL) | | | | |
|---|---|---|---|---|---|---|---|
| Reference | *N* | Response | *N* | ≤1000 | *N* | >1000 | *P* value |
| Marin et al. [10] | 84 | CMR | 43 | 23.3 % | 41 | 44.4 % | 0.14 |
| | | MMR | | 60.1 % | | 83.2 % | 0.02 |
| Takahashi et al. [41] | 254 | CCyR | 146 | 83.6 % | 108 | 88.9 % | 0.276 |
| | | MMR | | 58.9 % | | 74.1 % | 0.012 |
| Picard et al. [42] | 68 | MMR | 32 | 25.0 % | 36 | 72.2 % | 0.03 |
| Ishikawa et al. [42, 43] | 60 | MMR | 29 | 48.3 % | 31 | 77.4 % | 0.019 |

$C_0$ plasma trough concentration of imatinib

population pharmacokinetics (PK) and exposure-response relationship of nilotinib in patients with imatinib-resistant or imatinib-intolerant CML [44]. In this large cohort, patients with a lower concentration (<500 ng/mL) had a significantly longer time to CCyR ($P = 0.010$), a longer time to MMR ($P = 0.012$), and a shorter time to progression ($P = 0.009$).

Although the plasma imatinib concentration depends on daily dose, there is an interindividual variability that can be ignored. The distribution of plasma trough imatinib concentration varies widely from 140 to 3910 ng/mL in patients treated with 400 mg of the drug [41]. The interindividual variability is associated with several factors such as age, sex, liver function, renal function, drug-drug interactions [8, 9], adherence [10], and polymorphisms of drug metabolism or drug transport [6, 7].

### 5.3.2 TKIs and Drug Transporters

TKIs such as imatinib, nilotinib, and dasatinib are substrates of ATP-binding cassette (ABC) transporters such as P-glycoprotein (P-gp) encoded by the *ABCB1* gene and breast cancer resistance protein (BCRP) encoded by *ABCG2* gene [45–50] (Fig. 5.1). Imatinib is also a substrate of the uptake transporter, organic cation transporter 1 (OCT1), which is encoded by *SLC22A1* gene [51–53] (Fig. 5.1). Pharmacogenetic research on imatinib has focused in part on the relation between

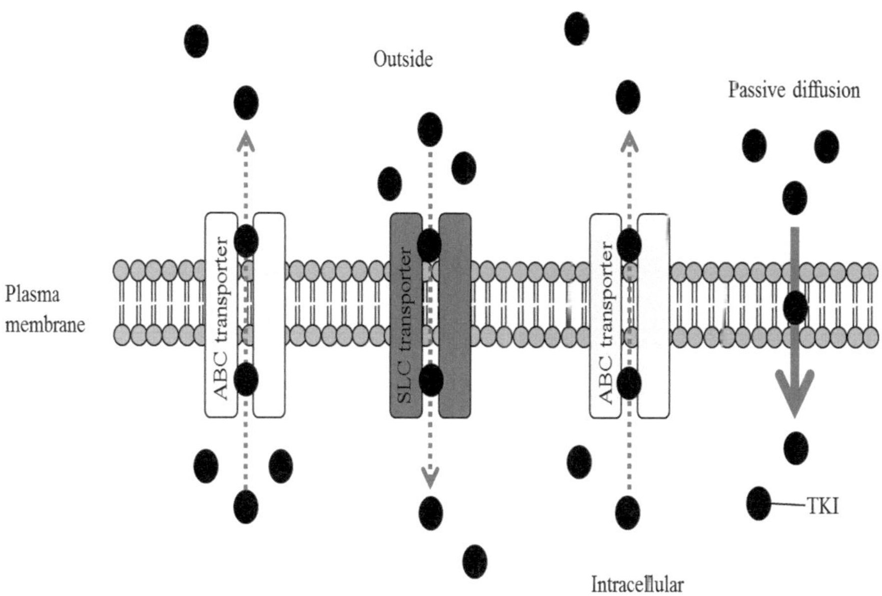


**Fig. 5.1** Schematic diagram of the transporters on the membrane of leukemia cells

**Table 5.2** Effect on pharmacokinetics or molecular response and *ABCG2* 421C > A for imatinib

| Reference | *N* | Genotype (*n*) | Effect on PK/response |
|---|---|---|---|
| Takahashi et al. [55] | 67 | 421 CC vs. 421 CA + AA [25] | $C_0$ increased |
| Petain et al. [56] | 46 | 421 CC vs. 421 CA [5] | CL/F decreased |
| Kim et al. [57] | 229 | 421 CC vs. 421 CA + AA (NA) | MMR/CMR increased |
| Sinohara et al. [58] | 152 | 421 CC vs. 421 CA + AA [59] | CMR increased |

*PK* pharmacokinetics, $C_0$ plasma trough concentration of imatinib, *CL/F* imatinib clearance, *MMR* major molecular response, *CMR* complete molecular response, *NA* not available

imatinib exposure and the clinical response to imatinib (pharmacodynamic effect) and the expression levels of these transporters.

Three single nucleotide polymorphisms (SNPs) in *ABCB1*, C1236T, G2677T/A, and C3435T can affect cellular transport of imatinib. The association between these SNPs and imatinib response in CML patients has been widely evaluated, but the results are inconsistent. To derive a conclusive assessment of the associations, we performed a meta-analysis using data from 12 reports including 1826 patients [54]. The presence of the 1236CC genotype, 2677T/A allele, or 3435C allele marks improved response to imatinib in CML patients.

We reported that the dose-adjusted imatinib plasma trough concentration was significantly lower in Japanese patients with the *ABCG2* 421C/C genotype than in patients with the C/A + A/A genotypes (Table 5.2) [55]. In addition, Petain et al. reported that imatinib clearance in patients carrying the *ABCG2* 421C/A genotype was significantly lower than in those with the 421C/C genotype [56]. Kim et al. reported that patients with the *ABCG2* 421A/A genotype achieved MMR and complete molecular response (CMR) much more than patients with *ABCG2* 421C/A + C/C [57]. It thus appears that among CML patients, the *ABCG2* 421A allele is associated with a higher imatinib exposure and a better response to imatinib in CML patients than the 421C allele. Moreover, the percentage of patients with CMR was significantly lower among those with the *ABCG2* 421C/C genotype than among those with the A allele [58]. This finding suggests that the *ABCG2* 421A allele is associated with higher intracellular retention and therefore higher imatinib exposure than the wild-type genotype. This finding is in agreement with the in vitro study by Imai et al. that demonstrated that protein expression levels of BCRP, which is encoded by *ABCG2*, were markedly decreased in patients with the *ABCG2* 421A allele compared with the 421C/C genotype [59].

OCT1 is primarily expressed in hepatocytes, suggesting that it plays a role in substrate uptake into the liver. Moreover, the level of OCT1 expression likely correlates with the intracellular imatinib concentration, as primary CML cells expressing high levels of OCT1 show greater drug uptake than those exhibiting more modest OCT1 expression [6, 51, 52] (Fig. 5.1). On the other hand, nilotinib and dasatinib are passively transported into cells without OCT1 activity and so are not affected by OCT1 activity on the surface of leukemia cells.

### 5.3.3 Immunological Biomarkers

Several studies have reported that patients treated with dasatinib developed large granular lymphocytosis and significantly optimal molecular responses [60, 61]. The large granular lymphocytosis was identified as natural killer (NK) cells or NK/T cells based on immunophenotypic profiles [62]. Mizoguchi et al. reported that the percentage of effector NK cell populations were significantly higher in patients with TFR than in those without TFR and control groups [63]. Moreover, European groups also showed the relationship between successful TFR and NK cells [64, 65].

In a German clinical study that evaluated a maintenance therapy regimen comprising interferon-alpha following combined imatinib and interferon-alpha therapy in CML-CP patients that achieved CMR, interferon-alpha therapy was associated with expansion of proteinase-3-specific cytotoxic T cells, and it may result in improved molecular response [66]. Shinohara et al. evaluated immunological parameters in CML-CP patients treated with imatinib and reported that regulatory T cells were significantly lower in patients with CMR than in those without CMR [58]. Barachandran et al. reported that imatinib therapy activated CD8+ T cells and induced regulatory T-cell apoptosis within gastrointestinal stromal tumors (GISTs). The number and activity of these T-cell populations are crucial to the antitumor effects of imatinib in GIST [67]. These results suggest that the immunological activation status of T cells and NK cells contributes to TFR or clinical outcomes in imatinib treatment. We are currently planning to evaluate immunophenotypic profiling as exploratory research in a prospective JALSG STIM213 study (UMIN000011971) that will elucidate the role of NK/T cells as a component of leukemia immune surveillance.

### 5.3.4 BIM

BCL2-like 11 (BIM) is a protein associated with apoptosis and is required to induce TKI-mediated apoptosis in tumor cells [68]. The common intron 2 deletion polymorphism of the *BIM* gene is found in 20 % of the Asian population and results in the expression of a BIM isoform lacking the BH3 domain. It was recently reported that this *BIM* polymorphism is involved in the poor response to TKIs in CML cell lines, but this resistance could be overcome with BH3-mimetic drugs. Additionally, individuals with CML harboring the polymorphism experienced significantly inferior responses to TKIs than individuals without the polymorphism [11]. A French group recently showed that the T allele of *BIM* c465C > T (rs724710) is associated with Sokal score and a longer time to MMR achievement [69]. The study suggested that polymorphisms in *BIM* might influence TKI treatment effects in non-Asians as well as Asians.

**Table 5.3** Clinical endpoints, surrogate endpoints, and biomarkers for CML treatment

| | Clinical endpoints | Surrogate endpoints | Candidate for biomarkers |
|---|---|---|---|
| TKI treatment | OS | MMR at 18 months (bcr-abl$^{IS}$ $<0.1$ %) | TKI concentration |
| | PFS | EMR at 3 months (bcr-abl$^{IS}$ $<10$ %) | OCT1 activity |
| | | EMR at 6 months (bcr-abl$^{IS}$ $<1$ %) | *ABCB1* C1236T |
| | | | *ABCB1* G2677T/A |
| | | | *ABCB1* C3435T |
| | | | *ABCG2* C421A |
| | | | LGL (NK cell/T cell) |
| | | | *BIM* common deletion polymorphism |
| TKI stop | OS | TFR at 6 months (bcr-abl$^{IS}$ $<0.0032$ %) | *ABCG2* C421A |
| | RFS | | Treg |
| | | | NK cell |

## 5.4 Conclusions

In this review, we discussed plasma concentration of TKIs, drug transporters, T/NK cells, and *BIM* polymorphisms as biomarkers for predicting the outcome in CML treatment (Table 5.3). As of now, these factors are still candidate biomarkers and will need to be evaluated in large prospective studies in the future.

## References

1. O'Brien SG, Guilhot F, Larson RA, Gathmann I, Baccarani M, Cervantes F, et al. Imatinib compared with interferon and low-dose cytarabine for newly diagnosed chronic-phase chronic myeloid leukemia. N Engl J Med. 2003;348(11):994–1004.
2. Druker BJ, Guilhot F, O'Brien SG, Gathmann I, Kantarjian H, Gattermann N, et al. Five-year follow-up of patients receiving imatinib for chronic myeloid leukemia. N Engl J Med. 2006;355(23):2408–17.
3. Gorre ME, Mohammed M, Ellwood K, Hsu N, Paquette R, Rao PN, et al. Clinical resistance to STI-571 cancer therapy caused by BCR-ABL gene mutation or amplification. Science. 2001;293(5531):876–80.
4. Radich JP, Dai H, Mao M, Oehler V, Schelter J, Druker B, et al. Gene expression changes associated with progression and response in chronic myeloid leukemia. Proc Natl Acad Sci U S A. 2006;103(8):2794–9.
5. Crossman LC, O'Brien SG. Imatinib therapy in chronic myeloid leukemia. Hematol Oncol Clin North Am. 2004;18(3):605–17. 3.
6. Thomas J, Wang L, Clark RE, Pirmohamed M. Active transport of imatinib into and out of cells: implications for drug resistance. Blood. 2004;104(12):3739–45.

7. White DL, Dang P, Engler J, Frede A, Zrim S, Osborn M, et al. Functional activity of the OCT-1 protein is predictive of long-term outcome in patients with chronic-phase chronic myeloid leukemia treated with imatinib. J Clin Oncol. 2010;28(16):2761–7.
8. Peng B, Hayes M, Resta D, Racine-Poon A, Druker BJ, Talpaz M, et al. Pharmacokinetics and pharmacodynamics of imatinib in a phase I trial with chronic myeloid leukemia patients. J Clin Oncol. 2004;22(5):935–42.
9. Cortes JE, Egorin MJ, Guilhot F, Molimard M, Mahon FX. Pharmacokinetic/pharmacodynamic correlation and blood-level testing in imatinib therapy for chronic myeloid leukemia. Leukemia. 2009;23(9):1537–44.
10. Marin D, Bazeos A, Mahon FX, Eliasson L, Milojkovic D, Bua M, et al. Adherence is the critical factor for achieving molecular responses in patients with chronic myeloid leukemia who achieve complete cytogenetic responses on imatinib. J Clin Oncol. 2010;28(14):2381–8.
11. Ng KP, Hillmer AM, Chuah CT, Juan WC, Ko TK, Teo AS, et al. A common BIM deletion polymorphism mediates intrinsic resistance and inferior responses to tyrosine kinase inhibitors in cancer. Nat Med. 2012;18(4):521–8.
12. BDW Group. Biomarkers and surrogate endpoints: preferred definitions and conceptual framework. Clin Pharmacol Ther. 2001;69(3):89–95.
13. Strimbu K, Tavel JA. What are biomarkers? Curr Opin HIV AIDS. 2010;5(6):463–6.
14. Sokal JE, Cox EB, Baccarani M, Tura S, Gomez GA, Robertson JE, et al. Prognostic discrimination in "good-risk" chronic granulocytic leukemia. Blood. 1984;63(4):789–99.
15. Hasford J, Pfirrmann M, Hehlmann R, Allan NC, Baccarani M, Kluin-Nelemans JC, et al. A new prognostic score for survival of patients with chronic myeloid leukemia treated with interferon alfa. Writing Committee for the Collaborative CML Prognostic Factors Project Group. J Natl Cancer Inst. 1998;90(11):850–8.
16. Hasford J, Baccarani M, Hoffmann V, Guilhot J, Saussele S, Rosti G, et al. Predicting complete cytogenetic response and subsequent progression-free survival in 2060 patients with CML on imatinib treatment: the EUTOS score. Blood. 2011;118(3):686–92.
17. Tao Z, Liu B, Zhao Y, Wang Y, Zhang R, Han M, et al. EUTOS score predicts survival and cytogenetic response in patients with chronic phase chronic myeloid leukemia treated with first-line imatinib. Leuk Res. 2014;38(9):1030–5.
18. Uz B, Buyukasik Y, Atay H, Kelkitli E, Turgut M, Bektas O, et al. EUTOS CML prognostic scoring system predicts ELN-based 'event-free survival' better than Euro/Hasford and Sokal systems in CML patients receiving front-line imatinib mesylate. Hematology. 2013;18 (5):247–52.
19. Tiribelli M, Bonifacio M, Calistri E, Binotto G, Maino E, Marin L, et al. EUTOS score predicts long-term outcome but not optimal response to imatinib in patients with chronic myeloid leukaemia. Leuk Res. 2013;37(11):1457–60.
20. Hoffmann VS, Baccarani M, Lindoerfer D, Castagnetti F, Turkina A, Zaritsky A, et al. The EUTOS prognostic score: review and validation in 1288 patients with CML treated frontline with imatinib. Leukemia. 2013;27(10):2016–22.
21. Breccia M, Finsinger P, Loglisci G, Latagliata R, Mancini M, Salaroli A, et al. The EUTOS score identifies chronic myeloid leukaemia patients with poor prognosis treated with imatinib first or second line. Leuk Res. 2012;36(9):e209–10.
22. Bonifacio M, Binotto G, Calistri E, Maino E, Tiribelli M. EUTOS score predicts early optimal response to imatinib according to the revised 2013 ELN recommendations. Ann Hematol. 2014;93(1):163–4.
23. Iriyama N, Hatta Y, Kobayashi S, Uchino Y, Miura K, Kurita D, et al. The European Treatment and Outcome Study score is associated with clinical outcomes and treatment response following European LeukemiaNet 2013 recommendations in chronic-phase chronic myeloid leukemia. Int J Hematol. 2014;100(4):379–85.
24. Marin D, Ibrahim AR, Goldman JM. European Treatment and Outcome Study (EUTOS) score for chronic myeloid leukemia still requires more confirmation. J Clin Oncol [Letter]. 2011;29:3944–5.

25. Yamamoto E, Fujisawa S, Hagihara M, Tanaka M, Fujimaki K, Kishimoto K, et al. European Treatment and Outcome Study score does not predict imatinib treatment response and outcome in chronic myeloid leukemia patients. Cancer Sci. 2014;105(1):105–9.
26. Jabbour E, Cortes J, Nazha A, O'Brien S, Quintas-Cardama A, Pierce S, et al. EUTOS score is not predictive for survival and outcome in patients with early chronic phase chronic myeloid leukemia treated with tyrosine kinase inhibitors: a single institution experience. Blood. 2012;119(19):4524–6.
27. Baccarani M, Deininger MW, Rosti G, Hochhaus A, Soverini S, Apperley JF, et al. European LeukemiaNet recommendations for the management of chronic myeloid leukemia: 2013. Blood. 2013;122(6):872–84.
28. Saglio G, Kim DW, Issaragrisil S, le Coutre P, Etienne G, Lobo C, et al. Nilotinib versus imatinib for newly diagnosed chronic myeloid leukemia. N Engl J Med. 2010;362(24):2251–9.
29. Kantarjian HM, Hochhaus A, Saglio G, De Souza C, Flinn IW, Stenke L, et al. Nilotinib versus imatinib for the treatment of patients with newly diagnosed chronic phase, Philadelphia chromosome-positive, chronic myeloid leukaemia: 24-month minimum follow-up of the phase 3 randomised ENESTnd trial. Lancet Oncol. 2011;12(9):841–51.
30. Larson RA, Hochhaus A, Hughes TP, Clark RE, Etienne G, Kim DW, et al. Nilotinib vs imatinib in patients with newly diagnosed Philadelphia chromosome-positive chronic myeloid leukemia in chronic phase: ENESTnd 3-year follow-up. Leukemia. 2012;26(10):2197–203.
31. Kantarjian HM, Shah NP, Cortes JE, Baccarani M, Agarwal MB, Undurraga MS, et al. Dasatinib or imatinib in newly diagnosed chronic-phase chronic myeloid leukemia: 2-year follow-up from a randomized phase 3 trial (DASISION). Blood. 2012;119(5):1123–9.
32. Kantarjian HM, Shah NP, Cortes JE, Baccarani M, Agarwal MB, Undurraga MS, et al. Dasatinib or imatinib in newly diagnosed chronic-phase chronic myeloid leukemia: 2-year follow-up from a randomized phase 3 trial (DASISION). Blood. 2012;119(5):1123–9.
33. Hughes TP, Hochhaus A, Branford S, Muller MC, Kaeda JS, Foroni L, et al. Long-term prognostic significance of early molecular response to imatinib in newly diagnosed chronic myeloid leukemia: an analysis from the International Randomized Study of Interferon and STI571 (IRIS). Blood. 2010;116(19):3758–65.
34. Hanfstein B, Muller MC, Hehlmann R, Erben P, Lauseker M, Fabarius A, et al. Early molecular and cytogenetic response is predictive for long-term progression-free and overall survival in chronic myeloid leukemia (CML). Leukemia. 2012;26(9):2096–102.
35. Neelakantan P, Gerrard G, Lucas C, Milojkovic D, May P, Wang L, et al. Combining BCR-ABL1 transcript levels at 3 and 6 months in chronic myeloid leukemia: implications for early intervention strategies. Blood. 2013;121(14):2739–42.
36. Jabbour E, Kantarjian HM, Saglio G, Steegmann JL, Shah NP, Boque C, et al. Early response with dasatinib or imatinib in chronic myeloid leukemia: 3-year follow-up from a randomized phase 3 trial (DASISION). Blood. 2014;123(4):494–500.
37. Hughes TP, Saglio G, Kantarjian HM, Guilhot F, Niederwieser D, Rosti G, et al. Early molecular response predicts outcomes in patients with chronic myeloid leukemia in chronic phase treated with frontline nilotinib or imatinib. Blood. 2014;123(9):1353–60.
38. Mahon FX, Rea D, Guilhot J, Guilhot F, Huguet F, Nicolini F, et al. Discontinuation of imatinib in patients with chronic myeloid leukaemia who have maintained complete molecular remission for at least 2 years: the prospective, multicentre Stop Imatinib (STIM) trial. Lancet Oncol. 2010;11(11):1029–35.
39. Ross DM, Branford S, Seymour JF, Schwarer AP, Arthur C, Yeung DT, et al. Safety and efficacy of imatinib cessation for CML patients with stable undetectable minimal residual disease: results from the TWISTER study. Blood. 2013;122(4):515–22.
40. Rousselot P, Charbonnier A, Cony-Makhoul P, Agape P, Nicolini FE, Varet B, et al. Loss of major molecular response as a trigger for restarting tyrosine kinase inhibitor therapy in patients with chronic-phase chronic myelogenous leukemia who have stopped imatinib after durable undetectable disease. J Clin Oncol. 2014;32(5):424–30.

41. Takahashi N, Wakita H, Miura M, Scott SA, Nishii K, Masuko M, et al. Correlation between imatinib pharmacokinetics and clinical response in Japanese patients with chronic-phase chronic myeloid leukemia. Clin Pharmacol Ther. 2010;88(6):809–13.
42. Picard S, Titier K, Etienne G, Teilhet E, Ducint D, Bernard MA, et al. Trough imatinib plasma levels are associated with both cytogenetic and molecular responses to standard-dose imatinib in chronic myeloid leukemia. Blood. 2007;109(8):3496–9.
43. Ishikawa Y, Kiyoi H, Watanabe K, Miyamura K, Nakano Y, Kitamura K, et al. Trough plasma concentration of imatinib reflects BCR-ABL kinase inhibitory activity and clinical response in chronic-phase chronic myeloid leukemia: a report from the BINGO study. Cancer Sci. 2010;101(10):2186–92.
44. Giles FJ, Yin OQ, Sallas WM, le Coutre PD, Woodman RC, Ottmann OG, et al. Nilotinib population pharmacokinetics and exposure-response analysis in patients with imatinib-resistant or -intolerant chronic myeloid leukemia. Eur J Clin Pharmacol. 2013;69(4):813–23.
45. Burger H, Nooter K. Pharmacokinetic resistance to imatinib mesylate: role of the ABC drug pumps ABCG2 (BCRP) and ABCB1 (MDR1) in the oral bioavailability of imatinib. Cell Cycle. 2004;3(12):1502–5.
46. Burger H, van Tol H, Boersma AW, Brok M, Wiemer EA, Stoter G, et al. Imatinib mesylate (STI571) is a substrate for the breast cancer resistance protein (BCRP)/ABCG2 drug pump. Blood. 2004;104(9):2940–2.
47. Burger H, van Tol H, Brok M, Wiemer EA, de Bruijn EA, Guetens G, et al. Chronic imatinib mesylate exposure leads to reduced intracellular drug accumulation by induction of the ABCG2 (BCRP) and ABCB1 (MDR1) drug transport pumps. Cancer Biol Ther. 2005;4 (7):747–52.
48. Ozvegy-Laczka C, Hegedus T, Varady G, Ujhelly O, Schuetz JD, Varadi A, et al. High-affinity interaction of tyrosine kinase inhibitors with the ABCG2 multidrug transporter. Mol Pharmacol. 2004;65(6):1485–95.
49. Brendel C, Scharenberg C, Dohse M, Robey RW, Bates SE, Shukla S, et al. Imatinib mesylate and nilotinib (AMN107) exhibit high-affinity interaction with ABCG2 on primitive hematopoietic stem cells. Leukemia. 2007;21(6):1267–75.
50. Dohse M, Scharenberg C, Shukla S, Robey RW, Volkmann T, Deeken JF, et al. Comparison of ATP-binding cassette transporter interactions with the tyrosine kinase inhibitors imatinib, nilotinib, and dasatinib. Drug Metab Dispos. 2010;38(8):1371–80.
51. White DL, Saunders VA, Dang P, Engler J, Zannettino AC, Cambareri AC, et al. OCT-1-mediated influx is a key determinant of the intracellular uptake of imatinib but not nilotinib (AMN107): reduced OCT-1 activity is the cause of low in vitro sensitivity to imatinib. Blood. 2006;108(2):697–704.
52. Wang L, Giannoudis A, Lane S, Williamson P, Pirmohamed M, Clark RE. Expression of the uptake drug transporter hOCT1 is an important clinical determinant of the response to imatinib in chronic myeloid leukemia. Clin Pharmacol Ther. 2008;83(2):258–64.
53. Choi MK, Song IS. Organic cation transporters and their pharmacokinetic and pharmacodynamic consequences. Drug Metab Pharmacokinet. 2008;23(4):243–53.
54. Zheng Q, Wu H, Yu Q, Kim DH, Lipton JH, Angelini S, et al. ABCB1 polymorphisms predict imatinib response in chronic myeloid leukemia patients: a meta-analysis. Pharmacogenomics J. 2015;15(2):127–34.
55. Takahashi N, Miura M, Scott SA, Kagaya H, Kameoka Y, Tagawa H, et al. Influence of CYP3A5 and drug transporter polymorphisms on imatinib trough concentration and clinical response among patients with chronic phase chronic myeloid leukemia. J Hum Genet. 2010;55 (11):731–7.
56. Petain A, Kattygnarath D, Azard J, Chatelut E, Delbaldo C, Geoerger B, et al. Population pharmacokinetics and pharmacogenetics of imatinib in children and adults. Clin Cancer Res. 2008;14(21):7102–9.

57. Kim DH, Sriharsha L, Xu W, Kamel-Reid S, Liu X, Siminovitch K, et al. Clinical relevance of a pharmacogenetic approach using multiple candidate genes to predict response and resistance to imatinib therapy in chronic myeloid leukemia. Clin Cancer Res. 2009;15(14):4750–8.
58. Shinohara Y, Takahashi N, Nishiwaki K, Hino M, Kashimura M, Wakita H, et al. A multicenter clinical study evaluating the confirmed complete molecular response rate in imatinib-treated patients with chronic phase chronic myeloid leukemia by using the international scale of real-time quantitative polymerase chain reaction. Haematologica. 2013;98(9):1407–13.
59. Imai Y, Nakane M, Kage K, Tsukahara S, Ishikawa E, Tsuruo T, et al. C421A polymorphism in the human breast cancer resistance protein gene is associated with low expression of Q141K protein and low-level drug resistance. Mol Cancer Ther. 2002;1(8):611–6.
60. Kim DH, Kamel-Reid S, Chang H, Sutherland R, Jung CW, Kim HJ, et al. Natural killer or natural killer/T cell lineage large granular lymphocytosis associated with dasatinib therapy for Philadelphia chromosome positive leukemia. Haematologica. 2009;94(1):135–9.
61. Mustjoki S, Ekblom M, Arstila TP, Dybedal I, Epling-Burnette PK, Guilhot F, et al. Clonal expansion of T/NK-cells during tyrosine kinase inhibitor dasatinib therapy. Leukemia. 2009;23(8):1398–405.
62. Kreutzman A, Juvonen V, Kairisto V, Ekblom M, Stenke L, Seggewiss R, et al. Mono/oligoclonal T and NK cells are common in chronic myeloid leukemia patients at diagnosis and expand during dasatinib therapy. Blood. 2010;116(5):772–82.
63. Mizoguchi I, Yoshimoto T, Katagiri S, Mizuguchi J, Tauchi T, Kimura Y, et al. Sustained upregulation of effector natural killer cells in chronic myeloid leukemia after discontinuation of imatinib. Cancer Sci. 2013;104(9):1146–53.
64. Rea D, Dulphy N, Henry G, Guilhot J, Guilhot F, Nicolini FE, et al. Low Natural Killer (NK) cell counts and functionality are associated with molecular relapse after imatinib discontinuation in patients (pts) with chronic phase (CP)-chronic myeloid leukemia (CML) with undetectable BCR-ABL transcripts for at least 2 years: preliminary results From immunostim, on behalf of STIM investigators. Blood (ASH Annual Meeting Abstracts). 2013;122:865.
65. Ilander MM, Olsson-Strömberg U, Hanna Lähteenmäki H, Kasanen T, Koskenvesa P, Söderlund S, et al. Disease relapse after TKI discontinuation in CML is related both to low number and impaired function of NK-cells: data from Euro-SKI. Blood (ASH Annual Meeting Abstracts). 2013;122:379.
66. Burchert A, Muller MC, Kostrewa P, Erben P, Bostel T, Liebler S, et al. Sustained molecular response with interferon alfa maintenance after induction therapy with imatinib plus interferon alfa in patients with chronic myeloid leukemia. J Clin Oncol. 2010;28(8):1429–35.
67. Balachandran VP, Cavnar MJ, Zeng S, Bamboat ZM, Ocuin LM, Obaid H, et al. Imatinib potentiates antitumor T cell responses in gastrointestinal stromal tumor through the inhibition of Ido. Nat Med. 2011;17(9):1094–100.
68. Kuroda J, Puthalakath H, Cragg MS, Kelly PN, Bouillet P, Huang DC, et al. Bim and Bad mediate imatinib-induced killing of Bcr/Abl + leukemic cells, and resistance due to their loss is overcome by a BH3 mimetic. Proc Natl Acad Sci U S A. 2006;103(40):14907–12.
69. Augis V, Airiau K, Josselin M, Turcq B, Mahon FX, Belloc F. A single nucleotide polymorphism in cBIM is associated with a slower achievement of major molecular response in chronic myeloid leukaemia treated with imatinib. PLoS One. 2013;8(11):e78582.

# Chapter 6
# Updated European LeukemiaNet Recommendations for the Management of CML

Noriko Usui

**Abstract** After imatinib became the first approved BCR-ABL tyrosine kinase inhibitor (TKI) for chronic myelogenous leukemia (CML), more potent TKIs have been developed, and some of them (dasatinib, nilotinib, bosutinib) are now clinically available. Currently, it becomes rather complicated to select appropriate therapies among at least three effective management of CML, which are allogeneic stem cell transplantation (alloSCT), interferon, and TKIs. European LeukemiaNet (ELN) had proposed recommendations or guidelines for the management of CML in 2006, 2009, and 2013 that are occasionally called ELN2006, ELN2009, and ELN2013 for short.

Based upon results of clinical trials including pivotal phase III studies such as IRIS, DASISION, and ENESTnd as well as reported case studies, the panels of these ELN recommendations or guidelines have updated definitions of phases, relative risk, response, evaluation of response (especially molecular response), and treatment recommendations in management of CML. Although response evaluation of "optimal response" was not included in ELN2006, it was defined clearly in ELN2009 and updated more sophisticated in ELN2013. To understand how these ELN recommendations or guidelines for CML have been updated allows us to improve outcome of patients with CML.

**Keywords** Imatinib • Dasatinib • Nilotinib • ELN2013

## 6.1 Introduction

Chronic myelogenous leukemia (CML, also called chronic myeloid leukemia) is one of myeloproliferative neoplasms characterized by disorder of pluripotent bone marrow (BM) stem cell and by being associated with *BCR-ABL1* fusion gene located in the Philadelphia chromosome (Ph) [i.e., t (9;22) (q34;q11)] [1].

N. Usui, MD, PhD (✉)
Division of Clinical Oncology and Hematology, Department of Internal Medicine, The Jikei University Daisan Hospital, 4-11-1 Izumi-Honcho, Komae, Tokyo 201-8601, Japan
e-mail: usuin@jikei.ac.jp



M. Kizaki (ed.), *Molecular Pathogenesis and Treatment of Chronic Myelogenous Leukemia*, DOI 10.1007/978-4-431-55714-2_6

This abnormal fusion gene produces a unique protein named BCR-ABL, which is a constitutively active tyrosine kinase. It is this deregulated tyrosine kinase that is major cause of development of CML. Since the oral inhibitors of this tyrosine kinase have been developed [2], treatment of CML has dramatically changed.

The first clinical trials of tyrosine kinase inhibitors (TKIs) in CML were conducted in patients refractory to or intolerant of interferon therapy which had been the standard care before introduction of imatinib [3–7]. Effects of imatinib were observed not only chronic phase (CP) but also advanced phases, accelerated phase (AP) and blast phase (BP, also called blast crisis). Since imatinib had superb efficacy for chronic-phase CML (CP-CML) as salvage setting, the randomized IRIS (International Randomized Study of Interferon and STI571) trial subsequently compared imatinib with interferon therapy in newly diagnosed patients with CP-CML [8]. Imatinib produced higher efficacy in both hematologic and cytogenetic responses and much less toxicity. Because of the majority of patients allowed to change from interferon to imatinib, survival benefit of imatinib has not been demonstrated. However, results of long-term follow-up of patients registered in the imatinib arm in IRIS trial [9–11] and of interferon-α including treatment [12–14] have indicated that imatinib will provide better overall survival than interferon. Therefore, imatinib became the first approved TKI for CML. Since then, more potent TKIs have been developed, and some of them (dasatinib, nilotinib, bosutinib) are now clinically available.

Currently, we have at least three effective therapies for management of CML, which are allogeneic stem cell transplantation (alloSCT), interferon, and TKIs. In order to select appropriate therapies among these therapeutic modalities, European LeukemiaNet (ELN) had proposed recommendations or guidelines for the management of CML in 2006, 2009, and 2013 [15–17]. To understand recent dramatic improvement of outcome of CML by imatinib and other TKIs, these ELN recommendations or guidelines are reviewed and evaluated how to be updated.

## 6.2 Time Line of Proposing ELN Recommendations or Guidelines

The first recommendation or guideline of management of CML was started to be made by an expert panel that included hematologists and oncologists from the United States, England, France, Germany, and Italy convened by the American Society of Hematology (ASH) in 1996. The ASH expert panel proceeded evidence-based analysis of effect of busulfan, hydroxyurea, interferon, and alloSCT in treating CP-CML by end of 1998 and published evidence-based guideline in 1999 [18]. In the first guideline, TKIs were not considered because imatinib has just developed and started clinical trials [2–4].

ELN convened 19-member panel that recognized clinical and research expert in CML from European Union countries, Switzerland, the United States, and Australia and to review treatment of CML since 1998. Then, new treatment recommendations or guidelines were published as ELN 2006 recommendations for management of CML (ELN2006) based upon computerized literature search in April and November 2005, and relevant abstracts presented at the 2004 and 2005 meetings of ASH, the American Society of Clinical Oncology (ASCO), the European Group for Blood and Marrow Transplantation (EBMT), the European Hematology Association (EHA), and the International Society for Experimental Hematology (ISEH) [15]. In the ELN2006, the vast majority of clinical results of imatinib for all phases of CML were included even though there were some results of IFN or alloSCT updated, and the establishment of superiority of imatinib over IFN combined low-dose cytarabine in the IRIS trial played an important role.

Development and clinical introduction of second-generation TKIs as salvage therapy for failure to imatinib made ELN 2006 update to ELN 2009 recommendations (ELN2009). The panel reviewed the relevant papers after 2005 up to February 2009 and relevant abstracts presented at the 2008 meetings EHA and ASH and published recommendations in December 2009 [16].

Two prospective randomized trials comparing second-generation TKIs (nilotinib and dasatinib) to imatinib for newly diagnosed CP-CML were started in middle of 2007. The ENESTnd trial, testing nilotinib 300 mg twice daily vs imatinib 400 mg once daily, reported a significantly higher rate of durable cytogenetic and molecular response [19–21]. The DASSION trial, testing dasatinib 100 mg once daily vs imatinib 400 mg once daily, also reported a significantly higher rate of durable cytogenetic and molecular response [22, 23]. Based upon these two trials, nilotinib and dasatinib can be used as first-line therapy as well as imatinib. In addition, nilotinib and dasatinib have been widely used as second- or third-line TKIs and development and clinical introduction of other new TKIs (bosutinib and ponatinib) made recommendations about appropriate management with TKIs. The composition of the ELN panel for recommendations in CML was increased to include 32 experts from Europe, America, and the Asia-Pacific areas. The panel reviewed relevant papers after 2009 up to February 2013 and abstracts presented at the latest meetings of the EHA (June 2012) and of the ASH (December 2012) before published ELN 2013 recommendations (ELN 2013) in August 2013 [17].

## 6.3 Updating Definitions

### *6.3.1 Criteria of Advanced Phases and Relative Risk (Table 6.1)*

The criteria of AP-CML were defined in both ELN2006 [15] and ELN2013 [17] together with World Health Organization (WHO) criteria [1, 24]. The criteria of BP-CML were defined in ELN2013 with WHO criteria. These criteria slightly

**Table 6.1** Definition of advanced phases of CML

| Disease phase | ELN (2006) | WHO (2008) | ELN (2013) |
|---|---|---|---|
| Accelerated phase | Blast cells in blood or bone marrow 15–29 %, or blasts + promyelocyte in blood or marrow >30 %, with blasts <30 % | Blast cells in blood or bone marrow 10–19 % | Blast cells in blood or bone marrow 15–29 %, or blasts + promyelocyte in blood or marrow >30 %, with blasts <30 % |
| | Basophils in blood ≥20 % | Basophils in blood ≥20 % | Basophils in blood ≥20 % |
| | Persistent thrombocytopenia ($<100 \times 10^9$/L) unrelated to therapy | Persistent thrombocytopenia ($<100 \times 10^9$/L) unrelated to therapy | Persistent thrombocytopenia ($<100 \times 10^9$/L) unrelated to therapy |
| | | Thrombocytosis ($>1000 \times 10^9$/L), unresponsive to therapy | Clonal chromosome abnormalities in Ph+ cells (CCA/Ph+), major route, on treatment |
| | | Persistent or increasing WBC ($>10 \times 10^9$/L) count and/or persisting or increasing splenomegaly unresponsive to therapy | |
| | | Clonal cytogenetic evolution occurring after initial diagnostic karyotype | |
| Blast phase | Not referred | Blasts in blood or marrow ≥20 % | Blasts in blood or marrow ≥30 % |
| | | Extramedulary blast proliferation, apart from the spleen | Extramedulary blast proliferation, apart from the spleen |

*ELN* European LeukemiaNet, *WHO* World Health Organization

differ between ELN and WHO. For patients in AP-CML, the proportion of blasts in blood or bone marrow is defined as 15–29 % in ELN2006 and ELN2013 while that is 10–19 % in WHO2008. For BP-CML, blasts in blood or bone marrow are defined greater than 30 % in ELN2013 while greater than 20 % in WHO2008 (Table 6.1). Comparing to ELN2006 and ELN2013 criteria of AP-CML, a factor of clonal chromosome abnormalities was added, which is considered as a sign of progression of disease.

The panel used a term of early chronic-phase (ECP) patients with CML. ECP-CML included patients diagnosed as CP-CML within 1 year without heavily treated with interferon because these patients can receive better efficacy of imatinib compared to patients classified as late chronic phase (LCP) who were resistant or intolerant to interferon αtherapy. However, the majority of patients with CP-CML have been treated by imatinib as the first-line therapy after ELN2006; terms of ECP and LCP in CP-CML were disappeared in ELN2009 [16] or ELN2013 [17].

The relative risk (RR) of progression and death in treatment-naïve CP patients or newly diagnosed CP-CML is important for selection of therapy. Sokal and Hasford scores [25, 26] were both defined as relative risk (RR) evaluations in ELN2006 and ELN2009, and EUTOS score [27] was introduced in ELN2013.

### *6.3.2 Definition of Response*

Response to treatment for CP-CML has been defined by three categories, hematologic, cytogenetic, and molecular responses. Definition of hematologic response has not been changed since it was listed in ELN2006 [15]. However, definitions of cytogenetic and molecular responses have been updated since the majority of patients with newly diagnosed CP-CML have an excellent response to first-line treatment with a TKI after introduction of imatinib (Table 6.2).

In ELN2006, as only chromosome banding analysis (CBA) of marrow cell metaphases can be used to assess the degree of cytogenetic response (CgR or CyR), CBA of marrow cells should be performed before treatment, at least every 6 months until a complete CCyR (CCgR or CCyR) has been achieved and confirmed and then every 12 months. Fluorescence in situ hybridization (FISH) of blood interphase cell nuclei could substitute for CBA of marrow cell metaphases only for the assessment of CCyR, which is then defined by <1 % BCR-ABL1-positive nuclei of at least 200 nuclei, from ELN2009 [16] and ELN2013 [17].

The panel of ELN2006 indicated that it is necessary to measure the level of the *BCR-ABL1* transcripts to determine minimal residual disease (MRD) since the frequency of CCyR is very high in imatinib-treated patients. A 3-log reduction from a standard baseline or lower than 0.1 % of *BCR-ABL1* transcript level was defined as major molecular response (MMolR or MMR) in ELN2006, which was based on the data collected from IRIS trial and others [28–30]. Definition of MMR was supported but definitions of deeper MR were updated in ELN2009 and ELN2013 by progress of measuring of *BCR-ABL1* transcript and of standardizing internationally. The panel of ELN2013 [17] defined molecular response according to the International Scale (IS) as the ratio of *BCR-ABL1* transcripts to *ABL1* transcripts, or other internationally recognized control transcripts, and it is expressed and reported as *BCR-ABL1*% on a log scale, where 10 %, 1 %, 0.1 %, 0.01 %, 0.0032 %, and 0.001 % correspond to a decrease of 1, 2, 3, 4, 4.5, and 5 logs, respectively, below the standard baseline that was used in the IRIS trial [16, 30–33]. The panel proposed that the term complete molecular response should be avoided and substituted with the term molecularly undetectable leukemia, with specification of the number of the control gene transcript copies. The panel indicated that these definitions depend critically on the ability of testing laboratories to measure absolute numbers of control gene transcripts in a comparable manner, as well as their ability to achieve the polymerase chain reaction (PCR) sensitivity

**Table 6.2** Definitions of response

| | ELN 2006 | ELN 2009 | ELN 2013 |
|---|---|---|---|
| *Hematologic response* | | | |
| Complete (CHR) | Platelet count <450 × 10⁹/L | | |
| | WBC count <10 × 10⁹/L, differential | | |
| | Without immature granulocytes and with less than 5 % basophils | Same as definition of ELN 2006 | Same as definition of ELN 2006 |
| | Nonpalpable spleen | | |
| | *Cytogenetic response (is evaluated by morphologic cytogenetics of at least 20 marrow metaphases)* | | |
| | | | |
| Complete | CCgR: Ph+ 0 % | CCgR: no Ph+ metaphases | CCyR: no Ph+ metaphases, <1 % *BCR-ABL1*-positive nuclei of at least 200 nuclei |
| Partial | PCgR: Ph+ 1–35 % | PCgR: 1–35 % Ph+ metaphases | PCyR: 1–35 % Ph +metaphases |
| Minor | MinorCgR: Ph+ 36–65 % | mCgR: 35–65 % Ph+ metaphases | mCyR: 36–65 % Ph +metaphases |
| Minimal | MinCgR: Ph+ 66–95 % | minCgR: 66–95 % Ph+ metaphases | minCyR: 66–95 % Ph+ metaphases |
| None | None: Ph+ >95 % | noCgR: >Ph+ metaphases | noCyR: >Ph+ metaphases |
| Molecular response (BCR-ABL to control gene ratio according to International Scale) | | | (Is assessed according to the International Scale (IS) as ratio of *BCR-ABL1* transcripts to *ABL1* transcripts |
| Complete | Transcript nonquantifiable and nondetectable | CMolR: undetectable *BCR-ABL* mRNA transcripts by real-time quantitative and/or nested PCR in two consecutive blood samples of adequate quality (sensitivity >10⁴) | $MR^{4.5}$ <0.0032 % *BCR-ABL1* IS or undetectable disease in cDNA with >32,000 *ABL1* transcripts in the same volume of cDNA used to test for *BCR-ABL1* |
| | | | $MR^{4.0}$ <0.01 % *BCR-ABL*1 IS or undetectable disease in cDNA with >10.000 *ABL1* transcripts |
| Major | ≤0.10 | MMolR: ratio of *BCR-ABL* to *ABL* (or other housekeeping genes) ≤0.1 % on the International Scale | MMR: *BCR-ABL1* IS expression of ≤0.1 % |

required for *BCR-ABL1* detection [17]. Therefore, definitions of deeper MR will be updated in further recommendations or guidelines for management CML.

## 6.4 Updating Evaluation of Response

The goals of treatment for CML are to eradicate leukemic cells, to restore normal hematopoiesis, and to obtain durable best response without adverse effects. Criteria of evaluation of response were updated as listed in Table 6.3. Based upon long-term results of IRIS trial [9–11], imatinib can provide most patients their best response within the first year of treatment and some of patients continue to deepen their response more than several years. It is critically important to carefully follow patients using timepoint evaluation proposed by ELN recommendations. Data from IRIS trial suggested that early CyR is the most important response-related prognostic factor. However, since clinical efficacy of imatinib has not been fully established at time of ELN206 published, the panel avoided defining optimal response. Instead, the panel proposed to define the response to the treatment at different timepoints (at 3, 6, 12, 18 months) as failure, suboptimal, and warnings including implication for patients.

The concept of optimal response has been proposed from ELN2009 [16]. The panel of ELN2009 also proposed that monitoring the response to imatinib requires blood counts and differentials, cytogenetics, and molecular testing for *BCR-ABL1* transcript level and for *BCR-ABL1* kinase domain mutations as some research required [34–36]. Timepoint and methods for response evaluation are proposed comprehensively in ELN2009: (a) blood counts and differentials are required frequently during the first 3 months until a CHR; (b) cytogenetics, performed with CBA of marrow cell metaphases, is required at 3 and 6 months, then every 6 months until a CCgR, and then every 12 months if regular molecular monitoring cannot be assured, and always in instances of myelodysplastic features, suboptimal response, or failure; (c) marrow CBA is preferred to interphase fluorescent in situ hybridization (I-FISH), but I-FISH can be substituted after CCgR; (d) real-time, quantitative polymerase chain reaction should be performed on whole buffy-coat blood cells, and results should be expressed as a ratio of BCR-ABL to ABL (or other housekeeping genes) $\times$ 100 %; converted to the International Scale, the ratio $\leq$0.1 % defined MMolR (or MMR).

Response evaluation for CP-CML with TKIs as first-line treatment has updated in ELN2013 based upon collected data from some clinical trials of initial treatment with imatinib [10, 11, 37–45]. According to ELN2013 [17], total 4360 patients with CP-CML treated with imatinib (400–800 mg/day) as the first-line therapy were followed at more than 5 years; progression-free survival (PFS) ranged between 83 and 94 % (median 90 %) and overall survival (OS) ranged 83 and 97 % (median 89 %). The panel of ELN2013 also considered efficacy of nilotinib and dasatinib as the first-line therapy based upon ENESTnd [19–21] and DASISION trials [22, 23]. As the panel of ELN2013 indicated that nilotinib and dasatinib as well

**Table 6.3** Evaluation of overall Responses to TKIs as first-line therapy in chronic myeloid leukemia-chronic phase (CML-CP)

| ELN 2006 (evaluation of overall responses to imatinib first line in early CML-CP) | | | |
|---|---|---|---|
| Timepoint | Failure | Suboptimal response | Warnings |
| Diagnosis | NA | NA | High risk, del9q+, ACAs in Ph+ cells |
| 3 months after diagnosis | No HR (stable disease or disease progression) | No HR (stable disease or disease progression) | NA |
| 6 months after diagnosis | <CHR, no CgR (Ph+ >95 %) | <PCgR (Ph+ >35 %) | NA |
| 12 months after diagnosis | <PCgR (Ph+ >35 %) | <CCgR | <MMolR |
| 18 months after diagnosis | <CCgR (Ph+ = 0) | <MMolR | NA |
| Anytime | Loss of CHR[a], loss of CCgR[b], mutation[c] | ACA in Ph+ cells[d], loss of MMolR[d], mutation[e] | Any rise in transcript level; other chromosome abnormalities in Ph- cells |
| Implication for patients | Move to other treatments whenever available | Continue imatinib but long-term outcome is not likely to be optimal. Be eligible for other treatments | Monitor very carefully. Become eligible for other treatments |

| ELN 2009 (evaluation of overall responses to imatinib first line in CML-CP) | | | | |
|---|---|---|---|---|
| Evaluation Time (months) | Response | | | |
| | Optimal | Suboptimal | Failure | Warning |
| Baseline | NA | NA | NA | High risk, CCA/Ph+[f] |
| 3 | CHR and at least minor CgR (Ph+ ≤ 65 %) | No CgR (Ph + >95 %) | No CgR (Ph+ >95 %) | NA |
| 6 | At least PCgR (Ph+ ≤ 35 %) | <PCgR (Ph + >35 %) | No CgR (Ph+ >95 %) | NA |
| 12 | CCgR | PCgR (Ph+ 1–35 %) | <CCgR | <MMolR |
| 18 | MMolR | <MMolR | <CCgR | NA |
| Any time during treatment | Stable or improving MMolR[g] | Loss of MMolR[g] mutations[h] | Loss of CHR, loss of CCgR, mutations[i], CCA/Ph+ | Increase in transcript levels[j], CCA/Ph- |

| ELN 2013 (evaluation of overall responses to imatinib, dasatinib, or nilotinib first line in CML-CP) | | | |
|---|---|---|---|
| | Optimal | Warnings | Failure |
| Baseline | NA | High risk, or CCA/Ph+, major route | NA |

(continued)

**Table 6.3** (continued)

| ELN 2013 (evaluation of overall responses to imatinib, dasatinib, or nilotinib first line in CML-CP) | | | |
|---|---|---|---|
| | Optimal | Warnings | Failure |
| 3 months | *BCR-ABL1* ≤10 % and/or Ph+ ≤35 % | *BCR-ABL1* >10 % and/or Ph+ 36–95 % | Non-CHR and/or Ph+ >95 % |
| 6 months | *BCR-ABL1* <1 % and/or Ph+ 0 | *BCR-ABL1* 1–10 % and/or Ph+ 1–35 % | *BCR-ABL1* >10 % and/or Ph+ >35 % |
| 12 months | *BCR-ABL1* ≤0.1 % | BCR-ABL1 >0.1–1 % | *BCR-ABL1* >1 % and/or Ph+ >0 |
| At any time | *BCR-ABL1* ≤0.1 % | CCA/Ph− (−7 or 7q−) | Loss of CHR, loss of CCyR, confirmed loss of MMR[k], mutation, CCA/Ph+ |

After 12 months, if an MMR is achieved, the response can be assessed by real quantitative polymerase chain reaction (RQ-PCR) every 3–6 months, and cytogenetics is required only in case of failure or if standardized molecular testing is not available. Note that MMR (MR3.0 or better) is for survival but that a deeper response is likely to be required for a successful discontinuation of treatment.

*NA* not available, *ACAs* abnormal cytogenetic abnormalities, *HR* hematologic response, *CHR* complete hematologic response, *CgR* cytogenetic response, *PCgR* partial CgR, *CCgR* complete CgR, *MMolR* major molecular response, *CCA* clonal chromosome abnormalities, *Ph*+ Philadelphia chromosome positive, *Ph*− Philadelphia chromosome negative, *MMR* major molecular response, *BCR-ABL1*≤ 0.1 % = MR3.0 or better, *CCA/Ph*+ clonal chromosome abnormalities in Ph+ cells, *CCA/Ph*− clonal chromosome abnormalities in Ph− cells.

[a]To be confirmed on 2 occasions unless associated with progression to AP/BC
[b]To be confirmed on 2 occasions, unless associated with CHR loss or progression to AP/BC
[c]High level of insensitivity to imatinib
[d]To be confirmed on 2 occasions, unless associated with CHR or CCgR loss
[e]Low level of insensitivity to imatinib
[f]CCA/Ph+ two consecutive cytogenetic tests are required and must show the same CCA in at least two Ph+ cells
[g]MMolR indicates a ratio of BCR-ABL1 to ABL1 or other housekeeping genes of ≤0.1 % on the International Scale
[h]BCR-ABL1 kinase domain mutations still sensitive to imatinib
[i]BCR-ABL1 kinase domain mutations poorly sensitive to imatinib
[j]The significance of the increase may vary by a factor of 2–10, depending on the laboratories
[k]In 2 consecutive tests, of which one with a BCR-ABL1 transcript level ≥1 %

as imatinib could be selected as first-line TKIs, evaluation of response was updated to define as "optimal" or "failure." Optimal response is associated with the best long-term outcome and it indicates to continue treatment with the same TKI. Timepoint of optimal response was updated in ELN2013. Since second-generation TKI provided faster and deeper response, it should be obtained more than partial CyR (or *BCR-ABL1* ≤10 %) by 3 months, more than CCyR (or *BCR-ABL1* ≤1 %) by 6 months, and more than MMR (or *BCR-ABL1* ≤0.1 %) by 12 months.

Failure means that the patient should receive a different treatment to limit the risk of progression and death. The previous term of "suboptimal" was changed to "warning" which implies that the characteristics of the disease and the response to treatment require more frequent monitoring to permit timely changes in therapy in case of treatment failure.

## 6.5 Resistant to TKIs (Emergence of BCR-ABL1 Mutations)

Among various factors that cause for emergence of resistance to TKIs, clonal evolution and mutations are likely to be the most important factors and are related to each other. Relation between IC50 values and these BCR-ABL1 mutations has been summarized firstly about imatinib in ELN2006, secondary about nilotinib and dasatinib addition to imatinib in ELN2009, and currently about available TKIs adding bosutinib and ponatinib in ELN2013 (Table 6.4) [15–17]. Recently, ABL1 kinase domain point mutations have been detectable about 50 % of patients with TKI-failure and progression to advanced phases [46–55].

More than 80 amino acid substitutions have been reported in association with resistance to imatinib [48, 51, 52]. Dasatinib and nilotinib have much smaller spectra of resistant mutations, but neither inhibits the T315I. Patients relapsing while taking nilotinib were most frequently found to have acquired Y253H, E255K/V, F359V/C/I, or T315I mutations, whereas patients relapsing while taking dasatinib were most frequently found to have acquired V299L, F317L/V/I/C, T315A, or T315I mutations [50–54]. T315I is also resistant to bosutinib [56, 57], whereas ponatinib inhibits T315I in vitro and is effective in patients with T315 in vivo [58–60].

## 6.6 Updating Treatment Recommendations (Tables 6.5, 6.6, and 6.7)

### 6.6.1 *For CP-CML (Table 6.5)*

For treatment of CP-CML, imatinib 400 mg once daily was proposed to use as first line in ELN2006 because imatinib was only TKI at that time. Imatinib was also recommended to use as second line with increased dose (600–800 mg daily) even though alloSCT was always option for failure, suboptimal response, or intolerance to imatinib [15]. In ELN2009, imatinib was selected as the first-line therapy, but dasatinib or nilotinib was recommended to use as second line as well as higher dose of imatinib [16]. AlloSCT was recommended for patients in AP or BP or with the T315I mutation and for the patients who experience suboptimal response to or failure on these second-line TKIs. The panel of ELN2009 proposed [16] that hydroxyurea can be used only for a short period of time or in a patient in whom a TKI is not advised and that IFN-α is still an option in case of pregnancy, for which

**Table 6.4** IC50 values of BCR-ABL1 mutations observed in patients treated with TKIs according to three types of ELN recommendations

ELN2006

| *BCR-ABL* | Imatinib IC50 nM Biochemical | Cellular |
|---|---|---|
| Wild type | 300 | 260-500 |
| M244V | 380 | 2 000 |
| P-loop | | |
| L248V | NA | 1 500 |
| G250E | 1 000 | 1 350-3 900 |
| Q252H | NA | 1 200-2 800 |
| Y253F | > 5 000 | 3 475 |
| Y253H* | > 5 000 | > 10 000 |
| E255K | 2 800 | 4 400-8 400 |
| E255V | > 5 000 | > 5 000 |
| D276G | NA | 1 500 |
| T277A | NA | NA |
| F311L | 775 | 480 |
| F311I | NA | NA |
| T315I* | > 5 000 | > 10 000 |
| F317L* | 900 | 810-1 500 |
| M343T | NA | NA |
| Catalytic domain | | |
| M351T | 820 | 930 |
| M351V | NA | NA |
| E355D | NA | NA |
| E355G | NA | 400 |
| F359V* | 4 700 | 1 200 |
| Activation loop | | |
| V379I | 800 | 1 630 |
| A380T* | 340 | 2 450 |
| F382L | NA | NA |
| L387M | 1 500 | 1 000 |
| L387F | NA | 1 100 |
| H396P | 340-800 | 850-4 200 |
| H396R | 1 950 | 1 750 |
| S417Y | NA | NA |
| E459K | NA | NA |
| F486S | 1 230 | 2 800 |

IC50 indicates the concentration that inhibits by 50% the biochemical TK activity of BCR-ABL and suppresses by 50% the growth of Ph+ cell lines; NA, not available.* IM contact sites.

ELN2009

| *BCR-ABL* Gene Mutation | IC50 Range by Agent (ng/mL) Imatinib | Nilotinib | Dasatinib |
|---|---|---|---|
| Unmutated | 153-400 | < 5-13 | 0.4-0.9 |
| M244V | 944-1,829 | 20.1-20.6 | 0.7 |
| L248V | 1,101-5,900 | 26-486 | 4.7 |
| G250E | 796 to > 11,800 | 25-116 | 0.9-4.1 |
| Q252H | 433-1,841 | 8-37 | 1.7-2.8 |
| Y253F | 1,114-5,274 | 30-66 | 0.7-1.5 |
| Y253H | > 3,800-10,442 | 238-688 | 1.3-10 |
| E255K | 1,873 to > 5,900 | 63-299 | 2.8-6.6 |
| E255V | 3,605-5,282 | 96-384 | 3.2-5.6 |
| D276G | 677 | 19 | 1.3 |
| E279K | 1,104 | 19-40 | 1.5 |
| V299L | 319-480 | 13 | 8-9.1 |
| F311L | 283-767 | 12 | 0.7 |
| T315I | > 3,800 to > 11,800 | 369 to > 5,300 | 69.3 to > 500 |
| T315A | 448 | NA | 63 |
| F317L | 620-4,425 | 21-48 | 3.7-9.1 |
| F317V | 207-295 | 185 | 27 |
| F317C | 708 | NA | NA |
| M351T | 519-2,891 | 4.1-20.1 | 0.6-0.8 |
| E355G | 1,404 | NA | NA |
| F359V | 826-1,077 | 48-93 | 1.1-1.4 |
| F359C | 708 | NA | NA |
| V379I | 590-962 | 27 | 0.4 |
| L384M | 398-1,652 | 21-22 | 2 |
| L387M | 590-649 | 26 | 1 |
| H396R | 1,032-3,186 | 22-29 | 0.7-1.5 |
| H396P | 850-2,537 | 22-23 | 0.3-1.0 |
| F486S | 1,609-5,369 | 17-46 | 2.8 |

Abbreviations: IC50, 50% inhibitory concentration, NA, not available or applicable.

ELN2013

| *BCR-ABL1* | IC50 Range by Agent (nM) Imatinib | Nilotinib | Dasatinib | Bosutinib | Ponatinib |
|---|---|---|---|---|---|
| Unmutated | 260-678 | <10-25 | 0.8-1.8 | 41.6 | 0.5 |
| M244V* | 1600-3100 | 38-39 | 1.3 | 147.4 | 2.2 |
| L248V | 1866-10 000 | 49.5-919 | 9.4 | NA | NA |
| G250E* | 1350 to >20 000 | 48-219 | 1.8-8.1 | 179.2 | 4.1 |
| Q252H | 734-3120 | 16-70 | 3.4-5.6 | 33.7 | 2.2 |
| Y253F | >6400-8953 | 182-725 | 6.3-11 | 40 | 2.8 |
| Y253H* | >6400-17 700 | 450-1300 | 1.3-10 | NA | 6.2 |
| E255K* | 3174-12 100 | 118-566 | 5.6-13 | 394 | 14 |
| E255V | 6111-8953 | 430-725 | 6.3-11 | 230.1 | 36 |
| D276G | 1147 | 35.3 | 2.6 | 25 | NA |
| E279K | 1872 | 36.5-75 | 3 | 39.7 | NA |
| V299L | 540-814 | 23.7 | 15.8-18 | 1086 | NA |
| F311L | 480-1300 | 23 | 1.3 | NA | NA |
| T315I* | >6400 to >20 000 | 697 to >10 000 | 137 to >1000 | 1890 | 11 |
| T315A | 125 | N.A. | 760 | NA | 1.6 |
| F317L* | 810-7500 | 39.2-91 | 7.4-18 | 100.7 | 1.1 |
| F317V | 500 | 350 | NA | NA | 10 |
| M351T* | 880-4900 | 7.8-38 | 1.1-1.6 | 29.1 | 1.5 |
| F359V* | 1400-1825 | 91-175 | 2.2-2.7 | 38.6 | 10 |
| V379I | 1000-1,630 | 51 | 0.8 | NA | NA |
| L384M* | 674-2800 | 39-41.2 | 4 | 19.5 | NA |
| L387M | 1000-1100 | 49 | 2 | NA | NA |
| H396R* | 1750-5400 | 41-55 | 1.3-3 | 33.7 | NA |
| H396P | 850-4300 | 41-43 | 0.6-2 | 18.1 | 1.1 |
| F486S | 2728-9100 | 32.8-87 | 5.6 | 96.1 | NA |
| Plasma drug concentration | | | | | |
| Cmin | 2062 ± 1334 | 1923 ± 1233 | 5.5 ± 1.4 | 268 (30-1533) | 64.3 ± 29.2 |
| Cmax | 4402 ± 1272 | 2329 ± 772 | 133 ± 73.9 | 392 (80-1858) | 145.4 ± 72.6 |

NA, not available.

* Representative of the 10 most frequent mutations.

**Table 6.5** Treatment recommendation proposed in three types of ELN – for chronic phase

| ELN 2006 | |
|---|---|
| *Chronic phase* | |
| First line | Imatinib 400 mg daily |
| | Discuss choice between IM or AlloHSCT if a patient with high disease risk and low EBMT risk score |
| Second line | |
| Failure to imatinib | AlloHSCT or imatinib 600–800 mg daily |
| Suboptimal to imatinib | Imatinib 600–800 mg daily, AlloHSCT could be offered |
| Intolerance to imatinib | AlloHSCT or rIFNα ± LD-Ara-C or apply for new agent trials |
| ELN2009 | |
| *Chronic phase* | |
| First line | |
| All patients | Imatinib 400 mg daily |
| Second line | |
| Imatinib intolerant | Dasatinib or nilotinib |
| Imatinib suboptimal response | Continue imatinib same dose; or test high-dose imatinib, dasatinib, or nilotinib |
| Imatinib failure | Dasatinib or nilotinib; alloHSCT in the patients who have experienced progression to AP/BP and in patients who carry the T315I mutation |
| Third line | |
| Dasatinib or nilotinib suboptimal response | Continue dasatinib or nilotinib, with an option for alloHSCT in patients with warning features (i.e., prior hematologic resistance to imatinib, mutations) and in patients with an EBMT risk score ≤2 |
| Dasatinib or nilotinib failure | AlloHSCT |
| ELN2013 | |
| *Chronic phase* | |
| First line | Imatinib or nilotinib or dasatinib |
| | HLA-type patients and siblings only in case of baseline warnings (high risk, major route CCA/Ph+) |
| Second line, intolerance to the first TKI | Anyone of the other TKIs approved first line (imatinib, nilotinib, dasatinib) |
| Second line, failure of imatinib first line | Dasatinib or nilotinib or bosutinib or ponatinib |
| | HLA-type patients and siblings |
| Second line, failure of nilotinib first line | Dasatinib or bosutinib or ponatinib |
| | HLA-type patients and siblings; search for an unrelated stem cell donor; consider alloSCT |
| Second line, failure of dasatinib first line | Nilotinib or bosutinib or ponatinib |
| | HLA-type patients and siblings; search for an unrelated stem cell donor; consider alloSCT |
| Third line, failure of and/or intolerance to 2 TKIs | Anyone of the remaining TKIs; alloSCT recommended in all eligible patients |

(continued)

**Table 6.5** (continued)

| ELN2013 | |
|---|---|
| Any line, T315I mutation | Ponatinib |
| | HLA-type patients and siblings; search for an unrelated stem cell donor; consider alloSCT |

*Abbreviations*: *LD-Ara-C* low-dose cytarabine, *AP* accelerated phase, *AlloHSCT* allogeneic hematopoietic stem cell transplantation, *alloSCT* allogeneic stem cell transplantation, *BP blast phase EBMT* European Group for Blood and Marrow Transplantation, *TKI* tyrosine kinase inhibitor

imatinib should not be administered either at conception or during gestation [61] and in some patients, mainly low-risk patients, for whom imatinib may be not appropriate because of comorbidities or concomitant medications.

In ELN2013, the first-line treatment of CP-CML can be use any of the 3 TKIs that have been approved for this indication and are available nearly worldwide, which are imatinib (400 mg once daily), nilotinib (300 mg twice daily), and dasatinib (100 mg once daily) [17]. These three TKIs can also be used in second or subsequent lines, at the standard or at a higher dose (imatinib 400 mg twice daily, nilotinib 400 mg twice daily, and dasatinib 70 mg twice daily or 140 mg once daily). Bosutinib (500 mg once daily) has been approved in the United States, European countries, and Japan for patients resistant or intolerant to prior therapy. Ponatinib (45 mg once daily) has only been approved in the United States for patients resistant or intolerant to prior TKI therapy. As we can use second-generation TKIs as second line, the panel of ELN2009 started to propose response definition of TKI as a second-line therapy for CP-CML and ELN2013 was updated and indicated in Table 6.6. Currently, treatment strategy of CP-CML was referred to ELN2013 that updated ELN2006 and ELN2009.

### 6.6.2 *For AP/BP-CML (Table 6.7)*

There are two types of advanced phases of CML; one is initially diagnosed in AP or BP, and another is progressed from chronic phase treated with TKIs. Therapeutic strategy of AP/BP is fundamentally same every ELN, and patients with AP or BC are to be treated initially with TKIs including imatinib, dasatinib, and nilotinib (selected based on mutational analysis) and then to proceed to alloSCT. For more detail, treatment recommendations for AP and BP in ELN2013 are indicated in Table 6.7 as well as addition to ELN2006 and ELN2009 [15–17, 62–70].

## 6.7 Usage of ELN in Japan (Fig. 6.1)

After imatinib has been available in Japan from November 2001 for newly diagnosed CP-CML, we conducted phase II study to evaluate efficacy of imatinib as the first-line therapy for Japanese patients. Among 489 patients treated with imatinib

**Table 6.6** Response definitions of response to TKIs as a second-line therapy of patients with CP-CML

| ELN 2009 recommendations | | | |
|---|---|---|---|
| Evaluation Time (months) | Response | | |
| | Suboptimal | Failure | Warnings |
| Baseline | NA | NA | Hematologic resistance to imatinib; CCA/Ph+ (i.e., clonal progression); mutations[a] |
| 3 | Minor CgR (Ph+ 36–65 %) | No CgR (Ph+ >95 %); new mutations[a] | Minimal CgR (Ph+ 66–95 %) |
| 6 | PCgR $6# (Ph+ 1–35 %) | Minimal CgR (Ph+ 66–95 %); new mutations[a] | Minor CgR (Ph+ 36–65 %) |
| 12 | Less than MMolR[b] | Less than PCgR (Ph+ >35 %); new mutations[a] | |
| **ELN 2013 recommendations** | | | |
| Evaluation Time (months) | Optimal | Warning | Failure |
| Baseline | NA | No CHR or loss of CHR on imatinib or lack of CyR to first-line TKI or high risk | NA |
| 3 months | BCR-ABL1≤ 10 % and/or Ph+ < 65 % | BCR-ABL1 >10 % and/or Ph+ 65–95 % | No CHR or Ph+ >95 % or new mutations |
| 6 months | BCR-ABL1 ≤10 % and/or Ph+ < 35 % | Ph+ 35–65 % | BCR-ABL1 >10 % and/or Ph+ >65 % and/or new mutations |
| 12 months | BCR-ABL1 <1 % and/or Ph + 0 | BCR-ABL1 1–10 % and/or Ph+ 1–35 % | BCR-ABL1 >10 % and/or Ph+ >35 % and/or new mutations |
| At any time | BCR-ABL1 ≤0.1 % | CCA/Ph− (−7 or 7q−) or BCR-ABL1 >0.1 % | Loss of CHR<br>or loss of CCyR or PCyR<br>New mutations<br>Confirmed loss of MMR[c]<br>CCA/Ph+ |

*Abbreviations*: *TKIs* tyrosine kinase inhibitors, *NA* not applicable or not available *CCA* clonal chromosome abnormalities, *Ph+* Philadelphia chromosome positive, *CgR* cytogenetic response, *PCgR* partial cytogenetic response, *MMolR* major molecular response, MMR, BCR-ABL1 ≥0.1 % = MR3.0 or better, *CCA/Ph+* clonal chromosome abnormalities in Ph+ cells, *CCA/Ph−* clonal chromosome abnormalities in Ph− cells.

[a]BCR-ABL1 kinase domain mutations poorly sensitive to TKIs (Table 6.4)

[b]Ratio of BCR-ABL1 to ABL1 or to other housekeeping genes ≤0.1 % on the International Scale

[c]In 2 consecutive tests, of which one with a BCR-ABL transcript level ≥1 %

**Table 6.7** Treatment recommendation proposed in three types of ELN – for advanced phase

| ELN2006 treatment recommendation for CML in AP or BP | |
|---|---|
| *Accelerated phase* | |
| First line | Imatinib |
| Blast phase (blastic crisis) | |
| Early BP | Imatinib or other TKIs followed by AlloHSCT if possible |
| **ELN2009 treatment recommendation for CML in AP or BP** | |
| *Accelerated and blast* | |
| First line | AlloHSCT, preceded by imatinib 600 or 800 mg, dasatinib, or nilotinib, in case of mutations poorly sensitive to imatinib |
| Patients who are TKI naïve | |
| Second line | |
| Patients with prior treatment of imatinib | AlloHSCT, preceded by dasatinib or nilotinib |
| **ELN2013 treatment strategy for CML in AP or BP** | |
| AP and BP in newly diagnosed | Imatinib 400 mg BID or dasatinib 70 mg BID or 140 mg QD |
| TKI-naïve patients | Stem cell donor search |
| | Then, alloSCT is recommended for all BP patients and for the AP patients who do not achieve an optimal response |
| | Chemotherapy may be required before alloSCT, to control the disease |
| AP and BP as a progression | Anyone of the TKIs that were not used before progression (ponatinib in case of T315I mutation) and then alloSCT in all patients |
| From CP in TKI-pretreated patients | Chemotherapy is frequently required to make patients eligible for alloSCT |

*Abbreviations*: *AlloHSCT* allogeneic hematopoietic stem cell transplantation, *AP* accelerated phase, *BP*:blast phase, *EBMT* European Group for Blood and Marrow Transplantation, *TK* tyrosine kinase inhibitor, *QD* once daily administration, *BID* divide twice daily administration

400 mg once daily, 481 patients were assessable for efficacy. The majority of patients obtained CHR (96 %), CCyR (90 %), MMR (79 %) by 7 years, and 7-year OS, PFS, and EFS were 93 %, 93 %, and 87 %, respectively [71]. Since these results are similar to IRIS trial [8–10], and second-generation TKIs have been clinically available from 2009, we have used ELN 2006 and 2009 in daily practice. After nilotinib and dasatinib have been allowed to use as the first-line therapy in 2010, Japanese Society of Hematology (JSH) started to make guideline for management of hematologic malignancies including CML and published it in 2013 [72]. To make treatment algorithm of CML shown in Fig. 6.1, we fully used ELN2013.

In conclusion, ELN recommendations or guidelines to appropriate management of CML will be kept updating according to new data, new drugs, and new methods to evaluate residual CML cells and new essential information to improve outcome of patients with CML.

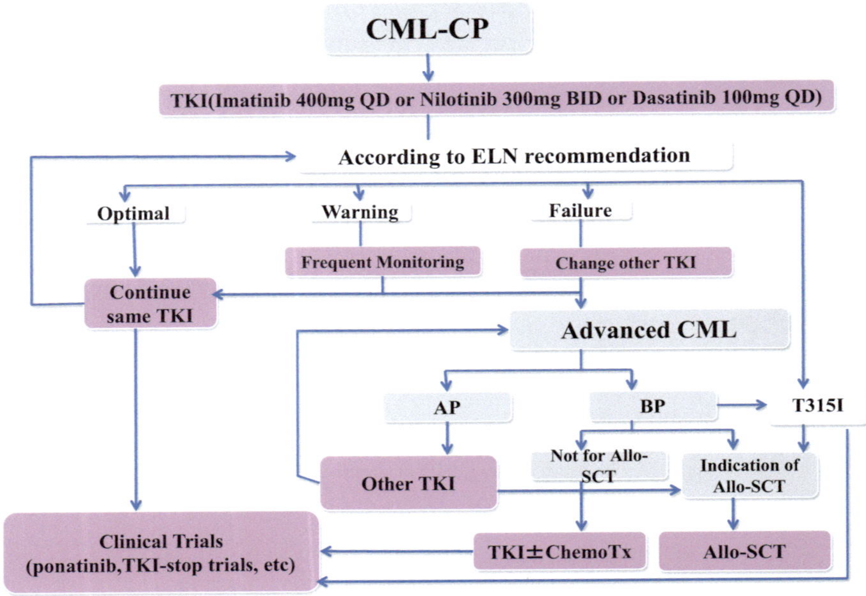


**Fig. 6.1** Treatment algorithm of CML-JSH2013cml guideline

## References


1. Vardiman JW, Melo JV, Baccarani M, Thiele J. Chronic myelogenous leukemia BCR-ABL1 positive. In: Swerdlow SH, Campo E, Harris NL, et al., editors. WHO classification of tumors of hematopoietic and lymphoid tissues. Lyon: IARC; 2008. p. 32–7.
2. Druker BJ, Tamura S, Buchdunger E, et al. Effects of a selective inhibitor of the Abl tyrosine kinase on the growth of Bcr-Abl positive cells. Nat Med. 1996;2:561–6.
3. Druker BJ, Talpaz M, Resta DJ, et al. Efficacy and safety of a specific inhibitor of the BCR-ABL tyrosine kinase in chronic myeloid leukemia. N Engl J Med. 2001;344:1031–7.
4. Druker BJ, Sawyers CL, Kantarjian H, et al. Activity of a specific inhibitor of the BCR-ABL tyrosine kinase in the blast crisis of chronic myeloid leukemia and acute lymphoblastic leukemia with the Philadelphia chromosome. N Engl J Med. 2001;344:1038–42.
5. Kantarjian H, Sawyers C, Hochhaus A, et al. Hematologic and cytogenetic responses to imatinib mesylate in chronic myelogenous leukemia. N Engl J Med. 2002;346:645–52.
6. Sawyers CL, Hochhaus A, Feldman E, et al. Imatinib induces hematologic and cytogenetic responses in patients with chronic myelogenous leukemia in myeloid blast crisis: results of a phase 2 study. Blood. 2002;99:3530–9.
7. Talpaz M, Silver RT, Druker BJ, et al. Imatinib induces durable hematologic and cytogenetic responses in patients with accelerated phase chronic myeloid leukemia: results of a phase 2 study. Blood. 2002;99:1928–37.
8. O'Brien SG, Guilhot F, Larson RA, et al. Imatinib compared with interferon and low-dose cytarabine for newly diagnosed chronic-phase chronic myeloid leukemia. N Engl J Med. 2003;348:994–1004.
9. Druker BJ, Guilhot F, O'Brien SG, et al.; IRIS Investigators. Five-year follow-up of patients receiving imatinib for chronic myeloid leukemia. N Engl J Med. 2006;355(23):2408–17.

10. Hochhaus A, O'Brien SG, Guilhot F, et al.; IRIS Investigators. Six-year follow-up of patients receiving imatinib for the first-line treatment of chronic myeloid leukemia. Leukemia. 2009;23(6):1054–61.
11. Deininger M, O'Brien S, Guilhot F, et al. International randomized study of interferon and STI571 (IRIS) 8-year follow-up: sustained survival and low risk for progression in patients with newly diagnosed chronic myeloid leukemia in chronic phase treated with imatinib. [abstract]. Blood. 2009;114:22(abstr 126).
12. Roy L, Guilhot J, Krahnke T, et al. Survival advantage from imatinib compared with the combination interferon-alpha plus cytarabine in chronic-phase chronic myelogenous leukemia: historical comparison between two phase 3 trials. Blood. 2006;108(5):1478–84.
13. Kantarjian HM, Talpaz M, O'Brien S, et al. Survival benefit with imatinib mesylate versus interferon-alpha-based regimens in newly diagnosed chronic-phase chronic myelogenous leukemia. Blood. 2006;108(6):1835–40.
14. Kantarjian H, O'Brien S, Jabbour E, et al. Improved survival in chronic myeloid leukemia since the introduction of imatinib therapy: a single-institution historical experience. Blood. 2012;119(9):19811987.
15. Baccarani M, Saglio G, Goldman J, et al.; European LeukemiaNet. Evolving concepts in the management of chronic myeloid leukemia: recommendations from an expert panel on behalf of the European LeukemiaNet. Blood. 2006;108(6):1809–20.
16. Baccarani M, Cortes J, Pane F, et al.; European LeukemiaNet. Chronic myeloid leukemia: an update of concepts and management recommendations of European LeukemiaNet. J Clin Oncol. 2009;27(35):6041–51.
17. Baccarani M, Deininger MW, Rosti G, et al.; European LeukemiaNet recommendations for the management of chronic myeloid leukemia: 2013. Blood. 2013;122:872–84.
18. Silver RT, Woolf SH, Hehlmann R, et al. An evidence-based analysis of the effect of busulfan, hydroxyurea, interferon, and allogeneic bone marrow transplantation in treating the chronic phase of chronic myeloid leukemia: developed for the American Society of Hematology. Blood. 1999;94:1517–36.
19. Saglio G, Kim DW, Issaragrisil S, et al.; ENESTnd Investigators. Nilotinib versus imatinib for newly diagnosed chronic myeloid leukemia. N Engl J Med. 2010;362(24):2251–59.
20. Kantarjian HM, Hochhaus A, Saglio G, et al. Nilotinib versus imatinib for the treatment of patients with newly diagnosed chronic phase, Philadelphia chromosome-positive, chronic myeloid leukaemia: 24-month minimum follow-up of the phase 3 randomised ENESTnd trial. Lancet Oncol. 2011;12(9):841–51.
21. Larson RA, Hochhaus A, Hughes TP, et al. Nilotinib vs imatinib in patients with newly diagnosed Philadelphia chromosome-positive chronic myeloid leukemia in chronic phase: ENESTnd 3-year follow-up. Leukemia. 2012;26(10):2197–203.
22. Kantarjian H, Shah NP, Hochhaus A, et al. Dasatinib versus imatinib in newly diagnosed chronic-phase chronic myeloid leukemia. N Engl J Med. 2010;362(24):2260–70.
23. Kantarjian HM, Shah NP, Cortes JE, et al. Dasatinib or imatinib in newly diagnosed chronic-phase chronic myeloid leukemia: 2-year follow-up from a randomized phase 3 trial (DASISION). Blood. 2012;119(5):1123–9.
24. Vardiman JW, Pierre R, Thiele J. Chronic myelogenous leukaemia. In: Jaffe ES, Harris NL, Stein H, et al., editors. World Health Organization Classification of Tumours: Pathology and Genetics of Tumours of Hematopoietic and Lymphoid Tissues. Lyon: IARC Press; 2001. p. 920–6.
25. Sokal JE, Cox EB, Baccarani M, et al. Prognostic discrimination in "good-risk" chronic granulocytic leukemia. Blood. 1984;63:789–99.
26. Hasford J, Pfirrmann M, Hehlmann R, et al. A new prognostic score for survival of patients with chronic myeloid leukemia treated with interferon alfa. J Natl Cancer Inst. 1998;90:850–8.
27. Hasford J, Baccarani M, Hoffmann V, et al. Predicting complete cytogenetic response and subsequent progression-free survival in 2060 patients with CML on imatinib treatment: the EUTOS score. Blood. 2011;118(3):686–92.

28. Hughes TP, Kaeda J, Branford S, et al. Frequency of major molecular responses to imatinib or interferon alfa plus cytarabine in newly diagnosed chronic myeloid leukemia. N Engl J Med. 2003;349:1421–32.
29. Müller MC, Gattermann N, Lahaye T, et al. Dynamics of BCR-ABL mRNA expression in first-line therapy of chronic myelogenous leukemia patients with imatinib or interferon alpha/ara-C. Leukemia. 2003;17:2392–400.
30. Cortes J, Talpaz M, O'Brien S, et al. Molecular responses in patients with chronic myelogenous leukemia in chronic phase treated with imatinib mesylate. Clin Cancer Res. 2005;11:3425–32.
31. Branford S, Fletcher L, Cross NC, et al. Desirable performance characteristics for BCR-ABL measurement on an international reporting scale to allow consistent interpretation of individual patient response and comparison of response rates between clinical trials. Blood. 2008;112:3330–8.
32. Müller MC, Cross NC, Erben P, et al. Harmonization of molecular monitoring of CML therapy in Europe. Leukemia. 2009;23:1957–63.
33. Cross NC, White HE, Müller MC, Saglio G, Hochhaus A. Standardized definitions of molecular response in chronic myeloid leukemia. Leukemia. 2012;26:2172–5.
34. Baccarani M, Pane F, Saglio G, et al. Monitoring treatment of chronic myeloid leukemia. Haematologica. 2008;92:161–9.
35. Kantarjian H, Scheffer C, Jones D, et al. Monitoring the response and course of chronic myeloid leukemia in the modern era of BCR-ABL tyrosine kinase inhibitors: Practical advice on the use and interpretation of monitoring methods. Blood. 2008;111:1774–9.
36. Jabbour E, Cortes JE, Kantarjian HM. Molecular monitoring in chronic myeloid leukemia. Cancer. 2008;112:2112–8.
37. de Lavallade H, Apperley JF, Khorashad JS, et al. Imatinib for newly diagnosed patients with chronic myeloid leukemia: incidence of sustained responses in an intention-to-treat analysis. J Clin Oncol. 2008;26(20):3358–63.
38. Marin D, Milojkovic D, Olavarria E, et al. European LeukemiaNet criteria for failure or suboptimal response reliably identify patients with CML in early chronic phase treated with imatinib whose eventual outcome is poor. Blood. 2008;112(12):4437–44.
39. Cortes JE, Kantarjian HM, Goldberg SL, et al.; Rationale and Insight for Gleevec High-Dose Therapy (RIGHT) Trial Study Group. High-dose imatinib in newly diagnosed chronic-phase chronic myeloid leukemia: high rates of rapid cytogenetic and molecular responses. J Clin Oncol. 2009;27(28):4754–59.
40. Cervantes F, López-Garrido P, Montero MI, et al. Early intervention during imatinib therapy in patients with newly diagnosed chronic-phase chronic myeloid leukemia: a study of the Spanish PETHEMA group. Haematologica. 2010;95(8):1317–24.
41. Preudhomme C, Guilhot J, Nicolini FE. et al; SPIRIT Investigators, France Intergroupe des Leucémies Myéloïdes Chroniques (Fi-LMC). Imatinib plus peginterferon alfa-2a in chronic myeloid leukemia. N Engl J Med. 2010;363(26):2511–21.
42. Gugliotta G, Castagnetti F, Palandri F, et al.; Gruppo Italiano Malattie Ematologiche dell'Adulto CML Working Party. Frontline imatinib treatment of chronic myeloid leukemia: no impact of age on outcome, a survey by the GIMEMA CML Working Party. Blood. 2011;117(21):5591–99.
43. Faber E, Mužík J, Koza V, et al. Treatment of consecutive patients with chronic myeloid leukaemia in the cooperating centres from the Czech Republic and the whole of Slovakia after 2000—a report from the population-based CAMELIA Registry. Eur J Haematol. 2011;87(2):157–68.
44. Hehlmann R, Lauseker M, Jung-Munkwitz S, et al. Tolerability-adapted imatinib 800 mg/d versus 400 mg/d versus 400 mg/d plus interferon-α in newly diagnosed chronic myeloid leukemia. J Clin Oncol. 2011;29(12):1634–42.
45. Kim DW, Goh HG, Kim SH, Choi SY, Park SH, Jang EJ, Kim DW. Comprehensive therapeutic outcomes of frontline imatinib mesylate in newly diagnosed chronic phase chronic

myeloid leukemia patients in Korea: feasibility assessment of current ELN recommendation. Int J Hematol. 2012;96(1):47–57.
46. Shah NP, Nicoll JM, Nagar B, et al. Multiple BCR-ABL kinase domain mutations confer polyclonal resistance to the tyrosine kinase inhibitor imatinib (STI571) in chronic phase and blast crisis chronic myeloid leukemia. Cancer Cell. 2002;2:117–25.
47. Al-Ali HK, Heinrich MC, Lange T, et al. High incidence of BCR-ABL kinase domain mutations and absence of mutations of the PDGFR and KIT activation loops in CML patients with secondary resistance to imatinib. Hematol J. 2004;5:55–60.
48. Apperley JF. Part I: mechanisms of resistance to imatinib in chronic myeloid leukaemia. Lancet Oncol. 2007;8(11):1018–29.
49. Apperley JF. Part II: management of resistance to imatinib in chronic myeloid leukaemia. Lancet Oncol. 2007;8(12):1116–28.
50. Soverini S, Gnani A, Colarossi S, et al. Philadelphia-positive patients who already harbor imatinib-resistant Bcr-Abl kinase domain mutations have a higher likelihood of developing additional mutations associated with resistance to second- or third-line tyrosine kinase inhibitors. Blood. 2009;114(10):2168–71.
51. Soverini S, Hochhaus A, Nicolini FE, et al. BCR-ABL kinase domain mutation analysis in chronic myeloid leukemia patients treated with tyrosine kinase inhibitors: recommendations from an expert panel on behalf of European LeukemiaNet. Blood. 2011;118(5):1208–15.
52. Bixby D, Talpaz M. Seeking the causes and solutions to imatinib-resistance in chronic myeloid leukemia. Leukemia. 2011;25(1):7–22.
53. Gruber FX, Ernst T, Porkka K, et al. Dynamics of the emergence of dasatinib and nilotinib resistance in imatinib-resistant CML patients. Leukemia. 2012;26(1):172–7.
54. Hochhaus A, Saglio G, Larson RA, et al. Nilotinib is associated with a reduced incidence of BCR-ABL mutations vs imatinib in patients with newly diagnosed chronic myeloid leukemia in chronic phase. Blood. 2013;121(18):3703–8.
55. Parker WT, Ho M, Scott HS, Hughes TP, Branford S. Poor response to second-line kinase inhibitors in chronic myeloid leukemia patients with multiple low-level mutations, irrespective of their resistance profile. Blood. 2012;119(10):2234–8.
56. Cortes JE, Kim DW, Kantarjian HM, et al. Bosutinib versus imatinib in newly diagnosed chronic-phase chronic myeloid leukemia: results from the BELA trial. J Clin Oncol. 2012;30 (28):3486–92.
57. Jabbour E, Jones D, Kantarjian HM, et al. Long-term outcome of patients with chronic myeloid leukemia treated with second-generation tyrosine kinase inhibitors after imatinib failure is predicted by the in vitro sensitivity of BCR-ABL kinase domain mutations. Blood. 2009;114 (10):2037–43.
58. O'Hare T, Shakespeare WC, Zhu X, et al. AP24534, a pan-BCR-ABL inhibitor for chronic myeloid leukemia, potently inhibits the T315I mutant and overcomes mutation-based resistance. Cancer Cell. 2009;16(5):401–12.
59. Cortes JE, Kantarjian H, Shah NP, et al. Ponatinib in refractory Philadelphia chromosome-positive leukemias. N Engl J Med. 2012;367(22):2075–88.
60. Cortes J, Kim DW, Pinilla-Ibarz J, et al. A phase 2 trial of ponatinib in Philadelphia chromosome-positive leukemias. N Engl J Med. 2013;369(19):1783–96.
61. Pye SM, Cortes J, Ault P, et al. The effects of imatinib on pregnancy outcome. Blood. 2008;111:5505–8.
62. Cortes J, Kim DW, Raffoux E, et al. Efficacy and safety of dasatinib in imatinib-resistant or -intolerant patients with chronic myeloid leukemia in blast phase. Leukemia. 2008;22 (12):2176–83.
63. Apperley JF, Cortes JE, Kim DW, et al. Dasatinib in the treatment of chronic myeloid leukemia in accelerated phase after imatinib failure: the START a trial. J Clin Oncol. 2009;27(21):3472–9.

64. Kantarjian H, Cortes J, Kim DW, et al. Phase 3 study of dasatinib 140 mg once daily versus 70 mg twice daily in patients with chronic myeloid leukemia in accelerated phase resistant or intolerant to imatinib: 15-month median follow-up. Blood. 2009;113(25):6322–9.
65. Giles FJ, Abruzzese E, Rosti G, et al. Nilotinib is active in chronic and accelerated phase chronic myeloid leukemia following failure of imatinib and dasatinib therapy. Leukemia. 2010;24(7):1299–301.
66. Jabbour E, Cortes J, Santos FP, et al. Results of allogeneic hematopoietic stem cell transplantation for chronic myelogenous leukemia patients who failed tyrosine kinase inhibitors after developing BCR-ABL1 kinase domain mutations. Blood. 2011;117(13):3641–7.
67. Jiang Q, Xu LP, Liu DH, et al. Imatinib mesylate versus allogeneic hematopoietic stem cell transplantation for patients with chronic myelogenous leukemia in the accelerated phase. Blood. 2011;117(11):3032–40.
68. Nicolini FE, Basak GW, Soverini S, et al. Allogeneic stem cell transplantation for patients harboring T315I BCR-ABL mutated leukemias. Blood. 2011;118(20):5697–700.
69. Giles FJ, Kantarjian HM, le Coutre PD, et al. Nilotinib is effective in imatinib-resistant or -intolerant patients with chronic myeloid leukemia in blastic phase. Leukemia. 2012;26(5):959–62.
70. le Coutre PD, Giles FJ, Hochhaus A, et al. Nilotinib in patients with Ph+ chronic myeloid leukemia in accelerated phase following imatinib resistance or intolerance: 24-month follow-up results. Leukemia. 2012;26(6):1189–94.
71. Ohnishi K, Nakaseko C, Takeuchi J, et al. Long-term outcome following imatinib therapy for chronic myelogenous leukemia, with assessment of dosage and blood levels: the JALSG CML202 study. Cancer Sci. 2012;103(6):1071–8.
72. Japanese Society of Hematology. Chronic myelogenous leukemia/Myeloproliferative neoplasms. Guideline of management of hematologic malignancies-2013. Tokyo: Kanehara-shuppan; 2013. p. 71–104.

# Chapter 7
# Optimal Monitoring of CML Treatment: Molecular and Mutation Analysis

**David T. Yeung and Susan Branford**

**Abstract** With successful tyrosine kinase inhibitor treatment, the vast majority of chronic myeloid leukaemia patients diagnosed in chronic phase achieve long-term leukaemia-free survival as well as deep molecular responses. Accurate assessment of residual disease by RT-qPCR not only allows patients at risk of treatment failure to be segregated for treatment intensification but also identify patients with deep molecular responses for treatment cessation studies in the future. Specificity, sensitivity and accuracy of the RT-qPCR assay depend on optimised methodology and high-quality specimens with minimal RNA degradation. International standardisation projects allow for RT-qPCR results to be compared across laboratories and in clinical studies. For patients who fail to achieve a desired treatment outcome, mutational analysis allows for optimised selection of subsequent line therapies.

**Keywords** *BCR-ABL1* RT-qPCR • Molecular response • *BCR-ABL1* mutation analysis

---

D.T. Yeung
Centre for Cancer Biology and Department of Genetics and Molecular Pathology, SA Pathology, PO Box 14, Rundle Mall, Adelaide, SA 5000, Australia

Department of Haematology, SA Pathology, Adelaide, Australia

Discipline of Medicine, School of Medicine, University of Adelaide, Adelaide, Australia

S. Branford (✉)
Centre for Cancer Biology and Department of Genetics and Molecular Pathology, SA Pathology, PO Box 14, Rundle Mall, Adelaide, SA 5000, Australia

Discipline of Medicine, School of Medicine, University of Adelaide, Adelaide, Australia

School of Molecular and Biomedical Science, University of Adelaide, Adelaide, Australia

School of Pharmacy and Medical Science, University of South Adelaide, Adelaide, Australia
e-mail: susan.branford@health.sa.gov.au

 
M. Kizaki (ed.), *Molecular Pathogenesis and Treatment of Chronic Myelogenous Leukemia*, DOI 10.1007/978-4-431-55714-2_7

## 7.1 Introduction

With the introduction of imatinib and other tyrosine kinase inhibitors (TKIs) for the treatment of CML, most patients diagnosed in chronic phase disease now enjoy excellent leukaemia-free survival not achievable with previously available therapies such as hydroxyurea (hydroxycarbamide), busulfan and interferon. TKIs modify the underlying risk of disease progression by reducing overall tumour burden through their specific inhibitory activity against ABL1. Residual disease comprising of Philadelphia (Ph)-positive cells in a patient can be estimated by cytogenetics or molecular assays. As demonstrated in previous chapters, assessment of residual disease or demonstration of milestone responses by either methods is correlated with clinical outcome such as progression-free survival, event-free and failure-free survival [1–3].

Although the cytogenetic result is associated with important clinical prognostic information, this test is laborious, time consuming and entails significant discomfort for patients with serial examinations. Conventionally, 20–40 metaphases are examined per specimen, resulting in a test sensitivity of ~5 %. Fluorescent in situ hybridisation allows 200 metaphases to be screened by an experienced cytogeneticist, improving sensitivity to ~1 %. These tests are unable to reproducibly detect the presence of tumour if the number of residual Ph + cells falls below 1:100. With increasing numbers of patients achieving minimal residual disease levels below the limit of cytogenetic detection, molecular methods have become widely adopted as a more sensitive and convenient method of monitoring. With an optimised RT-qPCR method and a good-quality specimen, a limit of detection as low as 0.001 % has become the standard of care.

## 7.2 Sensitive and Specific RT-qPCR: Technical Aspects

The *BCR-ABL1* RT-qPCR (reverse transcription quantitative polymerase chain reaction) assay is based on the basic principal of the PCR, in which DNA templates are amplified exponentially by DNA polymerase in a reaction containing primers specific to the sequence of interest. In the quantitative PCR reaction (qPCR), a hydrolysis probe is annealed to each of the DNA templates present in the reaction, downstream of the primer. These probes are comprised of a reporter fluorophore in close proximity to a quencher dye, both situated on an oligonucleotide with complementary sequences to the DNA template. As the PCR reaction proceeds, the annealed primer is extended by the DNA polymerase, which also degrade the annealed probe into constituent nucleotides by its $5' > 3'$ exonuclease activity. The reporter fluorophore, thus liberated, can be detected. The relative fluorescence detected at the end of each cycle of PCR represents the number of DNA templates present in the reaction in that PCR cycle. In *BCR-ABL1* RT-qPCR, *BCR-ABL1* mRNA transcripts are first synthesised into complementary DNA (cDNA) in a stoichiometric, reverse transcription (RT) reaction. The cDNA is then used as template for the subsequent qPCR. Thus, the assay is commonly referred to as, RT-qPCR or RQ-PCR. The steps from reverse transcription to the qPCR may be performed in the same tube with no extra manual input in a "one-step" reaction with the necessary reagents and enzymes for both being added altogether at the beginning of the reaction. Alternatively, the RT and the qPCR reactions may be performed on separate protocols in separate tubes in a "two-step" reaction.

*BCR-ABL1* mRNA is a preferred starting material for a qPCR reaction even if it entails an extra RT step, as its sequence is well known and relatively uniform. Most CML patients acquire the *BCR-ABL1* fusion gene when either exon 13 or exon 14 of the *BCR* gene is juxtaposed to exon 2 of *ABL1*. The genomic DNA breakpoints are highly individualised and occur in large intronic regions [4] and spliced out in transcription. The resultant Ph + clone may produce either the e13a2 or e14a2 transcript depending on the breakpoint [5]. The two transcripts may coexist in the same patient through alternative splicing of the 75 bp *BCR* exon 14 [6]. An assay using mRNA as starting material can amplify the two most common transcripts using a single primer pair, greatly simplifying assay design and standardisation across laboratories. In contrast, an assay using DNA will require identification of the breakpoints for each individual patient before appropriate patient specific primers can be designed and inter-patient differences in PCR efficiencies adjusted.

Apart from the common e13a4 and e14a2 *BCR-ABL1* transcripts, others are also occasionally encountered. The most common of these atypical transcripts is e1a2, most commonly seen in Ph + acute lymphoblastic leukaemia but also in some CML cases. Other transcripts that may be encountered include e19a2 (common in the variant of CML associated with thrombocytosis), e6a2, e8a2, e13a3 and e14a2 amongst others (Fig. 7.1).

The general workflow starts with either anticoagulated blood or marrow from the patient. Both blood and bone marrow correlate equally well with the amount of residual leukaemic cells, and either tissue type is acceptable for longitudinal monitoring of treatment response. However, occasional patients have significantly discordant results between marrow and blood *BCR-ABL1* transcript numbers, and sequential analysis should rely on results from one tissue type. This is usually peripheral blood as it is more readily available [7]. Specimen quality is of paramount importance in maximising the sensitivity and minimising the variability of a *BCR-ABL1* RT-qPCR result. RNA is labile and subjected to degradation by enzymatic (endogenous RNAses) and nonenzymatic processes. After 72 h at room temperature, mRNA transcripts of interest such as *ABL1* may have fallen to 13 % of its original value [8]. Delays in specimen transport therefore lead to decreased test sensitivity and false-negative results. Specimens should therefore be transported to the laboratory as soon as practicable in a suitable anticoagulant such as EDTA. Carry over heparin may interfere with downstream enzymatic processes and this anticoagulant should be avoided [9]. Specimens should ideally be shipped with cool packs, but not frozen. Alternatively, the specimen may be collected into tubes containing an anticoagulant as well as additives that inhibit RNA degradation. These tubes are commercially available (e.g. PAXgene™) which

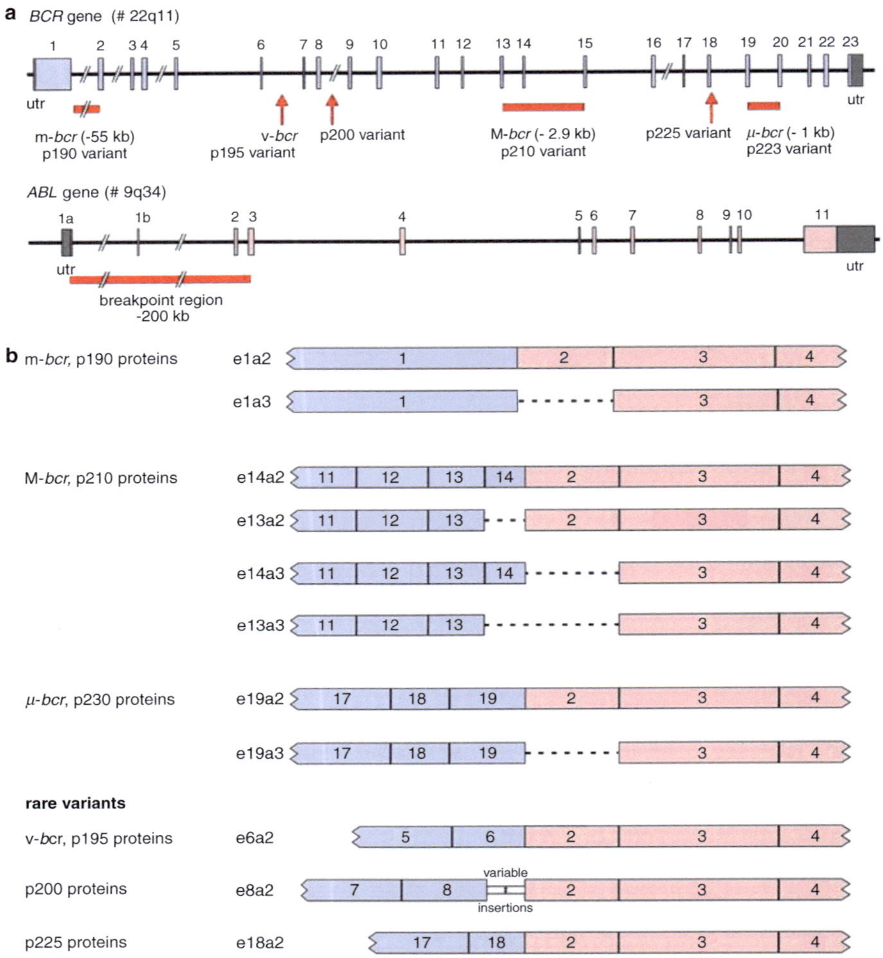


**Fig. 7.1** Structure of the *BCR-ABL1* fusion gene. Panel (**a**) illustrates the common breakpoints of the *BCR* and *ABL1* genes; panel (**b**) shows the common transcipt types. The most common *BCR-ABL1* transcripts encountered in CML are e13a2 and e14a2, leading to production of a 210 kDa BCR-ABL1 protein (p210). Occasionally, a patient may have both transcripts. Breakpoints are highly individualised and occur in the introns within the M-BCR region between exons 13 and 15 of the *BCR* gene and within a large 200 KB region before exon 2 of *ABL1*. Intronic breakpoints of the *BCR* gene between exons 1 and 2 and between exons 19 and 20 are called the m-BCR and μ-BCR regions, respectively, and give rise to the e1a2 transcript common in Ph + ALL and e19a2 transcript common in the thrombophilic variant of CML. Other breakpoints (v-*BCR*) are also occasionally encountered (figure originally published in Weerkamp et al. [54]. Reproduced with permission. © by the Nature Publishing Group)

may also provide proprietary RNA extraction methods [8, 10, 11] and are particularly attractive for centralised molecular monitoring (e.g. in a clinical trial setting). The PAXgene system is, however, more bulky (each PAXgene tube accommodates

2.5 mL of blood) and may be more expensive for routine use. RNA extraction from the PAXgene system is also inferior to the Trizol™ method (see below) for stabilisation and extraction of RNA in terms of assay sensitivity [12–14].

On sample receipt, erythrocytes are lysed (or removed by Ficoll centrifugation) and RNA is extracted from the resulting leucocytes pellet. This is frequently done using the guanidinium thiocyanate-phenol-chloroform method (with commercially available reagent such as TRIzol™ or Triagent™) [15]. Guanidinium thiocyanate and phenol inhibit protein activity; RNA in this solution is stable and can be stored for long periods without degradation, allowing for extraction to be batched. Using this method, DNA from the same samples may also be extracted with additional steps if desired. Both chloroform and phenol are toxic, however, and need specialised handling. RNA can also be extracted using column methods, a more convenient but expensive alternative.

Prior to qPCR, cDNA is first synthesised from RNA. The RT reaction is probably the greatest contributor to the variability of the RT-qPCR assay results, and optimisation of RT efficiency is a critical determinant of the overall sensitivity of the assay [7, 16]. A modified MMLV (Moloney Murine Leukaemia Virus) derived reverse transcriptase enzyme (such as Superscript™ from Invitrogen) is most commonly used, with the reaction primed with random hexamers. Studies have demonstrated that random pentadecamers may improve cDNA yield, though this is not commonly used [17, 18]. Gene-specific primers increase the specificity of the reaction and are favoured in one-step assays [19]. An RNAase inhibitor is commonly used to enhance reaction yield.

To maximise the specificity of the qPCR assay, probes and primers may be designed to bind across exon boundaries to avoid amplification of genomic DNA. Laboratories may optimise their individual primer and probe design or alternatively adopt primers and probe sequences as published by the Europe Against Cancer (EAC) standardisation and quality control project (Fig. 7.2). These primers are designed to quantify both e13a2 and e14a2 in the same reaction with a forward primer situated in *BCR* exon 13. In some laboratories (such as ours), the e13a2 and e14a2 transcripts are quantified in separate reactions (and added arithmetically in patients known who express both transcripts to derive the total *BCR-ABL1*). A set of standards with known concentrations of the target and control genes are run alongside patient samples. These may be RNA templates, though DNA plasmids are more commonly used as it has greater stability, and may include sequences of both target and the control gene within the same plasmid [20]. Many laboratories use standards derived from custom produced plasmid mixtures in serial dilutions, though standards calibrated to WHO reference materials are increasingly available through manufacturers of RT-qPCR kits (see below). The standard curve should be constructed from data points spanning the entire reported range of the assay using tenfold dilutions and should not be extrapolated to interpret assay results falling outside of either extremes. Linearity of each standard curve should be verified with correlation coefficients of >0.98 [7]. The coefficient of variation (CV) of results for standards with the lower copy numbers may be quite high, and it is our practice to include some dilutions of the standard as replicates in each assay to avoid ill-fitting

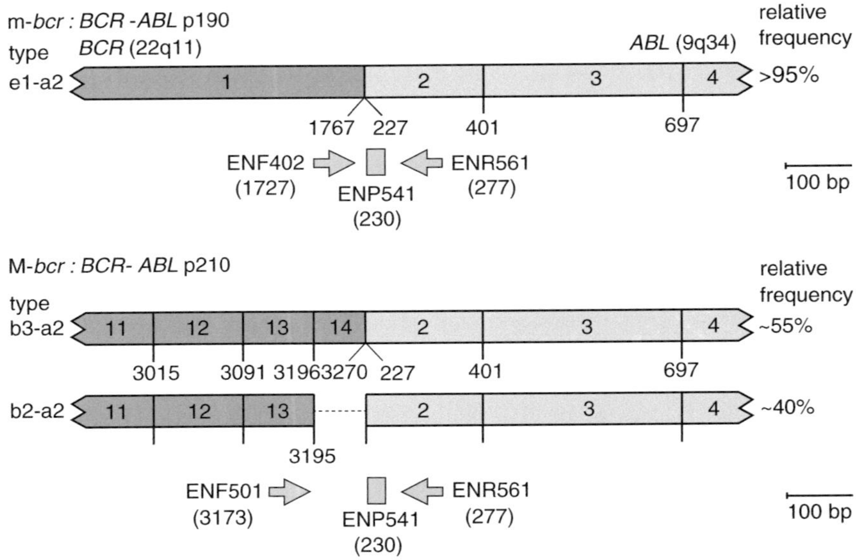


**Fig. 7.2** Standardised primers and hydrolysis probes for *BCR-ABL1* RT-qPCR used in the Europe Against Cancer project (Figure originally published in Gabert et al. [30]. Reproduced with permission. © by the Nature Publishing Group)

curves. The transcript numbers of unknown samples are then calculated from their Ct values via the standard curve.

Known negative and positive controls are included as quality control with each batch of samples processed, including all the steps from RNA extraction right through to calculation of the *BCR-ABL1* ratio. For instance, in our laboratory, a high control and a low control are included with each batch, being mixtures of *BCR-ABL1* positive cell lines Molm-1, K562 and SUP-B15 diluted in HeLa to give ratios of about 10 and 0.1 %. HeLa is used as a negative control. When these results are tracked longitudinally, characteristics of the assay, such as accuracy, precision, linearity, sensitivity, specificity and reportable range, may then be determined for the specific laboratory. Assay results from these controls also determine if results from a batch should be accepted when measured against predetermined assay tolerances (such as those suggested by Westgard) [21].

It is important to recognise that even with an optimised method and best quality assurance practices, there is an underlying variability inherent to RT-qPCR assays due both to technical factors and biological factors. Performing duplicate analyses is one way to minimise the effect of errors and variability due to technical factors. A study was undertaken in our laboratory where a sample was analysed repeatedly on 198 occasions, from the RT step through qPCR to result reporting. The mean of the results was 0.08 % (0.1 % IS). The two standard deviation range of results was 0.02–0.14 %, implying a CV of 35.1 %. However, when results were calculated as the mean of duplicate analyses, the CV fell to 25.6 % [7].

Detection of very low copy numbers using qPCR is challenging and the probability of obtaining an assay result that accurately reflects the true number of starting templates follows a Poisson distribution. For instance, using this distribution, one can predict that repeated testing performed on a sample with one known copy of *BCR-ABL1* will not only return a result of one copy, but some assays will also return a result of either 0 or 2 by chance. The lower limit of detection and the lower limit of quantification should be set for each laboratory individually based on local experience of reproducibility, though in general we would not regard copy numbers $<3$ as being reproducible and would calculate test sensitivity based on a minimum detectable *BCR-ABL1* of $\geq 3$ [22].

A significant problem for qPCR assays is the potential for contamination leading to false positives, and it is important to minimise this risk through good laboratory practice. This include the spatial separation of working areas where specimen preparation, RNA preparation and qPCR are performed and dedicated areas where reagents are kept and assays are set up. Use of disposable gloves and filtered pipette tips are recommended, and workers should change gloves and gowns when transiting between different areas. Laboratory surfaces should be regularly cleansed with appropriate chemical agents and critical areas should be exposed to UV radiation to breakdown contaminating nucleic acids. The replacement of thymidine with uracil and the use of uracil-N-glycosylase may prevent contamination from carry-over of previous amplicons [23].

### 7.2.1 Control Gene Measurement

Aside from the accurate measurement of *BCR-ABL1* transcript numbers within each sample, a control gene is also quantified routinely. The term housekeeping gene is not preferred. Control gene measurement is crucial in demonstrating RNA quantity and quality and ensuring specimen acceptability by highlighting any potential RNA degradation. It allows for the *BCR-ABL1* transcript numbers to be reported as a ratio and also helps to establish the sensitivity of each assay. All things being equal, the sensitivity of an assay increases with the number of measurable control gene transcripts [24] (Fig. 7.3 and Table 7.1).

Consensus recommendations have been published with regard to the essential characteristics of good candidates of a control gene [7, 16, 23, 25–27]. These include (i) similar level of expression between different individuals and between different cell types, including tumour versus non-tumour cells; (ii) expression levels at similar levels to the target gene (in this case, *BCR-ABL1* at diagnosis); (iii) similar rate of stability and degradation as the target gene (i.e. constancy of the ratio of target to control); and (iv) lack of similar sequences (such as pseudo-genes in genomic DNA) that may be amplified with primers used in the proposed assay.

In the context of *BCR-ABL1* measurement, *BCR*, *ABL1* and *GUSB* (β-glucuronidase) are the most commonly used control genes. *BCR* has similar expression levels and stability to *BCR-ABL1* [28] and was the control gene used in

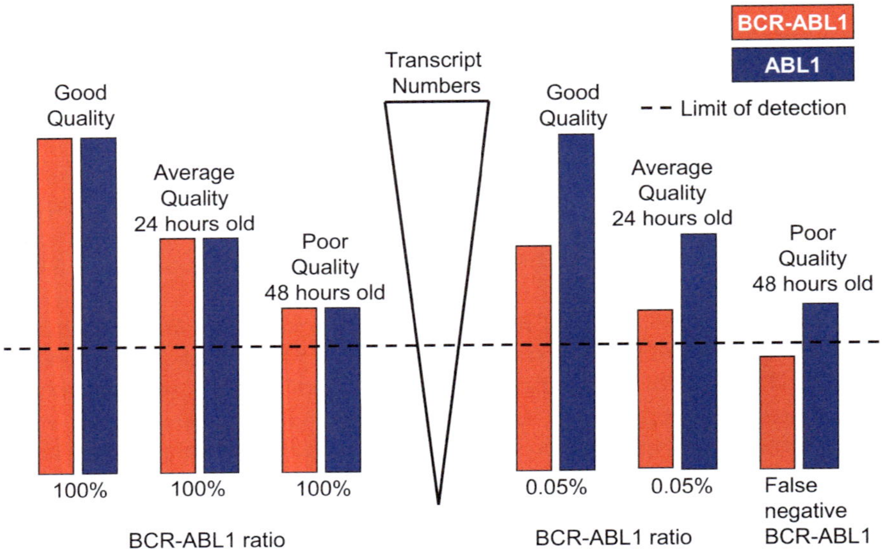


**Fig. 7.3** The effect of specimen quality on measured transcript numbers and *BCR-ABL1* result subsequently reported can be judged from the control gene transcript numbers. (Height of the bars approximates a logarithmic scale.) A specimen from a patient with newly diagnosed CML is simulated on the left. Measurement of the specimen soon after collection showed *BCR-ABL1*: *ABL1* ratio to be 100 %, with adequate copies of both target and control gene transcripts. With specimen degradation over time, both *BCR-ABL1* and *ABL1* transcripts degrade at the same rate, and the ratio remains the same. A specimen with a *BCR-ABL1* ratio of 0.05 % is simulated on the right. Specimen quality is adequate for *BCR-ABL1* quantification at the time of collection. After 24 h, the *BCR-ABL1* transcripts are barely detectable, though the ratio of *BCR-ABL1*:*ABL1* remains the same. After 48 h, the *BCR-ABL1* transcripts had fallen to an undetectable level leading to a false-negative result

the molecular assays that accompanied the IRIS study – the first phase III study using imatinib in CML treatment [29]. *ABL1* is the recommended control gene of the EAC and is the most commonly used of the three [30]. Laboratories may use primers that amplify exons 2 and 3 of *ABL1* in qPCR reactions, which may lead to a loss of linearity at high levels of *BCR-ABL1* (Fig. 7.4). This issue becomes important when one wishes to calculate the velocity of *BCR-ABL1* reduction in the initial months following commencement of TKI treatment [31]. However, for most specimens, the underestimation of *BCR-ABL1*/*ABL1* at the high end of the scale is of no clinical consequence. *BCR-ABL1* transcript numbers are usually significantly lower than *ABL1*, especially for the important cut-off of MMR at 0.1 % IS. Similarly, *GUSB* transcripts have been demonstrated to have similar stability to *BCR-ABL1*, and it has the advantage of not being involved in the formation of the *BCR-ABL1* rearrangement, and some authors would favour using this as their control gene [23].

**Table 7.1** Correlation between control gene copy numbers and test sensitivity and subsequent categorisation of molecular response for samples with low copy numbers

| | BCR-ABL1 copies (a) | ABL1 copies (b) | RT-qPCR result (c) (%) | Response | Minimum detectable BCR-ABL1 (d) (%) | Sensitivity (e) |
|---|---|---|---|---|---|---|
| A | 3 | 300,000 | 0.001 | MR5 | 0.001 | 5.0 |
| B | 4 | 160,000 | 0.002 | MR4.5 | 0.002 | 4.7 |
| C | 3 | 30,000 | 0.01 | MR4 | 0.01 | 4.0 |
| D | 30 | 300,000 | 0.01 | MR4 | 0.001 | 5.0 |
| E | 0 | 5000 | 0.0 | MR3 | 0.06 | 3.2 |
| F | 30 | 30,000 | 0.1 | MR3 | 0.01 | 4.0 |
| G | 3 | 3000 | 0.1 | Inadequate | 0.1 | 3.0 |

*BCR-ABL1* ratios are reported in two significant figures and down to four decimal places. All calculations are done assuming an International Scale conversion factor of 1.0. As discussed in the text, most laboratories would regard ≥3 copies as being the lower limit of detection, based on the Poisson statistics. Sample A meets the criteria for an achievement of $MR^5$, with a *BCR-ABL1*:*ABL1* ratio of 0.001 % and a test sensitivity of 5.0 logs below the standardised baseline. Sample C has the same number of *BCR-ABL1* transcripts as sample A, but the control gene number is 10-fold lower. The ratio is 10-fold higher, corresponding to a molecular response of $MR^4$. Even though the reported ratio is the same in samples C and D, both 0.01 %, the difference in test sensitivity is directly correlated to the number of control gene transcripts in these samples. In sample E, *BCR-ABL1* is undetectable and reported as 0.0 %. However, the minimum detectable *BCR-ABL1* ratio is 3/5000, not 0/5000, based on the Poisson statistics, equivalent to 0.06 %, and one cannot confidently exclude residual disease below this level based on this sample. Sensitivity of the test is $\log_{10}(0.0006)$, or 3.2 log below baseline. So even though sample E is reported as 0.0 % and sample A is reported as 0.001 %, the latter is a technically preferable result. The low number of control gene transcripts detectable in sample G indicates RNA degradation and unsuitable for assessment of deep molecular responses. Calculations (i) RT-qPCR result: $c\% = a/b*100$; (ii) minimum detectable *BCR-ABL1*: $d\% = m/b*100$, where m is the minimum reproducible copy number, in this case, 3; (iii) sensitivity: $e = [\log_{10}(d/100)]*-1$.

### 7.2.2 Standardisation Material

One important analytical variable affecting the measured transcript numbers is the determination of the standard curve, as generated for each RT-qPCR assay through accurately quantified calibration standards. The limited availability of stable biological material able to act as a reference standard to calibrate local assays has hampered both the development of international external quality assurance programmes and further enhancements of assay comparability. An ideal reference material should be available in adequate quantities to allow easy access, be stable in transport and storage, homogenous across batches, and yet replicate the characteristics of the primary test material as closely as possible under assay conditions. No material currently meet all these criteria as far as *BCR-ABL1* testing is concerned. In the absence of an internationally recognised calibration standard, laboratories produce standards individually or in collaboration with others, using serially diluted plasmid mixtures of known quantity.

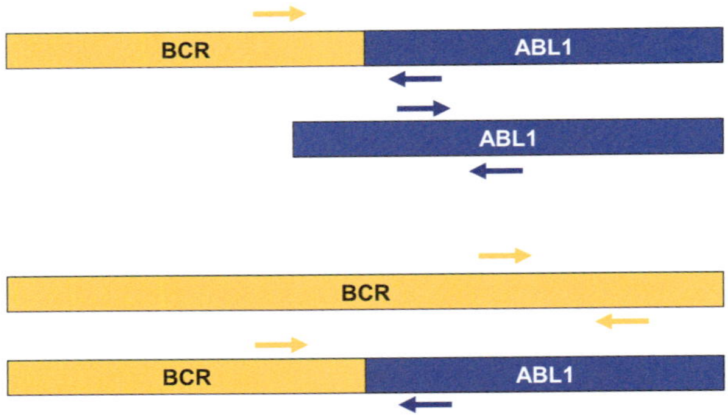


**Fig. 7.4** Schematic drawing showing the location of primers for amplification of *BCR-ABL1* and control genes commonly in use. The primer set used in the Europe Against Cancer project consist of a forward primer for *BCR-ABL1* in exon 13 (common to both e13a2 and a14a2 transcripts) and a reverse primer in *ABL1* exon 2. For the *ABL1* control gene, the forward primer is situated in exon 2 and reverse primer in exon 3. (Placing the forward primer in *ABL1* exon 1 is a problem, as exon 1a and exon 1b are alternately expressed.) Placing primers in this configuration, the *ABL1* qPCR will prime off templates from genetic sequences of both *ABL1* and *BCR-ABL1*, such that the target/control gene ratio is not *BCR-ABL1*:*ABL1* but actually *BCR-ABL1*: (*BCR-ABL1* + *ABL1*) leading to an underestimation when *BCR-ABL1* transcript numbers are high. However, this is of no clinical significance. In contrast, primers for *BCR* may be placed distal to the breakpoint and in this configuration only amplify native *BCR* and not the *BCR* sequence in *BCR-ABL1*. Using this control gene, linearity has recently been demonstrated to be preserved over the dynamic range of the assay [43]. Drawing is not to scale

The WHO International Genetic Reference Panel first released a reference material in 2009, consisting of freeze-dried K562 cells positive for the e14a2 transcript diluted in *BCR-ABL1* negative HL-60 cells in four different dilutions. Each is assigned a reference *BCR-ABL1* IS value after repeated testing [32]. However, the small quantity of the material available is released mainly to the manufacturers of secondary reference materials. Although plasmids cannot simulate the relevant biological test material at the RT stage, it is relatively easy to produce in larger quantities, and recent interest has increased in using this in substitution for cells. The performance characteristics of a certified plasmid reference material had recently been described [20]. This plasmid, pIRMM0099, contains sequences of *BCR-ABL1* e14a2, *BCR*, *ABL1* and *GUSB*. Six tenfold serial dilutions on a panel called ERM-AD623a-f had been independently quantified and assigned values by digital PCR before being tested in 63 laboratories and are currently distributed by the Institute for Reference Materials and Measurements in Belgium. An alternative to plasmids involves the use of *BCR-ABL1* RNA. One proprietary product developed by Asuragen is called Armored RNA Quant or ARQ. RNA is usually labile and subjected to degradation from ubiquitous RNAses present in the environment and biological materials. This may be minimised by packaging RNA molecules inside protective protein envelops. The use of stabilised RNA as a reference material allows the efficiency of the RT step to be included in the overall quality assessment. Preliminary results of a validation project have been recently published [33].

### 7.2.3 Results Standardisation: Reporting on the International Scale

The lack of internationally recognised suitable standard materials not only leads to difficulties for laboratories to assign values to their standards, but has also hampered direct comparability of results between different laboratories. Variations in reagents, machine platforms, control genes, primer/probe sequences and calibration standards lead to different values being reported by different laboratories for the same specimen [34]. One study demonstrated that, even when common primer/probe sets and plasmid standards were used with optimised methods, significant variation in reported *BCR-ABL1* values still occurred when testing the same sample amongst 37 European laboratories [35]. Thus, longitudinal comparisons of treatment response within the same individual were not possible when results came from different laboratories. Furthermore, correlation of survival outcomes with achievement of particular molecular treatment milestones would not be possible without inter-laboratory and inter-patient comparability.

A number of efforts have been made to standardise pre-analytical and analytical variables in order to minimise assay variability. These include the use of published consensus primer and probes sets from the EAC for targets and control genes [16, 30], as well as a set of consensus recommendations intended to harmonise other aspects of *BCR-ABL1* RT-qPCR methodology [23] (Fig. 7.2). One key proposal involved the development of laboratory specific conversion factors that allowed results to be adjusted and reported on a common International Scale (IS), enabling valid comparisons across individuals and laboratories [36, 37].

The initial steps of standardised RT-qPCR reporting first began with the IRIS study, the first to report molecular results following treatment with a TKI. Baseline samples from the same 30 patients were measured independently by three laboratories in London, Seattle and Adelaide, and the median value was taken to be the standardised diagnostic baseline and given a value of 100 %. Reduction in *BCR-ABL1* values for subsequent results from all IRIS patients was measured as $\log_{10}$ reductions from this value and expressed as a ratio of *BCR-ABL1*: *BCR* [29]. Achievement of major molecular response (MMR) was designated for patients who achieved a 3-log reduction in transcript numbers from this standardised baseline and is equivalent to a *BCR-ABL1* value of 0.1 %. Subsequent major international standardisation efforts involved sample exchanges between a number of central laboratories and peripheral laboratories who performed assays in parallel. Peripheral laboratories were expected to have optimised their methods and minimised assay variations prior to participation in the project, which led to the determination of a conversion factor, permitting participating laboratories to report results on the International Scale [36, 37]. Through this process, concordance between the central laboratory and a participating laboratory on whether a sample has *BCR-ABL1* $\leq 0.1$ % (MMR) reached 91 % at best, although only about half of the participating laboratories were deemed to meet the desirable performance characteristics [36]. Inherent variability of the assay or suboptimal method development was responsible for discordance in the remaining laboratories.

Currently, conversion factors only enable e13a2 and e14a2 results to be adjusted for reporting on the IS, and a mechanism to report atypical transcripts such as e1a2 and e19a2 using a similar scale does not yet exist.

### 7.2.4 Clinical Aspects: Indications and Interpretation of Results

RT-qPCR testing is currently recommended for all patients at diagnosis. The type of transcript expressed should be documented at diagnosis using an assay that can identify atypical transcripts in cases that do not express the more common e13a2 and e14a2. Thereafter, RT-qPCR should be performed every 3 months until MMR is achieved. Loss of MMR or CCyR is rare for patients with *BCR-ABL1* $\leq 0.1$ % [2], and RT-qPCR monitoring every 3–6 months for these patients is adequate [3]. Management decisions based on molecular monitoring should be made only when the inherent variability of an optimised RT-qPCR assay had been considered. The technical variability is potentially equivalent to a 2-fold variation of the reported result for a sample with 0.1 % *BCR-ABL1*. At the higher level of 10 % *BCR-ABL1*, the CV is slightly lower (~18 %), and at 0.0032 % the variation approaches ~5-fold (both unpublished observations within our laboratory). Although these CVs may be wide when compared to more commonly used diagnostic assays such as haemoglobin or serum sodium, this degree of variability is expected given the dynamic range of the assay and the clinical context (i.e. a very small change in the expression of *BCR-ABL1* does not have the same physiological significance as an out of range serum sodium). Changes in a patient's *BCR-ABL1* value should be interpreted within this context to determine whether a change is within the measurement reliability of the assay or a true biological change [7]. A repeat assay should be performed when the significance of a *BCR-ABL1* increase is unclear.

Several groups have explored the optimal cut-off in the *BCR-ABL1* increase most likely to predict for an adverse outcome, though a consensus value had not been reached. The different conclusions are related to differences in the performance characteristics of individual laboratory molecular assays, and although a common value cannot be agreed upon, clinically relevant rises in *BCR-ABL1* in many instances have been demonstrated to approximate the precision limit of the assay in the investigating laboratory. Furthermore, loss of MMR in the context of a rising *BCR-ABL1* level increases the clinical significance of the rise [38]. For instance, Press et al. demonstrated that in their cohort of 90 patients, a rise in the

*BCR-ABL1/G6PDH* ratio of >0.5 $\log_{10}$(~3.2-fold) was associated with a loss of CCyR. Using a lower cut-off in the *BCR-ABL1* rise led to a higher false-positive rate, as the contemporaneous variability in RT-qPCR in their laboratory due to technical variations was 0.46 log [39]. The same group subsequently concluded that a 2.6-fold increase in *BCR-ABL1* was the optimal cut-off for predicting the development of a concomitant kinase domain mutation and reported that a 2.6-fold change was the analytical precision limit for that particular analysis. In contrast, the Hammersmith group found that a rise of *BCR-ABL1/ABL1* was predictive of loss of CCyR and progression to advanced phase, providing that the resultant *BCR-ABL1* was >0.05 % [40]. We would regard a rise in the *BCR-ABL1* of >2-fold in our laboratory as significant and in line with current recommendations would proceed to mutation analysis if this results in a loss of MMR [38]. Other aspects that can lead to therapeutic failure should also be addressed, such as compliance or concomitant drug interactions (see mutation analysis below). Patients with a >2-fold rise, but not associated with loss of MMR, should be monitored more closely.

Patients who fail to achieve time-dependent molecular targets are at higher risk of disease transformation and death. According to the current recommendations of two most widely used CML treatment guidelines, both the ELN and the NCCN would regard the failure to achieve *BCR-ABL1* ≤ 10 %, ≤1 % and ≤0.1 % at 3, 6 and 12 months, respectively, after a CML-CP patient commences treatment with a TKI to be associated with inferior outcomes [3, 41] (Fig. 7.5). The evidence with regard to the 3-month time point is particularly strong, and patients with *BCR-ABL1* > 10 % at this time point have inferior overall and progression-free survival as well as inferior achievement of molecular responses, regardless of the TKI chosen for treatment [42]. The level of uncertainty with regards to *BCR-ABL1* measurement is of particular importance when an individual patient's molecular result is measured against recommended milestone responses. In particular, even though the guidelines are specific as to the cut-offs that segregate high-risk patients from good-risk patients, in reality the association between the *BCR-ABL1* ratio and the degree of risk exists as a continuum. For instance, a patient with *BCR-ABL1* of 1 % 3 months after starting TKI therapy clearly has a lower risk of disease progression compared to a patient with a result of 10.5 % at 3 months. However, it is unclear if a patient with 9.5 % has a clearly different level of risk to a patient with 10.5 %, yet the response level and risk are assessed as different using an absolute cut-off. Taking into account the underlying inherent assay variability, a reported *BCR-ABL1* of 9.5 % may actually reflect a true value that ranges between 6 and 12 % (given a CV of 18 %). Consequently, many would urge caution when making clinical decisions based on one single *BCR-ABL1* result, and a patient's history should be considered when management decisions are made. Furthermore, the ELN cautioned that a single measurement at 3 months is insufficient for decisions regarding a change of treatment. The ELN recommends repeat testing at up to monthly for patients with *BCR-ABL1* > 10 % at 3 months and changing treatment for patients who are still >10 % at 6 months [3].

The speed at which a patient achieves milestone responses had been demonstrated to add valuable prognostic information. This is encapsulated in the concept

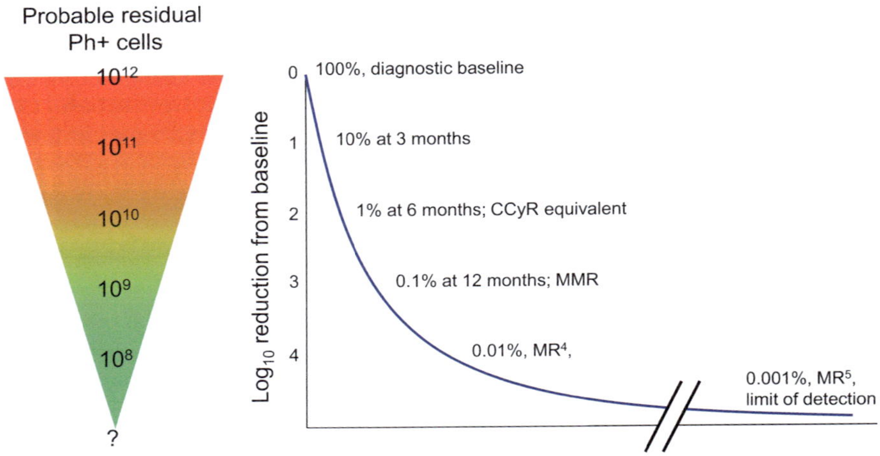


**Fig. 7.5** Idealised trajectory of time-dependent molecular responses and corresponding residual leukaemic burden. At diagnosis, a patient may harbour as many as $10^{12}$ leukaemic cells. The median RT-qPCR value of *BCR-ABL1* at diagnosis is set at 100 % using 30 patients who participated in the IRIS study. After 3 months of treatment, the RT-qPCR should have fallen by 10-fold (1-log reduction from the standardised baseline) to 10 % on the International Scale (IS). At 6 months, most patients achieve a *BCR-ABL1* $\leq 1$ % IS, a convenient surrogate marker for complete cytogenetic response (CCyR). CCyR is associated with long-term progression-free survival. By 12 months, the majority of patients achieve a 3-log reduction in *BCR-ABL1*, equivalent to 0.1 % IS, also called major molecular response (MMR) or MR$^3$. Patients who achieve MMR are unlikely to lose this response, provided that they are compliant with therapy. Deeper molecular responses are termed MR$^4$, MR$^{4.5}$ and MR$^5$, equivalent to 0.01 %, 0.0032 % and 0.001 % IS, respectively. A 5-log reduction is the limit of detection for most *BCR-ABL1* RT-qPCR assays. Patients with disease at this level may still harbour up to $10^7$ Ph + cells

of the "*BCR-ABL1* halving time" which the Adelaide group has used to further refine prognosis in patients with *BCR-ABL1* > 10 % at 3 months. This takes into account both the magnitude of the fall in *BCR-ABL1* transcript numbers and duration over which this occurred. The initial fall in *BCR-ABL1* transcripts after TKI commencement is linear when *BCR* is used as the control gene, and a slope can be calculated using these two parameters. From their cohort of 500+ imatinib-treated patients, the number of days necessary for the *BCR-ABL1* to reduce by 50 % can be calculated providing both results at baseline and 3 months are available. Patients with *BCR-ABL1* > 10 % at 3 months and a halving time of >76 days are at particularly high risk of treatment failure [43]. The German CML study group arrived at the same conclusion that the velocity of *BCR-ABL1* transcript elimination in the early months of treatment is correlated with treatment outcomes and concluded that failure to achieve a half-log decrease in transcript numbers is associated with inferior progression-free and overall survival [31].

The ELN and NCCN guidelines also set down time-dependent cytogenetic responses which correlate with clinical outcomes. If cytogenetic results are unavailable (either for technical or clinical reasons), molecular responses can be used as a surrogate. A *BCR-ABL1* ratio of <10 % is generally considered to be equivalent to major cytogenetic response (Ph + metaphases 1–35 %; MCyR), whereas patients with *BCR-ABL1* < 1 % have almost certainly achieved complete cytogenetic response (0 % Ph + metaphases; CCyR) [7, 44–46].

Given the stated CVs and measurement uncertainty with molecular assays, some have argued that cytogenetics should be the preferred method for monitoring treatment response in CML, especially because of the perceived greater certainty of cytogenetic responses. This is an erroneous assumption, however, as cytogenetics has actually been demonstrated to be associated with an even greater level of measurement uncertainty, especially with regard to cut-offs important for clinical decision making [47]. Given this context, molecular and cytogenetic data should be used in combination, especially when the limited dynamic range of cytogenetic analysis is considered.

## 7.3 Emergent Methods of Molecular Monitoring

### *7.3.1 Digital PCR*

Conventional qPCR techniques allow for robust, sensitive and specific quantification of *BCR-ABL1* RNA transcripts in a diagnostic setting. Further refinements, made possible with improvements in biomaterial engineering and microfluidics, have led to the development of digital quantitative PCR (dqPCR) techniques. In conventional qPCR, amplicons of interest increase exponentially with each cycle of PCR. Each of the amplicons in a reaction contributes to a unit of fluorescence from a corresponding hydrolysed probe. The fluorescence detected is a combined output from the entire reaction and increases exponentially with each PCR cycle until it reaches a plateau. The resultant signal output is analogue in nature.

With dqPCR, the sample and the reagents usually used in a conventional qPCR reaction are partitioned into much smaller reaction chambers by microfluidics, such that on average some wells will only have one starting template whilst others will have none. These reactions occur either in wells etched onto the surface of a chip (e.g. Fluidigm™) [48, 49] or alternatively occur into droplets formed by emulsion [50]. The resultant signal is "digital" in nature – a well can either be positive (contain one starting template) or negative. The number of starting templates within the sample is equivalent to the number of positive reactions, on a background of negative reactions. The level of uncertainty can again be estimated using the Poisson distribution.

Several groups have demonstrated a good correlation between conventional qPCR and dqPCR for measurement of *BCR-ABL1* transcripts [48–50]. Whilst these results are promising, increases in assay sensitivity with dqPCR have only been demonstrated with the inclusion of a pre-amplification step. Further sensitivity improvements may be possible with enhanced assay design and the full potential of this platform is yet to be explored.

### 7.3.2 GeneXpert

Although RT-qPCR is the standard of care for molecular monitoring in CML, it is difficult to perform this test and assure quality in smaller centres with low test volumes. In laboratories that lack specialised expertise or equipment, *BCR-ABL1* RT-qPCR may be routinely referred to larger laboratories (when transportation of specimen with minimal RNA degradation may be a problem). Alternatively, *BCR-ABL1* RT-qPCR may be performed using a benchtop machine called the GeneXpert manufactured by the Cepheid Corporation. Cepheid also offer other PCR assays (e.g. for the detection of antibiotic resistant microorganisms) using different single-use cartridges on the same platform, increasing its versatility and attractiveness to small laboratories. Minimum sample preparation is required before being added to a single-use cartridge which contains all necessary reagents for the assay [51]. Analysis is automated with a turnaround time of approximately 2 h, using internally developed standards calibrated against currently available WHO reference material.

The Xpert BCR-ABL Monitor™ system had been compared alongside RT-qPCR in a prospective study of newly diagnosed CML patients treated with nilotinib. Apart from a slight negative bias, there was a good concordance between the two methods at all levels above 0.01 % ($MR^4$) [52]. The cartridges gave less accurate results in samples with low number of *BCR-ABL1* transcripts, however. Based on current operating characteristics, the Xpert BCR-ABL Monitor™ is appropriate for most medium- to small-sized laboratories for rapid diagnosis of e13a2/e14a2 CML and for disease monitoring down to $MR^4$. Applicability and appeal will increase in the future assuming that any bias in GeneXpert results will be amenable to correction with a conversion factor to IS and that sensitivity for samples can be improved for samples below $MR^4$. However, this system currently cannot detect atypical transcripts, and a negative result does not rule out the diagnosis of Ph+ leukaemia. Furthermore, a separate RT-PCR is still required for patients needing mutational analysis. In addition, the extra cost of single-use cartridges may make this system uneconomical for the larger laboratories.

### 7.3.3 DNA PCR

As detailed previously, the majority of CML cases are a result of the e13a2 and e14a2 *BCR-ABL1* transcripts, a consequence of a rearrangement between chromosomes 9 and 22 fusing the gene *BCR* to *ABL1*. The breakpoints of this rearrangement occur in large intronic regions within each gene and are individualised to each patient [4]. Consequently, any attempts to use genomic DNA of the *BCR-ABL1* fusion oncogene as template for a molecular assay would first necessitate sequencing for the location of this breakpoint and making individual primer and probe sets suitable for the qPCR assay. Furthermore, it would be near impossible to ensure that all primer and probe sets perform with adequate efficiency to allow for standardised result reporting. However, DNA PCR does have advantages. Cross contamination and carry-over are much less significant problems for DNA PCR. Additionally, DNA is a much more stable biological material, less subjected to degradation during transport and storage, and directly correlate with the number of residual leukaemic cells. However, due to aforementioned technical challenges and the lack of correlated clinical significance, DNA qPCR for *BCR-ABL1* currently remains a research tool. So far, available results in small series suggest a lack of correlation between PCR results using RNA vs DNA as starting material for patients with minimal residual disease [53].

### *7.3.4 Flow Cytometry*

Apart from the use of PCR-based techniques, an in-principle demonstration of a flow-cytometry-based BCR-ABL1 assay had been described [54]. Anti-BCR antibodies bound to beads are added to a sample together with anti-ABL1 antibodies bound to a phycoerythrin (PE) fluorochrome. The presence of BCR-ABL1 fusion protein will bring the PE fluorochrome within close proximity to the beads. A flow cytometer is then used to enumerate the beads and detect the juxtaposed PE signal. If only normal BCR and ABL1 proteins are present, no PE fluorescence signal will be detected on the beads. Whilst this is an innovative method to detect BCR-ABL1, the results of these initial assays remain to be validated in larger cohorts, and the clinical correlation of these results remains to be determined. Furthermore, there seems to be little correlation between *BCR-ABL1* transcripts and BCR-ABL1 protein levels.

## 7.4 Mutation Analysis

### *7.4.1 Indications and Clinical Significance of Kinase Domain Mutations*

Although the majority of CML patients achieve excellent outcomes, a substantial number still experience treatment failure. For instance, of the patients that commenced frontline treatment with imatinib in the IRIS study, 40 % discontinued imatinib at 8 years, half having done so for disease resistance [55]. The most commonly identified cause of treatment resistance or loss of a previously achieved milestone response is *BCR-ABL1* kinase domain (KD) mutations, which may be detected in 30–40 % of CML-CP cases of treatment failure in some series by direct sequencing [56, 57]. The incidence of mutations is much higher for patients with treatment resistance in accelerated or blastic phase disease as well as relapsed Philadelphia-positive ALL [58, 59].

Over 100 different KD point mutations have now been reported, mostly in imatinib-treated patients. Although imatinib is susceptible to the widest range of KD mutations, second-generation TKIs do not uniformly lead to a decreased rate of KD mutation acquisition. For instance, in the randomised phase III study ENESTnd, where two doses of nilotinib were compared against imatinib in the treatment of newly diagnosed CML-CP patients, 3.9 % of nilotinib-treated patients acquired mutations with a 3-year minimum follow-up, as compared to 7.4 % in the imatinib arm [60]. There was no gross difference in the number of highly resistant mutations detected. In contrast, 3.8 % of patients acquired mutations in the phase III DASISION study, regardless of whether they were assigned treatment with imatinib versus dasatinib, though dasatinib-treated patients were more likely to have acquired highly resistant mutations [61]. It should be noted that the criteria that triggered mutation analysis in the two trials were slightly different, and the rate should not be directly compared.

Nucleic acid substitutions that result in KD mutations lead to changes in the amino acids sequences of the BCR-ABL1 protein and conformation of the ATP-binding pocket. TKI binding in the ATP pocket is compound specific and depends on the formation of a number of critical hydrogen bonds between particular amino acids and the drug. A changed ATP pocket resulting from KD mutations lead to less efficient TKI binding. Consequently, kinase activity is restored, leading to loss of response and re-capitulation of the disease phenotype. The tyrosine residue at position 315 is particularly important in its interaction with all first- and second-generation TKIs and is exchanged for isoleucine in the most commonly reported T315I mutation [62, 63]. This gatekeeper mutation confers resistance to all TKIs currently in use except for ponatinib [64]. Other commonly encountered mutations of clinical significance include E255K/V and Y253H which confer resistance to nilotinib and imatinib, and V299L and F317V/I mutations which confer resistance to dasatinib [65, 66]. Sensitivities of different KD mutations to various TKIs can be determined in vitro using BaF3 cells engineered to express the respective mutant BCR-ABL1. Most commonly encountered KD mutations and their relative sensitivities to dasatinib and nilotinib are illustrated in Fig. 7.6, which correlates with clinical experience for most but not all mutations [63].

The most commonly used method for mutation detection is direct Sanger sequencing. The technology and technical aspects have been extensively reviewed elsewhere [67, 68]. This technique can detect *BCR-ABL1* KD mutations when present at 10–20 % of total *BCR-ABL1*. Nested PCR is used to facility mutation detection in samples with low total *BCR-ABL1* copies. Both forward and reverse strands of *BCR-ABL1* should be sequenced to increase confidence for calling mutations. Standardised mutation reports should include information on the nucleotide exchange, the amino acid exchange, the estimated abundance of the mutant

| Dasatinib | | Nilotinib | |
|---|---|---|---|
| O'Hare et al[65] | Redaelli et al[66] | O'Hare et al[65] | Redaelli et al[66] |
| T315I | T315I | T315I | T315I |
| T315A* | V299L | Y253H | E255V |
| F317V | E255K | E255V | E255K |
| V299L | L248V | E255K | F359V |
| E255V | F317L | F359V | **G250E** |
| F317L | **G250E** | Y253F | Y253F |
| E255K | E255V | Q252H | **H396R** |
| Q252H | Q252H | T315A | L248V |
| F359V | F486S | V379I | Q252H |
| L387M | L384M | **F317L** | **H396P** |
| **G250E** | E279K | L387M | L384M |
| E355G | H396R | **G250E** | **F317L** |
| Y253F | Y253F | **H396R** | E279K |
| Y253H | F359V | **H396P** | D276G |
| M244V | D276G | M244V | F486S |
| H396R | H396P | F311L | V299L |
| F311L | M351T | M351T | G398R |
| M351T | G398R | | M351T |
| V379I | | | |
| H396P | | | |

**Fig. 7.6** Sensitivity of different kinase domain mutations to either dasatinib or nilotinib as determined by in vitro cellular proliferation assays. Colour shading runs from red to orange, yellow and then green from resistant to most sensitive (Originally appeared in Branford et al. [63]. Reproduced by agreement. © by the American Society of Hematology)

and the expected sensitivities to TKIs relevant for the clinical setting [23]. The numbering of nucleotide and amino acid residues is based on the Abl protein variant B (which includes ABL exon 1b but not exon 1a) [23].

Both the ELN [62] and the NCCN [41] currently recommend mutation analysis be performed in patients who have either failed to achieve a milestone response (primary failure) or experience a loss of previously achieved response (secondary failure). If mutation analysis is indicated, it should always be performed on a specimen taken prior to switching to the next line of therapy and prior to discontinuation of the previous line of therapy. Leukaemic clones bearing the KD mutations undergo expansion under the selective pressure of TKI treatment. With TKI discontinuation, clones with wild-type *BCR-ABL1* may rapidly expand, either leading to underestimation of the mutant clone abundance or a false-negative result

[69–71]. Performing mutational analysis after TKI switching may also lead to erroneous results from rapid deselection of mutants that expanded during the previous line treatment. Furthermore, one should always consider the mutation status before selecting the next line agent. It is important to note that when mutant clones become rapidly deselected in response to a change of TKI, that clone is usually dormant and may persist at low levels for many years and is likely to re-emerge if circumstances are favourable. For instance, if a Y253H mutation is detected with frontline imatinib failure in a patient who subsequently switched to dasatinib, the Y253H mutation may become undetectable with successful dasatinib treatment. However, if a V299L dasatinib-resistant mutation then develops, switching to nilotinib will likely lead to a re-emergence of the dormant Y253H clone, which is a known nilotinib-resistant mutation [69]. Thus, in patients switching to third or subsequent line therapies, one must also consider a patient's previous mutation history.

Mutation detection at diagnosis has a low yield in treatment-naïve early CP patients and is only indicated at baseline in advanced-phase disease (AP/BC) [62, 72]. For instance, in the 846 patient ENESTnd study, none of the baseline samples harboured a KD mutation [60]. In the setting of primary treatment failure, the likelihood of discovering a KD mutation relates a patient's best response achieved whilst on TKI therapy and is the highest in patients who fail to achieve even a complete haematological response, followed by patients who failed to achieve a cytogenetic response [59, 73]. In contrast, KD mutations are rarely responsible for failure to achieve MMR in patients who have already achieved CCyR. Similarly, KD mutations are much more commonly found in cases where secondary failure results in a high tumour burden, resulting in either a loss of CCyR of loss of haematological response [38, 59, 73, 74]. There is no consensus on the trigger for mutation analysis based solely on a rise in *BCR-ABL1*, and this threshold may be different for different laboratories. We and others have found a >2-fold increase in *BCR-ABL1* to be associated with a higher incidence of KD mutation acquisition [38, 75], though others have found a higher threshold [76]. The discrepancies are likely related to differences in measurement uncertainty between methods. For patients who have achieved MMR, the current recommendation is that *BCR-ABL1* increases should only be a trigger for mutation analysis if it results in a loss of MMR [62]. The yield of detectable mutations is highest with progression to AP/BC and for patients diagnosed in AP/BC who subsequently experience treatment resistance, and therefore mutation analysis should always be performed in these instances [38, 59, 77]. KD mutations observed in these cases are more likely to confer resistance to not only imatinib but also to a second-generation TKI, such as T315I, E255K/V and Y253F/H [63]. In all cases of treatment failure, it is important to consider mechanisms of resistance aside from KD mutations. These include clonal evolution [78], non-compliance [79], and other pharmacokinetic factors [80].

Occasionally, patients may have two or more concomitant detectable KD mutations. When these KD mutations occur on separate transcripts produced by separate *BCR-ABL1* clones, these are termed polyclonal mutations. When more than one KD mutation occurs on the same transcript, the term compound mutation is used. Changes in the protein structure at more than one amino acid residue may lead to greater level of resistance than is expected with either component alone [81]. As described previously, the gatekeeper mutation T315I confers resistance to imatinib and all second-generation TKIs. Ponatinib, a third-generation TKI, had been rationally designed to have activity against T315I and most other mutations when occurring singularly. This agent has completed its phase II registration study (PACE) and now may be used in patients with T315I. However, in vitro studies suggest that ponatinib is susceptible to certain compound mutations, especially those with E255K/V as one of the components [82]. Several compound mutations have recently been confirmed in vitro as conferring ponatinib resistance, using primary specimens from PACE patients who experienced treatment failure [83]. However, there is currently no recognised diagnostic method to easily identity compound mutations and distinguish them accurately from polyclonal mutations. Initial surveys suggested that the mutations detected in the majority of patients with ≥1 KD mutation were indeed compound mutations [84–86], though these reports used methods that have subsequently been demonstrated to lead to erroneous overestimations of clonal complexity, and the implausibly complex phylogenetic architectures reported have since been called into question [87]. Thus, the true prevalence and clinical impact of compound mutations are currently undetermined (Fig. 7.7).

### 7.4.2 Emergent Mutational Analysis Techniques

Sanger sequencing is currently regarded as the standard of care method for mutation analysis. It has a number of advantages: (i) it is commonly available: (ii) mutants detected are annotated with clinical correlations; (iii) it offers an unbiased interrogation of the KD (i.e. prior knowledge of mutations likely to be present in a sample is not necessary to perform this test). However, it also has a number of disadvantages: it has low sensitivity and is only semi-quantitative in its estimation of the mutant allele burden. It is also relatively labour intensive and does not lend itself to mass screening for mutations (e.g. in a clinical trial setting). A number of other techniques may offer technical improvements over Sanger sequencing. For instance, pyrosequencing [88] is another unbiased method which sequences by synthesis. Instead of using fluorescent terminating nucleotides to identify bases in sequence, pyrosequencing detects pyrophosphates released upon successful incorporation of a nucleotide complementary to the template. This method has improved sensitivity compared to direct sequencing (limit of detection ~5 %) but give shorter sequences (interrogation of the whole KD can only be done in multiple reads) and is more expensive.

Denaturing high-performance liquid chromatography (D-HPLC) provides a high-throughput method for mutation screening. Sample cDNA is first amplified in a nested PCR reaction, and the amplicons are run through a cartridge matrix. KD

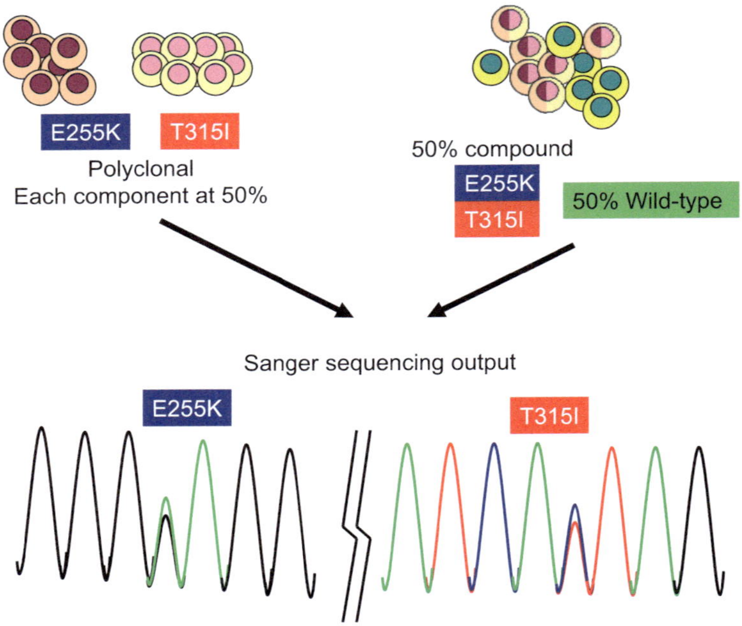


**Fig. 7.7** Sanger sequencing is the most commonly used method for mutation analysis in the diagnostic setting. It is widely available and allows for an unbiased interrogation of the kinase domain but has relatively low sensitivity. Furthermore, sequencing results reflect the average signal from all molecules within a sample mixture and are unable to differentiate polyclonal mutations from compound mutations. In these simulated sequencing chromatograms, the mutated base is present at 50 % on a wild-type background, leading to peaks with similar amplitudes for both samples

mutations present will lead to an altered electrical charge density reflected in the elution pattern [72]. Although D-HPLC is more sensitive than direct sequencing and can detect mutations present at >1–5 %, it will not characterise the mutant. D-HPLC-positive samples require direct sequencing subsequently to reveal the exact nucleotide exchange. Similarly, high-resolution melt (HRM) curve analysis also relies on changes in physical properties to screen for mutations, as the presence of a mutation leads to changes in the annealing or denaturing temperature. Like D-HPLC, HRM can only show if a mutation is present, but cannot reveal the identity of the mutant [89].

Allele-specific oligonucleotide PCR is both sensitive and specific. In this assay, oligonucleotides complementary to mutated *BCR-ABL1* may be used as the primer in a PCR assay. Mutant DNA templates will lead to exponential amplicon replication, whilst mismatched templates (wild-type *BCR-ABL1* in this case) will only amplify with significantly reduced efficiency. Whilst ASO-PCR can detect mutants with a sensitivity of 0.01–0.1 %, it is difficult to use this technique to screen for multiple mutations at once, especially for possible nucleotide exchanges in close proximity to each other. Furthermore, ASO-PCR will only reveal the presence of mutants complementary to oligonucleotide used and will not reveal any unexpected mutations [72, 90, 91]. Restriction fragment length polymorphism is now of historical interest only [72].

Newer techniques currently in development include mass spectrometry assays and massively parallel sequencing techniques. Mass spectrometry on the Sequenom platform has been used by the Adelaide group to demonstrate sensitive mutant detection in a multiplex reaction [92]. In this assay, a primer is annealed one nucleotide upstream from the suspected nucleotide exchange differentiating wild type from mutant. The primer is then allowed to extend by one nucleotide. Incorporation of a nucleotide complementary to the wild-type versus mutant template will result in a mass difference, which is detected using matrix-assisted laser desorption/ionisation mass spectrometry. Although this is a multiplexed assay which can screen for 31 of the most clinically relevant mutations with sensitivity down to 0.1 %, this technique cannot detect mutations not accounted for in the assay design. A more versatile approach may be to use next-generation sequencing techniques for mutation detection. This has been demonstrated to be feasible, though the clinical utility and assay characteristics (such as sensitivity, specificity, reproducibility and robustness) remain to be determined [93].

## 7.5 Conclusion

Molecular assays have become an indispensible tool in the management of CML, a disease in which the majority of patients enjoy excellent leukaemia-free survival. Time-dependent treatment responses as measured by RT-qPCR have been demonstrated in multiple clinical studies to be correlated with treatment outcomes and can segregate patients at high risk of treatment failure for additional therapeutic intervention. This forms the basis for inclusion of molecular treatment milestones into current treatment guidelines. RT-qPCR can also identify patients with deep molecular responses for future treatment cessation studies and surveillance for molecular relapse in this context. Reliable and sensitive RT-qPCR results reported on a standardised scale are routinely achieved in laboratories with optimised methodology and attention to good laboratory practice, when provided with good quality specimens.

In the setting of treatment failure, kinase domain mutations are the most commonly identified mechanism of resistance and interventions should be routinely preceded by mutation analysis, not only because the result will guide subsequent TKI selection but also because TKI switching or discontinuation will lead to rapid deselection of the clone associated with treatment resistance. Resistant clones lie dormant and may recur when favourable circumstances arise.

New technologies will lead to improvements in molecular assays for CML management, with the expectation that future tests will be more sensitive for minimal residual disease. These include assays based on digital PCR and next-generation sequencing platforms. They will also be more robust and accessible, with a benchtop RT-qPCR machine already available. Ongoing efforts at reference material development and standardisation will ensure result comparability between patients and laboratories. Increased sensitivity for low-level mutant detection and differentiation between polyclonal versus compound mutants are also in development, the clinical significance of which will be revealed in the future.

## References

1. Druker BJ, Guilhot F, O'Brien SG, Gathmann I, Kantarjian H, Gattermann N, et al. Five-year follow-up of patients receiving imatinib for chronic myeloid leukemia. N Engl J Med. 2006;355(23):2408–17. doi:10.1056/NEJMoa062867. 355/23/2408 [pii].
2. Hughes TP, Hochhaus A, Branford S, Muller MC, Kaeda JS, Foroni L, et al. Long-term prognostic significance of early molecular response to imatinib in newly diagnosed chronic myeloid leukemia: an analysis from the International Randomized Study of Interferon and STI571 (IRIS). Blood. 2010;116(19):3758–65.
3. Baccarani M, Deininger MW, Rosti G, Hochhaus A, Soverini S, Apperley JF, et al. European LeukemiaNet recommendations for the management of chronic myeloid leukemia: 2013. Blood. 2013;122(6):872–84. doi:10.1182/blood-2013-05-501569.
4. Ross DM, O'Hely M, Bartley PA, Dang P, Score J, Goyne JM, et al. Distribution of genomic breakpoints in chronic myeloid leukemia: analysis of 308 patients. Leukemia. 2013;27 (10):2105–7. doi:10.1038/leu.2013.116. leu2013116 [pii].
5. Goldman JM, Melo JV. Chronic myeloid leukemia-advances in biology and new approaches to treatment. N Engl J Med. 2003;349(15):1451–64. doi:10.1056/NEJMra020777. 349/15/1451 [pii].
6. Branford S, Hughes TP, Rudzki Z. Dual transcription of b2a2 and b3a2 BCR-ABL transcripts in chronic myeloid leukaemia is confined to patients with a linked polymorphism within the BCR gene. Br J Haematol. 2002;117(4):875–7.
7. Branford S, Cross NCP, Hochhaus A, Radich J, Saglio G, Kaeda J, et al. Rationale for the recommendations for harmonizing current methodology for detecting BCR-ABL transcripts in patients with chronic myeloid leukaemia. Leukemia. 2006;20(11):1925–30.
8. Muller MC, Merx K, Weisser A, Kreil S, Lahaye T, Hehlmann R, et al. Improvement of molecular monitoring of residual disease in leukemias by bedside RNA stabilization. Leukemia. 2002;16(12):2395–9.
9. Yokota M, Tatsumi N, Nathalang O, Yamada T, Tsuda I. Effects of heparin on polymerase chain reaction for blood white cells. J Clin Lab Anal. 1999;13(3):133–40. doi:10.1002/(SICI) 1098-2825(1999)13:3 < 133::AID-JCLA8 > 3.0.CO;2–0 [pii].
10. Rainen L, Oelmueller U, Jurgensen S, Wyrich R, Ballas C, Schram J, et al. Stabilization of mRNA expression in whole blood samples. Clin Chem. 2002;48(11):1883–90.
11. Chai V, Vassilakos A, Lee Y, Wright JA, Young AH. Optimization of the PAXgene blood RNA extraction system for gene expression analysis of clinical samples. J Clin Lab Anal. 2005;19(5):182–8. doi:10.1002/jcla.20075.
12. Thorn I, Olsson-Stromberg U, Ohlsen C, Jonsson A, Klangby U, Simonsson B, et al. Impact of RNA stabilization on minimal residual disease assessment in chronic myeloid leukemia. Haematologica. 2005;90(11):1350–5.
13. Kagedal B, Lindqvist M, Farneback M, Lenner L, Peterson C. Failure of the PAXgene blood RNA System to maintain mRNA stability in whole blood. Clin Chem Lab Med. 2005;43 (11):1190–2. doi:10.1515/cclm.2005.206.
14. Branford S, Prime J. Chronic myelogenous leukemia: monitoring response to therapy. Curr Hematol Malig Rep. 2011;6(2):75–81. doi:10.1007/s11899-011-0082-1.

15. Branford S, Hughes T. Diagnosis and monitoring of chronic myeloid leukemia by qualitative and quantitative RT-PCR. Methods Mol Med. 2006;125:69–92.
16. Beillard E, Pallisgaard N, van der Velden VH, Bi W, Dee R, van der Schoot E, et al. Evaluation of candidate control genes for diagnosis and residual disease detection in leukemic patients using 'real-time' quantitative reverse-transcriptase polymerase chain reaction (RQ-PCR) – a Europe against cancer program. Leukemia. 2003;17(12):2474–86.
17. Stangegaard M, Dufva IH, Dufva M. Reverse transcription using random pentadecamer primers increases yield and quality of resulting cDNA. Biotechniques. 2006;40(5):649–57.
18. Ross DM, Watkins DB, Hughes TP, Branford S. Reverse transcription with random pentadecamer primers improves the detection limit of a quantitative PCR assay for BCR-ABL transcripts in chronic myeloid leukemia: implications for defining sensitivity in minimal residual disease. Clin Chem. 2008;54(9):1568–71. doi:10.1373/clinchem.2008.105916.
19. Stanoszek LM, Crawford EL, Blomquist TM, Warns JA, Willey PF, Willey JC. Quality control methods for optimal BCR-ABL1 clinical testing in human whole blood samples. J Mol Diagn. 2013;15(3):391–400. doi:10.1016/j.jmoldx.2013.02.004.
20. White H, Deprez L, Corbisier P, Hall V, Lin F, Mazoua S, et al. A certified plasmid reference material for the standardisation of BCR-ABL1 mRNA quantification by real-time quantitative PCR. Leukemia. 2015;29(2):369–76. doi:10.1038/leu.2014.217. leu2014217 [pii].
21. Westgard JO, Barry PL, Hunt MR, Groth T. A multi-rule Shewhart chart for quality control in clinical chemistry. Clin Chem. 1981;27(3):493–501.
22. Armbruster DA, Pry T. Limit of blank, limit of detection and limit of quantitation. Clin Biochem Rev. 2008;29:S49–52.
23. Hughes T, Deininger M, Hochhaus A, Branford S, Radich J, Kaeda J, et al. Monitoring CML patients responding to treatment with tyrosine kinase inhibitors: review and recommendations for harmonizing current methodology for detecting BCR-ABL transcripts and kinase domain mutations and for expressing results. Blood. 2006;108(1):28–37.
24. Cross NC, White HE, Muller MC, Saglio G, Hochhaus A. Standardized definitions of molecular response in chronic myeloid leukemia. Leukemia. 2012;26(10):2172–5. doi:10.1038/leu.2012.104.
25. van der Velden VH, Hochhaus A, Cazzaniga G, Szczepanski T, Gabert J, van Dongen JJ. Detection of minimal residual disease in hematologic malignancies by real-time quantitative PCR: principles, approaches, and laboratory aspects. Leukemia. 2003;17(6):1013–34.
26. Mueller MC, Erben P, Saglio G, Gottardi E, Schenk T, Ernst T, et al. Harmonization of BCR-ABL mRNA quantification using an uniform control plasmid in 36 international laboratories. Blood (ASH Annual Meeting Abstracts). 2005;106:1991.
27. Lion T. Control genes in reverse transcriptase-polymerase chain reaction assays. Leukemia. 1996;10(9):1527–8.
28. Collins S, Coleman H, Groudine M. Expression of bcr and bcr-abl fusion transcripts in normal and leukaemic cells. Mol Cell Biol. 1987;7:2870.
29. Hughes TP, Kaeda J, Branford S, Rudzki Z, Hochhaus A, Hensley ML, et al. Frequency of major molecular responses to imatinib or interferon alfa plus cytarabine in newly diagnosed chronic myeloid leukemia. N Engl J Med. 2003;349(15):1423–32.
30. Gabert J, Beillard E, van der Velden VH, Bi W, Grimwade D, Pallisgaard N, et al. Standardization and quality control studies of 'real-time' quantitative reverse transcriptase polymerase chain reaction of fusion gene transcripts for residual disease detection in leukemia – a Europe against cancer program. Leukemia. 2003;17(12):2318–57.
31. Hanfstein B, Shlyakhto V, Lauseker M, Hehlmann R, Saussele S, Dietz C, et al. Velocity of early BCR-ABL transcript elimination as an optimized predictor of outcome in chronic myeloid leukemia (CML) patients in chronic phase on treatment with imatinib. Leukemia. 2014;28(10):1988–92. doi:10.1038/leu.2014.153. leu2014153 [pii].
32. White HE, Matejtschuk P, Rigsby P, Gabert J, Lin F, Lynn Wang Y, et al. Establishment of the first World Health Organization International Genetic Reference Panel for quantitation of

BCR-ABL mRNA. Blood. 2010;116(22):e111–7. doi:10.1182/blood-2010-06-291641. blood-2010-06-291641 [pii].

33. White HE, Hedges J, Bendit I, Branford S, Colomer D, Hochhaus A, et al. Establishment and validation of analytical reference panels for the standardization of quantitative BCR-ABL1 measurements on the international scale. Clin Chem. 2013;59(6):938–48. doi:10.1373/clinchem.2012.196477. clinchem.2012.196477 [pii].
34. Müller MC, Saglio G, Lin F, Pfeifer H, Press RD, Tubbs RR, et al. An international study to standardize the detection and quantitation of BCR-ABL transcripts from stabilized peripheral blood preparations by quantitative RT-PCR. Haematologica. 2007;92(7):970–3.
35. Müller MC, Erben P, Saglio G, Gottardi E, Nyvold CG, Schenk T, et al. Harmonization of BCR-ABL mRNA quantification using a uniform multifunctional control plasmid in 37 international laboratories. Leukemia. 2008;22(1):96–102.
36. Branford S, Fletcher L, Cross NCP, Muller MC, Hochhaus A, Kim D-W, et al. Desirable performance characteristics for BCR-ABL measurement on an international reporting scale to allow consistent interpretation of individual patient response and comparison of response rates between clinical trials. Blood. 2008;112(8):3330–8. doi:10.1182/blood-2008-04-150680.
37. Muller MC, Cross NCP, Erben P, Schenk T, Hanfstein B, Ernst T, et al. Harmonization of molecular monitoring of CML therapy in Europe. Leukemia. 2009;23(11):1957–63.
38. Branford S, Rudzki Z, Parkinson I, Grigg A, Taylor K, Seymour JF, et al. Real-time quantitative PCR analysis can be used as a primary screen to identify patients with CML treated with imatinib who have BCR-ABL kinase domain mutations. Blood. 2004;104(9):2926–32.
39. Press RD, Galderisi C, Yang R, Rempfer C, Willis SG, Mauro MJ, et al. A half-log increase in BCR-ABL RNA predicts a higher risk of relapse in patients with chronic myeloid leukemia with an imatinib-induced complete cytogenetic response. Clin Cancer Res. 2007;13(20):6136–43. doi:10.1158/1078-0432.ccr-07-1112.
40. Marin D, Khorashad JS, Foroni L, Milojkovic D, Szydlo R, Reid AG, et al. Does a rise in the BCR-ABL1 transcript level identify chronic phase CML patients responding to imatinib who have a high risk of cytogenetic relapse? Br J Haematol. 2009;145(3):373–5. doi:10.1111/j.1365-2141.2009.07646.x. BJH7646 [pii].
41. NCCN Clinical Practice Guidelines in Oncology Chronic Myelogenous Leukemia. Version 2.2014. http://www.nccn.org/professionals/physician_gls/f_guidelines.asp#site. Accessed 2 Jan 2014.
42. Yeung DT, Mauro MJ. Prognostic significance of early molecular response in chronic myeloid leukemia patients treated with tyrosine kinase inhibitors. Hematol Am Soc Hematol Educ Program. 2014;2014(1):240–3.
43. Branford S, Yeung DT, Parker WT, Roberts ND, Purins L, Braley JA, et al. Prognosis for patients with CML and >10% BCR-ABL1 after 3 months of imatinib depends on the rate of BCR-ABL1 decline. Blood. 2014;124(4):511–8. doi:10.1182/blood-2014-03-566323. blood-2014-03-566323 [pii].
44. Ross DM, Branford S, Moore S, Hughes TP. Limited clinical value of regular bone marrow cytogenetic analysis in imatinib-treated chronic phase CML patients monitored by RQ-PCR for BCR-ABL. Leukemia. 2006;20(4):664–70.
45. Branford S, Hughes TP, Rudzki Z. Monitoring chronic myeloid leukaemia therapy by real-time quantitative PCR in blood is a reliable alternative to bone marrow cytogenetics. Br J Haematol. 1999;107(3):587–99.
46. Lauseker M, Hanfstein B, Haferlach C, Schnittger S, Pfirrmann M, Fabarius A, et al. Equivalence of BCR-ABL transcript levels with complete cytogenetic remission in patients with chronic myeloid leukemia in chronic phase. J Cancer Res Clin Oncol. 2014;140(11):1965–9. doi:10.1007/s00432-014-1746-8.
47. Laneuville P. High risk of error in categorizing treatment response in individual CML patients by standard cytogenetic analysis or PCR assay with high CV: a Bayesian analysis blood. 2012;120(21):Abstract 3776.

48. Sanders R, Huggett JF, Bushell CA, Cowen S, Scott DJ, Foy CA. Evaluation of digital PCR for absolute DNA quantification. Anal Chem. 2011;83(17):6474–84. doi:10.1021/ac103230c.
49. Goh HG, Lin M, Fukushima T, Saglio G, Kim D, Choi SY, et al. Sensitive quantitation of minimal residual disease in chronic myeloid leukemia using nanofluidic digital polymerase chain reaction assay. Leuk Lymphoma. 2011;52(5):896–904.
50. Jennings LJ, George D, Czech J, Yu M, Joseph L. Detection and quantification of BCR-ABL1 fusion transcripts by droplet digital PCR. J Mol Diagn. 2014;16(2):174–9. doi:10.1016/j.jmoldx.2013.10.007. S1525-1578(13)00252-3 [pii].
51. Jobbagy Z, van Atta R, Murphy KM, Eshleman JR, Gocke CD. Evaluation of the Cepheid GeneXpert BCR-ABL assay. J Mol Diagn. 2007;9(2):220–7.
52. O'Dwyer ME, Swords R, Nagler A, McMullin MF, le Coutre PD, Langabeer SE, et al. Nilotinib 300 mg BID as frontline treatment of CML: prospective analysis of the Xpert BCR-ABL monitor system and significance of 3-month molecular response. Leuk Res. 2014;38(3):310–5. doi:10.1016/j.leukres.2013.11.016. S0145-2126(13)004 7-7 [pii].
53. Ross DM, Branford S, Seymour JF, Schwarer AP, Arthur C, Bartley PA, et al. Patients with chronic myeloid leukemia who maintain a complete molecular response after stopping imatinib treatment have evidence of persistent leukemia by DNA PCR. Leukemia. 2010;24 (10):1719–24. doi:10.1038/leu.2010.185. leu2010185 [pii].
54. Weerkamp F, Dekking E, Ng YY, van der Velden VH, Wai H, Bottcher S, et al. Flow cytometric immunobead assay for the detection of BCR-ABL fusion proteins in leukemia patients. Leukemia. 2009;23(6):1106–17. doi:10.1038/leu.2009.93. leu200993 [pii].
55. Deininger M, O'Brien SG, Guilhot F, Goldman JM, Hochhaus A, Hughes TP, et al. International randomized study of interferon Vs STI571 (IRIS) 8-year follow up: sustained survival and low risk for progression or events in patients with newly diagnosed chronic myeloid leukemia in chronic phase (CML-CP) treated with imatinib. ASH Annu Meet Abstr. 2009;114(22):Abstract 1126.
56. Branford S, Rudzki Z, Walsh S, Parkinson I, Grigg A, Szer J, et al. Detection of BCR-ABL mutations in patients with CML treated with imatinib is virtually always accompanied by clinical resistance, and mutations in the ATP phosphate-binding loop (P-loop) are associated with a poor prognosis. Blood. 2003;102(1):276–83.
57. Jabbour E, Kantarjian H, Jones D, Talpaz M, Bekele N, O'Brien S, et al. Frequency and clinical significance of BCR-ABL mutations in patients with chronic myeloid leukemia treated with imatinib mesylate. Leukemia. 2006;20(10):1767–73.
58. Soverini S, De Benedittis C, Papayannidis C, Paolini S, Venturi C, Iacobucci I, et al. Drug resistance and BCR-ABL kinase domain mutations in Philadelphia chromosome-positive acute lymphoblastic leukemia from the imatinib to the second-generation tyrosine kinase inhibitor era: the main changes are in the type of mutations, but not in the frequency of mutation involvement. Cancer. 2014;120(7):1002–9. doi:10 1002/cncr.28522.
59. Soverini S, Colarossi S, Gnani A, Rosti G, Castagnetti F, Poerio A, et al. Contribution of ABL kinase domain mutations to imatinib resistance in different subsets of Philadelphia-positive patients: by the GIMEMA Working Party on Chronic Myeloid Leukemia. Clin Cancer Res. 2006;12(24):7374–9. doi:10.1158/1078-0432.ccr-06-1516.
60. Hochhaus A, Saglio G, Larson RA, Kim D-W, Etienne G, Rosti G, et al. Nilotinib is associated with a reduced incidence of BCR-ABL mutations vs imatinib in patients with newly diagnosed chronic myeloid leukemia in chronic phase. Blood. 2013;121(18):3703–8. doi:10.1182/blood-2012-04-423418.
61. Kantarjian HM, Shah NP, Cortes JE, Baccarani M, Agarwal MB, Undurraga MS, et al. Dasatinib or imatinib in newly diagnosed chronic-phase chronic myeloid leukemia: 2-year follow-up from a randomized phase 3 trial (DASISION). Blood. 2012;119(5):1123–9. doi:10.1182/blood-2011-08-376087. blood-2011-08-376087 [pii].
62. Soverini S, Hochhaus A, Nicolini FE, Gruber F, Lange T, Saglio G, et al. BCR-ABL kinase domain mutation analysis in chronic myeloid leukemia patients treated with tyrosine kinase

inhibitors: recommendations from an expert panel on behalf of European LeukemiaNet. Blood. 2011;118(5):1208–15. doi:10.1182/blood-2010-12-326405.
63. Branford S, Melo JV, Hughes TP. Selecting optimal second-line tyrosine kinase inhibitor therapy for chronic myeloid leukemia patients after imatinib failure: does the BCR-ABL mutation status really matter? Blood. 2009;114(27):5426–35. doi:10.1182/blood-2009-08-215939.
64. Cortes JE, Kim DW, Pinilla-Ibarz J, le Coutre P, Paquette R, Chuah C, et al. A phase 2 trial of ponatinib in Philadelphia chromosome-positive leukemias. N Engl J Med. 2013;369 (19):1783–96. doi:10.1056/NEJMoa1306494.
65. O'Hare T, Eide CA, Deininger MWN. Bcr-Abl kinase domain mutations, drug resistance, and the road to a cure for chronic myeloid leukemia. Blood. 2007;110(7):2242–9. doi:10.1182/blood-2007-03-066936.
66. Redaelli S, Piazza R, Rostagno R, Magistroni V, Perini P, Marega M, et al. Activity of bosutinib, dasatinib, and nilotinib against 18 imatinib-resistant BCR/ABL mutants. J Clin Oncol. 2009;27(3):469–71. doi:10.1200/jco.2008.19.8853.
67. Alikian M, Gerrard G, Subramanian PG, Mudge K, Foskett P, Khorashad JS, et al. BCR-ABL1 kinase domain mutations: methodology and clinical evaluation. Am J Hematol. 2012;87 (3):298–304. doi:10.1002/ajh.22272.
68. Branford S, Hughes T. Detection of BCR-ABL mutations and resistance to imatinib mesylate. In: Illand H, Hertzgerg M, Marlton P, editors. Myeloid leukemia: methods and protocols, methods in molecular medicine. Totawa: Humana Press; 2006. p. 93–106.
69. Parker WT, Yeoman AL, Jamison BA, Yeung DT, Scott HS, Hughes TP, et al. BCR-ABL1 kinase domain mutations may persist at very low levels for many years and lead to subsequent TKI resistance. Br J Cancer. 2013;109(6):1593–8. doi:10.1038/bjc.2013.318.
70. Gruber FXE, Lamark T, Anonli A, Sovershaev MA, Olsen M, Gedde-Dahl T, et al. Selecting and deselecting imatinib-resistant clones: observations made by longitudinal, quantitative monitoring of mutated BCR-ABL. Leukemia. 2005;19(12):2159–65.
71. Hanfstein B, Muller MC, Kreil S, Ernst T, Schenk T, Lorentz C, et al. Dynamics of mutant BCR-ABL-positive clones after cessation of tyrosine kinase inhibitor therapy. Haematologica. 2011;96(3):360–6. doi:10.3324/haematol.2010.030999.
72. Willis SG, Lange T, Demehri S, Otto S, Crossman L, Niederwieser D, et al. High-sensitivity detection of BCR-ABL kinase domain mutations in imatinib-naive patients: correlation with clonal cytogenetic evolution but not response to therapy. Blood. 2005;106(6):2128–37.
73. Branford S, Goh H-G, Izzo B, Beppu L, Ortmann C-E, Duniec K, et al. A review of mutation analysis in the TOPS trial of standard dose versus high dose IM in CML suggests that refinements to the ELN recommendations for mutation screening may be appropriate. Blood. 2011;118(21):Abstract 889.
74. Sherbenou DW, Wong MJ, Humayun A, McGreevey LS, Harrell P, Yang R, et al. Mutations of the BCR-ABL-kinase domain occur in a minority of patients with stable complete cytogenetic response to imatinib. Leukemia. 2007;21(3):489–93.
75. Press RD, Willis SG, Laudadio J, Mauro MJ, Deininger MW. Determining the rise in BCR-ABL RNA that optimally predicts a kinase domain mutation in patients with chronic myeloid leukemia on imatinib. Blood. 2009;114(13):2598–605.
76. Wang L, Knight K, Lucas C, Clark RE. The role of serial BCR-ABL transcript monitoring in predicting the emergence of BCR-ABL kinase mutations in imatinib-treated patients with chronic myeloid leukemia. Haematologica. 2006;91(2):235–9.
77. Hochhaus A, La Rosee P. Imatinib therapy in chronic myelogenous leukemia: strategies to avoid and overcome resistance. Leukemia. 2004;18(8):1321–31.
78. Lahaye T, Riehm B, Berger U, Paschka P, Muller MC, Kreil S, et al. Response and resistance in 300 patients with BCR-ABL-positive leukemias treated with imatinib in a single center: a 4.5-year follow-up. Cancer. 2005;103(8):1659–69.

79. Ibrahim AR, Eliasson L, Apperley JF, Milojkovic D, Bua M, Szydlo R, et al. Poor adherence is the main reason for loss of CCyR and imatinib failure for chronic myeloid leukemia patients on long-term therapy. Blood. 2011;117(14):3733–6.
80. Apperley JF. Part I: Mechanisms of resistance to imatinib in chronic myeloid leukaemia. Lancet Oncol. 2007;8(11):1018–29.
81. Shah NP, Skaggs BJ, Branford S, Hughes TP, Nicoll JM, Paquette RL, et al. Sequential ABL kinase inhibitor therapy selects for compound drug-resistant BCR-ABL mutations with altered oncogenic potency. J Clin Invest. 2007;117(9):2562–9.
82. O'Hare T, Shakespeare WC, Zhu X, Eide CA, Rivera VM, Wang F, et al. AP24534, a pan-BCR-ABL inhibitor for chronic myeloid leukemia, potently inhibits the T315I mutant and overcomes mutation-based resistance. Cancer Cell. 2009;16(5):401–12. doi:10.1016/j.ccr.2009.09.028. S1535-6108(09)00339-0 [pii].
83. Zabriskie MS, Eide CA, Tantravahi SK, Vellore NA, Estrada J, Nicolini FE, et al. BCR-ABL1 compound mutations combining key kinase domain positions confer clinical resistance to ponatinib in Ph chromosome-positive leukemia. Cancer Cell. 2014;26(3):428–42. doi:10.1016/j.ccr.2014.07.006.
84. Khorashad JS, Kelley TW, Szankasi P, Mason CC, Soverini S, Adrian LT, et al. BCR-ABL1 compound mutations in tyrosine kinase inhibitor-resistant CML: frequency and clonal relationships. Blood. 2013;121(3):489–98. doi:10.1182/blood-2012-05-431379.
85. Soverini S, De Benedittis C, Machova Polakova K, Brouckova A, Horner D, Iacono M, et al. Unraveling the complexity of tyrosine kinase inhibitor-resistant populations by ultra-deep sequencing of the BCR-ABL kinase domain. Blood. 2013;122(9):1634–48. doi:10.1182/blood-2013-03-487728.
86. Smith CC, Brown M, Chin J, Kasap C, Salerno S, Damon LE, et al. Single molecule real time (SMRT™) sequencing sensitively detects polyclonal and compound BCR-ABL in patients who relapse on kinase inhibitor therapy. ASH Annu Meet Abstr. 2011;2011:Abstract 3752.
87. Parker WT, Phillis SR, Yeung DT, Hughes TP, Scott HS, Branford S. Many BCR-ABL1 compound mutations reported in chronic myeloid leukemia patients may actually be artifacts due to PCR-mediated recombination. Blood. 2014;124(1):153–5. doi:10.1182/blood-2014-05-573485. 124/1/153 [pii].
88. Khorashad JS, Anand M, Marin D, Saunders S, Al-Jabary T, Iqbal A, et al. The presence of a BCR-ABL mutant allele in CML does not always explain clinical resistance to imatinib. Leukemia. 2006;20:658–63.
89. Polakova KM, Lopotova T, Klamova H, Moravcova J. High-resolution melt curve analysis: initial screening for mutations in BCR-ABL kinase domain. Leuk Res. 2008;32(8):1236–43.
90. Roche-Lestienne C, Preudhomme C. Mutations in the ABL kinase domain pre-exist the onset of imatinib treatment. Semin Hematol. 2003;40(2 Suppl 2):80–2.
91. Roche-Lestienne C, Soenen-Cornu V, Grardel-Duflos N, Lai JL, Philippe N, Facon T, et al. Several types of mutations of the Abl gene can be found in chronic myeloid leukemia patients resistant to STI571, and they can pre-exist to the onset of treatment. Blood. 2002;100(3):1014–8.
92. Parker WT, Lawrence RM, Ho M, Irwin DL, Scott HS, Hughes TP, et al. Sensitive detection of BCR-ABL1 mutations in patients with chronic myeloid leukemia after imatinib resistance is predictive of outcome during subsequent therapy. J Clin Oncol. 2011;29(32):4250–9. doi:10.1200/JCO.2011.35.0934. JCO.2011.35.0934 [pii].
93. Li J, Liu W, Yan Z, Fang P, Darwanto A, Pelak K, et al. Next-generation sequencing of the BCR-ABL1 kinase domain and neighboring domains associated with therapy resistance. ASH Annu Meet Abstr. 2012;2012:Abstract 2549.

# Chapter 8
# Recommendations for the Management of CML in the Era of Second-Generation TKIs

**Alessandro Morotti, Carmen Fava, and Giuseppe Saglio**

**Abstract** Although imatinib 400 mg per day still represents the basic treatment for chronic myeloid leukemia (CML), the introduction of the second-generation tyrosine kinase inhibitors (TKIs) nilotinib and dasatinib and their subsequent registration as potential first- or second-line therapies are offering more options for the treatment of the CML patients. With respect to imatinib, nilotinib and dasatinib appear to offer some advantages in terms of efficacy as first-line treatment for newly diagnosed CML patients, like the capacity to induce very fast and deep molecular responses (MR4 and MR4.5) as well as to prevent part of the early progressions to AP/BC that may occur during the first two–three years from diagnosis. However their use has been associated with increased long-term toxicity, in particular in some groups of patients, and their high cost may represent a limitation to their use in countries where generic imatinib is or will soon become available. Potential long-term toxicity and a higher cost with respect to imatinib are also the factors that may influence the decision of the clinicians to switch the therapy to the use of a second-generation TKI in the cases showing a nonoptimal response to imatinib. All these elements are now animating an intense debate among hematologists on which could be the best therapeutic options to be used as first- and/or second-line therapies in the clinical management of CML patients.

**Keywords** CML • BCR-ABL • Ph chromosome • TK inhibitors

---

A. Morotti • C. Fava • G. Saglio, MD (✉)
Division of Hematology and Internal Medicine, Department of Clinical and Biological Sciences, University of Turin, "San Luigi Gonzaga", University Hospital, Orbassano, Turin 10043, Italy
e-mail: giuseppe.saglio@unito.it



M. Kizaki (ed.), *Molecular Pathogenesis and Treatment of Chronic Myelogenous Leukemia*, DOI 10.1007/978-4-431-55714-2_8

## 8.1 Introduction: Cytogenetic and Molecular End Points During CML Therapy

The better benefits of TKI therapy are observed in those patients who achieve and maintain complete cytogenetic remission (CCyR) for at least 2 years with a consequent similar OS to that of control healthy individuals [1]. On the other side, it was also shown that patients who do not achieve good cytogenetic or molecular responses (MR) to imatinib at defined time points have a worse outcome, associated with an increased risk of relapse, of progression, and of death [2, 3]. Following these observations, European LeukemiaNet (ELN) and National Comprehensive Cancer Network (NCCN) CML experts have revised treatment milestones to be achieved during TKI therapy of CML [4, 5]. In the attempt to optimize TKIs treatment of CML, an appropriate and timely follow-up with cytogenetic and standardized molecular methods of adequate reliability is mandatory [6–8]. In particular, molecular monitoring of BCR-ABL transcript levels by real-time quantitative PCR (RQ-PCR) represents the most useful and precise way to monitor CML patients. If compared to conventional cytogenetic analysis, RQ-PCR allows to prematurely monitor the reduction of the leukemic burden during TKI therapy and, on top, allows to estimate the amount of the residual disease once CCyR is achieved. Notably, when performed in a sample of good quality, the RQ-PCR sensitivity reaches the levels of $1\times10^{-4}/10^{-5}$, which corresponds to an amount between 2 and 3 logs below the threshold of CCyR achievement [6]. In line with the established international scale (IS), the TKI-induced BCR-ABL% targets to be achieved are 1 % (2 logs reduction with respect to the median BCR-ABL amount present at diagnosis and that roughly corresponds to the threshold of CCyR), 0.10 % BCR-ABL (MMR, major molecular response), and 0.01 % and 0.0032 % BCR-ABL, which are defined as MR4 (4 logs reduction) and MR4.5 (4.5 logs reduction), respectively [6–8].

Nowadays, the attainment of CCyR and the level of 1 % BCR-ABL$^{IS}$ represent the most significant responses to TKI therapy, which are associated with the highest probability of long-term survival for CML patients [9–11]. On the other side, a wealth of data does not clearly indicate that deeper responses, as the achievement of BCR-ABL$^{IS}$ $\leq$0.1 % (MMR), could increase the OS when compared to the achievement of CCyR without MMR [9, 10]. More recently, however, the 4-year analysis by the German CML-Study IV revealed that patients able to achieve a stable MR4.5 molecular response at 8 years showed a statistically significant better survival compared with those patients who have simply achieved CCyR, but not MMR [11]. If these results will be confirmed, MR4.5 will represent a new molecular predictor of long-term outcome. Moreover, several clinical studies demonstrated that a stable deep molecular response (at least MR4 or even better MR4.5) is mandatory to achieve a long-lasting treatment free remission (TFR), which is in turn the new treatment goal for CML patients [12, 13]. As a consequence, the MR4 and MR4.5 in addition to CCyR and MMR are appealing targets to pursuit. This recent essential concept, elucidated from many studies, highlights that the strongest

**Table 8.1** Recommendations during first-line and second-line treatment accordingly to ELN guidelines

| | First line | | Second line | |
|---|---|---|---|---|
| Time | Optimal response | Failure | Optimal response | Failure |
| *Baseline* | | | | |
| 3 months | BCR-ABL$^{IS}$ $\leq$10 % | No CHR | BCR-ABL$^{IS}$ $\leq$10 % | No CHR or Ph+ >95 % or mutations |
| | Ph+ $\leq$35 % | Ph+ >95 % | Ph+ <65 % | |
| 6 months | BCR-ABL$^{IS}$ <1 % | BCR-ABL$^{IS}$ >10 % | BCR-ABL$^{IS}$ $\leq$10 % | BCR-ABL$^{IS}$ >10 % |
| | Ph+ 0 % | Ph+ >35 % | Ph+ <35 % | Ph+ >65 %, mutations |
| 12 months | BCR-ABL$^{IS}$ $\leq$0.1 % | BCR-ABL$^{IS}$ >1 % | BCR-ABL$^{IS}$ <1 % | BCR-ABL$^{IS}$ >10 % |
| | | Ph+ >0 % | Ph+ 0 % | Ph+ >35 %, mutations |
| At any time | MMR | Loss of CHR, CCyR MMR, mutations | MMR | Loss of CHR, or CCyR or PCyR, or MMR |

prognostic parameters are represented by the early cytogenetic and molecular responses within the first year of TKI therapy [10, 14–16]. These end points regard OS, progression-free survival (PFS), or event-free survival (EFS) and, more importantly, allow to evaluate whether to discontinue TKI treatment without molecular relapse (TFR) [12]. Based on these observations, the last editions of the ELN and NCCN recommendations have substantially modified the time points at which optimal responses should be achieved (Table 8.1) [4, 5]. Whereas in the previous recommendations hematologic remission and some degree of cytogenetic response were exclusively expected after 3 months of TKI therapy and partial cytogenetic response (PCyR) after 6 months and CCyR after 1 year, in the last ELN and NCCN recommendations, the "optimal responders" patients should at least be in partial cytogenetic response (PCyR) and/or below the roughly corresponding 10 %$^{IS}$ BCR-ABL threshold after 3 months of therapy, at least in CCyR and/or below the 1 %$^{IS}$ BCR-ABL level after 6 months of therapy, and at least in MMR after 1 year of therapy and thereafter show a continuous decline of the BCR-ABL level until the achievement of deeper responses like MR4 or MR4.5 (Table 8.1) [4, 5]. As a consequence of these considerations, many studies suggest that the most clinically relevant target to be achieved during TKI therapy is represented by the reduction of the BCR-ABL$^{IS}$ transcript level below 10 % at 3 months [10, 14–16].

## 8.2 Imatinib as First-Line CML Therapy

The impressive complete cytogenetic responses (CCyR) and the consequent long-term overall survival (OS) together with a good tolerability have rapidly attributed to the first BCR-ABL tyrosine kinase inhibitor, imatinib at a dosage of 400 mg per day, the role of standard treatment, and the most widely frontline therapy for chronic phase CML patients [17, 18]. At the 8-year follow-up of the IRIS study, as confirmed by other studies and by independent retrospective analyses outside clinical trials, the cumulative CCyR rate was of 83 % with estimated overall survival (OS) rate of 85 %, which is far better from what was observed before the introduction of this drug [19–22]. These results are also associated with the substantial decrease in the number of the progressions to accelerated phase or blast crisis imatinib-treated patients. In all reports, the major cause of death for CML patients is indeed the progression to the accelerated or blast phase, being still incurable in most cases even with tyrosine kinase inhibitors (TKI) [23]. During imatinib therapy, the progression occurrence falls from an expected rate of approximately 15 % per year to a rate of 2–3 % per year. Furthermore, after the first 2–3 years of treatment, the progression rates drop dramatically [19]. The reduction of progression depends mostly on the astonishing leukemic mass reduction which is observed in most of the imatinib-treated patient. Notwithstanding, the inhibition of the BCR-ABL tyrosine kinase (TK) activity affects the ability of BCR-ABL to promote the genomic instability of the leukemic cells which is a cause of disease progression [24].

Based on the new ELN and NCCN criteria of TKI therapy response evaluation, one-third of newly diagnosed CML patients do not show an optimal response to the standard therapy with imatinib 400 mg, and they are therefore facing a statistically significant higher risk of an inferior outcome in terms of EFS, PFS, and also OS (approximately 80 % at 5 years with respect to >95 % of those below 10 % BCR-ABL$^{IS}$ at 3 months) [10, 14–16]. Actually we should consider that most of these patients (approximately 80 %) display only a delayed response to imatinib and that a switch to a second-generation TKI allows to achieve an optimal response in approximately 40–50 % of the cases [25, 26]. However, it should also be considered that approximately 15–20 % of them in a short time will progress to a more advanced phase of the disease and will die [10, 14–16]. In any case, several reports have shown that after 8 years from diagnosis, only approximately 55–60 % of the imatinib-treated patients are still on treatment with this drug [19, 20]. The reasons for imatinib discontinuation depend on failure, progression, and death; furthermore in about 10–12 % patients, adverse events (AEs) or intolerance to imatinib treatment required a switch to another TKI [19].

It is also noteworthy that the percentage of optimal response to imatinib may vary according to the initial clinical and hematological features of CML patients and their initial risk category, as established by the Sokal's, Euro, and also the more recent EUTOS score [27–29]. In the IRIS study, patients with low-, intermediate-, or high-risk Sokal's score showed significantly different response rates as 5-year CCyR (89 %, 82 %, and 69 %, respectively, $P < 0.001$) and progression to advanced disease (3 %, 8 %, and 17 %, respectively, $P = 0.002$) [17].

Based on all these considerations, several clinical trials aiming to improve first-line treatment of patients with chronic phase CML have been performed or are currently under recruiting. In particular, the first-line administration of the second-generation TKIs, or modified imatinib-based regimens, as higher dosages of imatinib from the start, or combinations of imatinib with other drugs, namely, interferon-alpha (IFN-α), have been evaluated. Currently, the only approved and registered first-line therapy regiments are the use of the second-generation TKIs nilotinib, at the dosage of 300 mg BID, and of dasatinib 100 mg OD. These two novel strategies are also included in the ELN and NCCN recommendations, whereas the other two quoted options still remain investigational [4]. Since CP-CML patients show a very long survival, very long follow-ups are mandatory to assess whether these alternative treatments promote a better OS. Meanwhile, the investigation of the efficacy of these regimens relies on important surrogate markers, as the rates of CCyR, MMR, MR4, and MR4.5; the early molecular response (EMR); and the more traditional event-free survival (EFS) and progression-free survival (PFS). However, it is important to consider that the methods to asses and to report the rate of responses can sometimes vary and that the definitions of the EFS and PFS may change substantially according to the protocol in different trials. This situation can therefore introduce bias that render difficult to compare the results [30, 31]. Considering this potential limitation, we will now review the currently available main treatment options to imatinib 400 mg OD as first-line therapy for CP-CML patients.

## 8.3 Second-Generation Tyrosine Kinase Inhibitors in First-Line Treatment

Following the success of imatinib, three different more potent second-generation BCR-ABL inhibitors have been developed and tested as first-line therapy to overcome the residual resistance observed in imatinib-treated patients and to further improve the outcome of CP-CML patients [32]. These TKI drugs were already approved as second-line therapy for imatinib-intolerant or imatinib-resistant patients, namely, dasatinib (Sprycel, Bristol-Myers Squibb) [33], a dual BCR-ABL and SRC inhibitor; nilotinib (Tasigna, Novartis) [34], a potent and more selective BCR-ABL inhibitor; and bosutinib (Bosulif, Pfizer) another potent dual BCR-ABL and SRC inhibitor [35].

When administrated as second-line therapy, all these drugs showed a substantially good toxicity profile and were able to induce a CCyR rate of 40–50 % in patients with primary or secondary resistance to imatinib [25, 26]. Notably, these results were achieved even in those patients expressing BCR-ABL mutations able to confer resistance to imatinib, with some notable exceptions like the T315I mutation [36].

The efficacy and the toxicity of nilotinib and dasatinib as first-line therapy were initially assessed in phase 2 studies and their rather long follow-up [37–39]. In the GIMEMA CML Working Party, obtained in 73 newly diagnosed CP-CML patients treated with nilotinib 400 mg twice a day, the CCyR achievement was observed in 78 % of patients at 3 months and in 96 % at 6 months, whereas the MMR rates observed were 52 % and 66 %, respectively, at the same time points and 85 % at 12 months [37]. Similarly, in 100 newly diagnosed CML patients treated at the MD Anderson Cancer Center with nilotinib 400 mg twice daily (BID), with a median follow-up of 29 months (range 1–73), the cumulative CCyR rate was 93 %, the MMR rate was 73 %, and the CMR rate (defined according to the previous ELN criteria as undetectable hybrid transcripts with a sensitivity of at least $10^{-4/-5}$) was 33 % [37]. At the same institution, 86 newly diagnosed patients were also treated with dasatinib 50 mg twice daily (BID) or 100 mg QD [39]. With a median follow-up of 24 months, most patients achieved a rapid CCyR (94 % at 6 months), with a cumulative CCyR ratio of 98 %. After 12 and 18 months, MMR was achieved by 71 % and 79 % of patients [39]. The toxicity profile with dasatinib was also favorable, with a better tolerability with dasatinib QD versus BID dosing.

ENESTnd is a phase 3, randomized, open-label, multicenter study comparing the efficacy and safety of nilotinib with imatinib in patients with newly diagnosed CML that has now reached the fifth year of follow-up [40, 41]. The trial included 846 patients randomly assigned 1:1:1 to nilotinib 300 mg BID ($n = 282$), nilotinib 400 mg BID ($n = 281$), or imatinib 400 mg/day ($n = 283$). The primary end point was the achievement of MMR at 12 months. Patients were stratified by Sokal's score with equal distributions of low-, intermediate-, and high-risk Sokal's scores in each arm of the trial. Efficacy results were presented in the intent-to-treat (ITT) population. The MMR rate at 12 months was significantly higher for nilotinib 300 mg BID (44 %, $P < .0001$) and nilotinib 400 mg BID (43 %, $P < .0001$) than for imatinib (22 %). As this was the primary end point of the study, nilotinib 300 mg BID was approved by the FDA and EMA as first-line therapy. Responses were rapidly achieved with nilotinib, with 6-month MMR rates of 33 %, 30 %, and 12 % for nilotinib 300 mg BID, nilotinib 400 mg BID, and imatinib, respectively. Nilotinib treatment was also associated with less AP/BC progressions than in imatinib-treated arm [39]. After a minimum follow-up of 5 years, rates of MMR and MR4.5 continue to be significantly higher in both nilotinib arm and the imatinib arm (MMR 77 and 77.2 % vs. 60 % and MR4.5 53.5 and 52.3 % vs. 31.4 %), with more than half of the nilotinib-treated patients achieving MR4.5 by 5 years [40]. Notably, the rates of freedom from progression to AP/BC in nilotinib-treated patients remain statistically higher (96.3 % and 97.8 % for nilotinib vs. 92.1 % imatinib), when considering progression events occurring during treatment and after treatment discontinuation. However, although estimated rates of OS are higher in both nilotinib arms versus the imatinib arm (93.7 % nilotinib 300 mg BID, 96.2 % nilotinib 400 mg BID, and 91.7 % imatinib), the moment the difference is barely statistically significant only for nilotinib 400 mg BID versus imatinib. The frequency of adverse events (AEs) causing treatment discontinuation was lowest in the nilotinib 300 mg BID arm (12.2 %), followed by the imatinib arm (13.9 %) and the nilotinib 400 mg BID arm (19.9 %) [40]. However, the occurrence of cardiovascular events, which have been frequently reported in association with nilotinib therapy, has been observed in both nilotinib and imatinib arms, although these events (including all definitions of different gravity and also cerebrovascular events and peripheral arterial disease (PAD)) are definitely more frequent in the 400 mg BID arm than in the 300 mg BID arm (7.5 % in the nilotinib 300 mg BID arm, 13.4 % in the nilotinib 400 mg BID arm vs. 91.7 % in the imatinib arm) [40]. In conclusion, the 5-year follow-up data confirm the sustained efficacy of frontline nilotinib over imatinib as frontline therapy including the achievement of earlier and deeper molecular responses and increased freedom from progression to AP/BC. The relevance of these responses relies also on the option for some patients reaching the MR4.5 to discontinue the therapy without recurrence of the disease at least for a relevant period of time [19]. It is also relevant that, comparing only nilotinib 300 mg BID and imatinib 400 mg OD at 3 months, 91 % of patients in the nilotinib arm versus 67 % in the imatinib arm achieved BCR-ABL$^{IS}$ transcript levels $\leq$10 % and 56 % and only 16 % of patients achieved already BCR-ABL$^{IS}$ transcript levels $\leq$1 % [15]. This rapid decrease of the leukemic mass correlates with progression to AP/BC and with OS in both treatment arms. Among patients who achieved $\leq$10 % BCR-ABL$^{IS}$ at 3 months, only three progressed on treatment whereas nine of 111 patients who achieved >10 % at 3 months progressed. These results clearly show the relevance to evaluate early molecular response at 3 months [15].

DASISION is a phase 3, randomized, open-label, multicenter study comparing the efficacy and safety of dasatinib 100 mg OD as first-line therapy with respect to that of imatinib [42]. Also this study has now achieved a minimum follow-up of 5 years [43]. All newly diagnosed CP-CML were stratified according to the Euro score and randomly assigned to dasatinib 100 mg/day or imatinib 400 mg/day. The primary end point was the CCyR by 12 months. After 1 year of treatment, dasatinib (83 %, $P < .001$) induces a higher response compared to imatinib (72 %), allowing this drug to be approved as first-line therapy by FDA and EMA. The best cumulative MMR rate by 12 months was also significantly higher for dasatinib (46 %, $P < .0001$) than for imatinib (28 %) [42]. Fewer progressions to accelerated phase or blast crisis (AP/BC) with dasatinib (1.9 %) than with imatinib (3.5 %) were already observed in the first report of these data [42]. Currently, after 5 years of follow-up, the rates of molecular response continue to be higher for dasatinib compared with imatinib (rates of MMR 76 % vs. 64 %, $P = .002$, and rates of MR4.5 42 % vs. 33 %, $P = .025$). As a consequence of these observations, the AP/BP progressions were lower with dasatinib ($n = 12/259$; 4.6 %) compared with imatinib ($n = 19/260$; 7.3 %). However 5-year PFS and OS rates were similar across treatment arms (PFS 85 % dasatinib, 86 % imatinib; OS 91 % dasatinib, 90 % imatinib) [43]. A higher proportion of patients on dasatinib achieved BCR-ABL$^{IS}$ $\leq$10 % at 3 months (84 %) compared with those on imatinib (64 %). Patients who achieved BCR-ABL$^{IS}$ $\leq$10 % versus >10 % at 3 months showed improved PFS, OS, and lower rates of transformation to AP/BP (PFS 89 % vs. 72 %, $P = .0014$; OS 94 % vs. 81 %, $P = .0028$; transformation $n = 6/198$ [3 %] vs. $n = 5/37$ [14 %]) and imatinib (PFS 93 % vs. 72 %, $P < .0001$; OS 95 % vs. 81 %, $P = .0003$;

transformation $n = 5/154$ 3 % vs. $n = 13/85$, 15 %) [16]. Regarding the total incidence of AEs, dasatinib was associated with pleural effusion in 29 %, but most cases were grade 1 or 2 (67 out of 74), and discontinuation of dasatinib due to pleural effusion occurred in only 15 patients (6 % overall and 20 % of patients who experienced a pleural effusion). Arterial ischemic events were uncommon, occurring in 12 patients (5 %) on dasatinib and 6 patients (2 %) on imatinib [43]. More recently, however, one investigator-initiated study comparing dasatinib 100 mg OD with imatinib 400 mg OD, although showing that the proportion of patients achieving CCyR was superior with dasatinib (84 % vs. 69 %) as well as the 12-month molecular responses (MMR 53 % vs. 35 %, $P = 0.049$; MR4 25 % vs. 10 %, $P = 0.038$), did not show any advantage in terms PFS as well as in terms of OS [44].

Finally, BELA is a phase 3 multicenter study comparing the efficacy and safety of bosutinib 500 mg OD with that of imatinib 400 mg OD [45]. The primary end point of this study was the CCyR by 12 months. Notably, bosutinib did not induce higher CCyR by 12 months (70 %), when compared with imatinib (68 %), and this did not allow bosutinib to be approved as first-line therapy. The high rate of bosutinib discontinuation mainly due to nonhematologic drug-related AEs may have jeopardized these results. In particular, the discontinuation rates were 19 % in the bosutinib arm with respect to 5 % in the imatinib arm and were associated with diarrhea on bosutinib. However, MMR rates by 12 months were significantly higher for bosutinib (39 % bosutinib vs. 26 % imatinib, $P = 0.002$), and there were numerically fewer progressions to AP/BC with bosutinib (2 %) than with imatinib (4 %) [45].

In conclusion, the first-line therapy with second-generation TKIs, due to their strongest inhibitory activity of the BCR-ABL kinase, displays superior features when compared to imatinib 400 mg OD. This is revealed by a faster time to cytogenetic and molecular responses, with more patients achieving BCR-ABL$^{IS}$ $\leq$10 % at 3 months and by sustained higher cumulative responses, particularly by higher rates of very deep molecular responses like MR4 and MR4.5. The immediate clinical advantage of their use as frontline therapy could be represented by a lower rate of transformation, whereas on a longer run, the advantage could be represented by a faster achievement of conditions allowing to reach and maintain a TFR state. However, a relevant observation is that after a 5-year follow-up, the OS rates are not statistically different with respect to imatinib while, on the contrary, few long-term toxicity effects, like a higher rate of cardiovascular events, could raise concerns for their use, particularly in some categories of patients [46].

## 8.4 Parameters for TKI Therapy Switch

The reasons underlying the decision of changing TKI therapy may be different. Besides imatinib treatment failure, which is associated with a high risk of progression and death, in general, 10–12 % of patients may show adverse events (AEs) and become intolerant to treatment with a given TKI and switch treatment with another drug [10]. Notably, after 8 years of TKI treatment, only 55–60 % of patients who started with imatinib are still on treatment with this drug [21]. Interestingly, a similar discontinuation rate was observed among patients who started therapy with second-generation TKIs as first-line therapy [40, 42]. Therefore the availability of several TKIs with different characteristics and different toxicity profiles, which are registered as first-, second-, or third-line therapy, represents a great step forward in CML treatment.

However the most difficult decision to be taken is when to change therapy in case of "nonoptimal response." If we consider the 10 % BCR-ABL1$^{IS}$ threshold at 3 months as a target for optimal response (Table 8.1), approximately one-third of imatinib-treated CML patients are facing a statistically significant higher risk of an inferior outcome in terms of EFS, PFS, and also OS (approximately 80 % at 5 years with respect to >95 % of those below 10 % BCR-ABL1 at 3 months) [10, 15, 16, 47]. This percentage is much lower (approximately 10–15 %) in patients treated with second-generation TKIs as first-line therapy, but the outcome of these patients is probably even worse with respect to those who do not obtain the response with imatinib [15, 16].

Regarding this aspect, the last versions of the ELN and of the NCCN guidelines offer discordant indications [4, 5]. In the NCCN guidelines, those patients who do not achieve the 10 % BCR-ABL1$^{IS}$ cutoff at 3 months should be treated with a different TKI drug, while in the ELN recommendations, a more delaying position is suggested. From the practical point of view, the ELN recommendations suggest simply to look more carefully by increasing the frequency of the RQ-PCR tests and to change therapy only if at 6 months, the percentage of BCR-ABL1$^{IS}$ is above 10 %, at this time considered failure [4].

Actually it should be noted that most of these patients (approximately 80 % of those first-line treated with imatinib) will only show a delayed response to TKI and that, in case of an overt failure, they will simply require a switch to treatment with a second-generation TKI to achieve a good response in at least 40–50 % of the cases [25, 26]. However, approximately 15–20 % of them in a short time will progress to a more advanced phase of the disease and will die [10, 15, 16, 47]. Most of these progressions occur in patients classified as high or intermediate Sokal's risk group at diagnosis, and progressions are rare in the low Sokal's risk group in TKI-treated patients. This may be related to the fact that the percentage of patients who do not show an optimal response to imatinib may vary according to the initial clinical and hematological features that determine their initial risk category, as established by the Sokal's, Euro, and also the more recent EUTOS score [27–29]. More recently, it has been suggested that the evaluation of the so-called halving time at 90 days of therapy (i.e., at least a halving of the BCR-ABL1$^{IS}$ percentage at 3 months with respect to that observed at diagnosis) may help to discriminate among imatinib-treated patients those patients who are at real risk of failure during imatinib therapy and should therefore change TKI therapy from those who are simply late responders and can therefore remain on the same therapy [48]. Similar data have been reported by RQ-PCR analysis using GUS instead of ABL as control gene, in order to have a more exact evaluation of the real amount of the disease burden at the diagnosis [49]. In this case, however, the best discriminating cutoff at 3 months is to reach a value of approximately one-third with respect to that present at diagnosis.

Independently from the risk of progression and of death, those that at 3 months show values of BCR-ABL1$^{IS}$ above 10 % have very scanty possibility to subsequently achieve a deep molecular response (MR4 and MR4.5), which are conditions necessary to remain in TFR after TKI therapy discontinuation. This concept is also consistent in those patients with a good halving time but that remain above 10 % after 3 months of therapy [48]. Indeed, to obtain a high rate of deep molecular responses, BCR-ABL1$^{IS}$ should be already $\leq$1 % at 3 months, as also those patients who at 3 months are between 10 % and 1 % of BCR-ABL1$^{IS}$ have lower possibilities of achieving MR4 or MR4.5 in a reasonable period of time [15, 16].

In summary, CML treatment guidelines include EMR at 3 months as the first measurement of TKI responses, as BCR-ABL1$^{IS}$ levels at this time are key predictors of long-term outcomes for CML patients not only in terms of PFS and of OS but also in terms of the subsequent possibility to achieve deep molecular responses allowing to consider TKI therapy suspension.

Some authors, however, in agreement with the ELN recommendations, believe that the 6 months' time point is probably the more suitable time to change therapy for those who have not achieved PCyR and/or are above the 10 % BCR-ABL1$^{IS}$ threshold at 3 months. Indeed, the 6 months' RQ-PCR analysis on patients who are above 10 % BCR-ABL1$^{IS}$ at 3 months shows that very few of these patients achieve an optimal response (less than 1 % BCR-ABL1$^{IS}$) but that those (approximately 35–40 %) who remain in the warning category (between 1 % and 10 % BCR-ABL1$^{IS}$) do not show a bad outcome as those who remain above 10 % BCR-ABL1$^{IS}$ even at 6 months (failure category according to the ELN recommendations). This is the main reason whereby the ELN recommends to delay the decision to change therapy in the absence of an overt failure. Patients who remain in the warning category, however, even if in terms of OS and PFS behave as patients in optimal response, appear to achieve MMR only in less than 50 % of the cases and frequently change therapy. In summary, if we decide to continue the therapy with imatinib in those 30 % of patients who are above 10 % of BCR-ABL1$^{IS}$ at 3 months of therapy and to wait for the 6 months RQ-PCR results, we are really saving the change of therapy to only approximately one-third of them and therefore to approximately 10 % of all patients.

However, we have also to consider that the 3 months' BCR-ABL1$^{IS}$ levels are associated not only with an improved PFS and OS but also with an increased possibility of achieving MR [4] and MR$^{4.5}$. Importantly, these end points are more frequently obtainable with the use of second-generation TKIs with respect to imatinib. It is still unclear whether a change in therapy at 3 months, in particular from imatinib to second-generation TKIs, can substantially improve the rates of achievement of MR [4] and MR$^{4.5}$. Therefore, a more flexible position is advisable. The change of TKI therapy should be decided case by case considering the goal expected to be achieved, the probability of achieving that goal in a given patient, and the final balance between the possible advantages and disadvantages, including the risk of toxicity and the economical cost that the achievement of the goal may require.

## 8.5 Final Considerations

The choice of first-line treatment of CML in chronic phase is at the moment one of the most hot topics of debate among hematologists around the world. Imatinib has represented a fundamental step for the treatment of CML patients, totally changing their survival perspectives, and it has been able to save their lives. Worldwide, the cost of imatinib-based therapy is not low, and this has certainly reduced the use of this drug in some low-income countries. The impact of this problem has been in part alleviated by the action of international charity programs supported by pharma companies, like the GIPAP program by Novartis. As it already happened in some countries, the imatinib treatment will certainly become more widely accessible at the expiration of imatinib patent with the consequent introduction of generic compounds. In spite of this, we should truly consider that the standard dose of imatinib (400 mg/day) is not optimal in approximately one-third of the newly diagnosed CML patients [19]. Currently, trials aiming to improve the outcome by increasing the imatinib dosage or by combining imatinib with IFN have provided in part contradictory results. However, the results obtained by the use of a tolerability-adapted imatinib dosage observed in the German CML-Study IV are very promising and have been recently confirmed by another independent study.[58] On the other side, the use of the more potent second-generation TKIs dasatinib and nilotinib has been approved and registered by the FDA and EMA entities as alternatives to first-line therapy with imatinib. Although not producing a significantly better OS with respect to standard-dose imatinib therapy, second-generation TKIs are indeed associated with faster and deeper responses and with the prevention of early progressions to AP/BC that may still occur during the first two–three years from diagnosis [40, 42]. This latter point however, as mentioned, has not been confirmed for dasatinib in a second investigator-initiated study and needs to be further explored [44].

The approval of nilotinib 300 mg/day and of dasatinib 100 mg/day as first-line therapy has introduced different therapeutic options for clinicians to treat newly diagnosed CML patients. Currently, as specified in the 2013 ELN guidelines, there are no preferential indications and clinicians should choose among the three approved drugs to tailor the treatment according to patients' characteristics [4, 5]. Therefore, clinicians should prescribe the second-generation TKIs for all patients from the beginning or only for some subgroups of patients with high risk of progression or, again, to initially start with imatinib 400 mg and to switch to a second-generation TKI when a nonoptimal response is observed. Notably, these three options should take in consideration drug efficacy, toxicity, and affordable cost for each individual patient. Trials testing all possible therapeutic strategies are however presently ongoing, and their results will certainly help clinicians to further make their decision.

At the moment, in the choice of initial CML therapy, we may also consider the variability from patient to patient [50]. In particular, for an elderly patient, the achievement of an OS probability overlapping the one of the corresponding control population without CML is a sufficient target. Conversely, a younger patient certainly aims to eradicate the disease and therefore can also accept a more demanding therapeutic approach. This explains why CMR and the more precise definitions of molecular degrees of residual disease recently introduced (like MR4 and MR4.5) have become the primary end point of some clinical trials [51]. As a fast initial response may be highly predictive of the patients' final outcome, a more intense schedule for monitoring the response with cytogenetic and/or molecular analysis within the first 6 months of therapy is advisable even in common clinical practice, as clearly stated in the ELN and NCCN recommendations [4, 5].

**Declaration of Conflict of Interests (COI)**
The authors declare that they have no conflict of interest.

**Acknowledgments** This work has been supported by grants from Associazione Italiana contro le Leucemie (AIL) and Associazione Italiana per la Ricerca sul Cancro (AIRC).

## References

1. Gambacorti-Passerini C, Antolini L, Mahon FX, et al. Multicenter independent assessment of outcomes in chronic myeloid leukemia patients treated with imatinib. J Natl Cancer Inst. 2011;103:553–61.
2. Kantarjian H, O'Brien S, Shan J, et al. Cytogenetic and molecular responses and outcome in chronic myelogenous leukemia: need for new response definitions? Cancer. 2008;112:837–45.
3. Marin D, Milojkovic D, Olavarria E, et al. European LeukemiaNet criteria for failure or suboptimal response reliably identify patients with CML in early chronic phase treated with imatinib whose eventual outcome is poor. Blood. 2008;112:4437–44.
4. Baccarani M, Deininger MW, Rosti G, et al. European LeukemiaNet recommendations for the management of chronic myeloid leukemia: 2013. Blood. 2013;122:872–84.
5. NCCN Clinical Practice Guidelines in Oncology (NCCN Guidelines ®) Chronic myelogenous leukemia Version 3. NCCN.org 2014.
6. Hughes T, Deininger M, Hochhaus A, et al. Monitoring CML patients responding to treatment with tyrosine kinase inhibitors: review and recommendations for harmonizing current methodology for detecting BCR-ABL transcripts and kinase domain mutations and for expressing results. Blood. 2006;108:28–37.
7. Muller MC, Saglio G, Lin F, et al. An international study to standardize the detection and quantitation of BCR-ABL transcripts from stabilized peripheral blood preparations by quantitative RT-PCR. Haematologica. 2007;92:970–3.
8. Cross NC, White HE, Muller MC, Saglio G, Hochhaus A. Standardized definitions of molecular response in chronic myeloid leukemia. Leukemia. 2012;26:2172–5.
9. Jabbour E, Kantarjian H, O'Brien S, et al. The achievement of an early complete cytogenetic response is a major determinant for outcome in patients with early chronic phase chronic myeloid leukemia treated with tyrosine kinase inhibitors. Blood. 2011;118:4541–6; quiz 759.
10. Hanfstein B, Muller MC, Hehlmann R, et al. Early molecular and cytogenetic response is predictive for long-term progression-free and overall survival in chronic myeloid leukemia (CML). Leukemia. 2012;26(9):2096–102.

11. Hehlmann R, Muller MC, Lauseker M, et al. Deep molecular response is reached by the majority of patients treated with imatinib, predicts survival, and is achieved more quickly by optimized high-dose imatinib: results from the randomized CML-study IV. J Clin Oncol. 2014;32:415–23.
12. Mahon FX, Rea D, Guilhot J, et al. Discontinuation of imatinib in patients with chronic myeloid leukaemia who have maintained complete molecular remission for at least 2 years: the prospective, multicentre Stop Imatinib (STIM) trial. Lancet Oncol. 2010;11:1029–35.
13. Ross DM, Branford S, Seymour JF, et al. Safety and efficacy of imatinib cessation for CML patients with stable undetectable minimal residual disease: results from the TWISTER study. Blood. 2013;122:515–22.
14. Milojkovic D, Ibrahim AR, Foroni L, et al. Assessment of BCR-ABL1 transcript levels at 3 months is the only requirement for predicting outcome for patients with chronic myeloid leukemia treated with imatinib. ASH Annu Meet Abstr. 2011;118:1680.
15. Hughes TP, Saglio G, Kantarjian HM, et al. Early molecular response predicts outcomes in patients with chronic myeloid leukemia in chronic phase treated with frontline nilotinib or imatinib. Blood. 2014;123:1353–60.
16. Jabbour E, Kantarjian HM, Saglio G, et al. Early response with dasatinib or imatinib in chronic myeloid leukemia: 3-year follow-up from a randomized phase 3 trial (DASISION). Blood. 2014;123:494–500.
17. O'Brien SG, Guilhot F, Larson RA, et al. Imatinib compared with interferon and low-dose cytarabine for newly diagnosed chronic-phase chronic myeloid leukemia. N Engl J Med. 2003;348:994–1004.
18. Goldman JM. Chronic myeloid leukemia: a historical perspective. Semin Hematol. 2010;47:302–11.
19. Hughes TP, Hochhaus A, Branford S, et al. Long-term prognostic significance of early molecular response to imatinib in newly diagnosed chronic myeloid leukemia: an analysis from the International Randomized Study of Interferon and STI571 (IRIS). Blood. 2010;116:3758–65.
20. Hehlmann R, Lauseker M, Jung-Munkwitz S, et al. Tolerability-adapted imatinib 800 mg/d versus 400 mg/d versus 400 mg/d plus interferon-alpha in newly diagnosed chronic myeloid leukemia. J Clin Oncol Official J Am Soc Clin Oncol. 2011;29:1634–42.
21. De Lavallade H, Apperley JF, Khorashad JS, et al. Imatinib for newly diagnosed patients with chronic myeloid leukemia: incidence of sustained responses in an intention-to-treat analysis. J Clin Oncol. 2008;26:3358–63.
22. Kantarjian H, O'Brien S, Jabbour E, et al. Improved survival in chronic myeloid leukemia since the introduction of imatinib therapy: a single-institution historical experience. Blood. 2012;119:1981–7.
23. Hehlmann R, Saussele S. Treatment of chronic myeloid leukemia in blast crisis. Haematologica. 2008;93:1765–9.
24. Bolton-Gillespie E, Schemionek M, Klein HU, et al. Genomic instability may originate from imatinib-refractory chronic myeloid leukemia stem cells. Blood. 2013;121:4175–83.
25. Shah NP, Guilhot F, Cortes JE, et al. Long-term outcome with dasatinib after imatinib failure in chronic-phase chronic myeloid leukemia: follow-up of a phase 3 study. Blood. 2014;123:2317–24.
26. Le Coutre PD, Giles FJ, Pinilla-Ibarz J, et al. Nilotinib in imatinib-resistant or -intolerant patients (pts) with chronic myeloid leukemia in chronic phase (CML-CP): 48-month follow-up results of a phase 2 study. ASH Annu Meet Abstr. 2011;118:3770.
27. Sokal JE, Cox EB, Baccarani M, et al. Prognostic discrimination in "good-risk" chronic granulocytic leukemia. Blood. 1984;63:789–99.
28. Hasford J, Pfirrmann M, Hehlmann R, et al. A new prognostic score for survival of patients with chronic myeloid leukemia treated with interferon alfa. Writing Committee for the Collaborative CML Prognostic Factors Project Group. J Natl Cancer Inst. 1998;90:850–8.

29. Hasford J, Baccarani M, Hoffmann V, et al. Predicting complete cytogenetic response and subsequent progression-free survival in 2060 patients with CML on imatinib treatment: the EUTOS score. Blood. 2011;118:686–92.
30. Kantarjian H, O'Brien S, Jabbour E, et al. Impact of treatment End point definitions on perceived differences in long-term outcome with tyrosine kinase inhibitor therapy in chronic myeloid leukemia. J Clin Oncol. 2011;29(23):3173–8.
31. Guilhot J, Baccarani M, Clark RE, et al. Definitions, methodological, and statistical issues for phase III clinical trials in chronic myeloid leukemia: a proposal by the European LeukemiaNet. Blood. 2012;119(25):5963–71.
32. Giles FJ. New directions in the treatment of imatinib failure and/or resistance. Semin Hematol. 2009;46:S27–33.
33. Doggrell SA. BMS-354825: a novel drug with potential for the treatment of imatinib-resistant chronic myeloid leukaemia. Expert Opin Investig Drugs. 2005;14:89–91.
34. Weisberg E, Manley P, Mestan J, Cowan-Jacob S, Ray A, Griffin JD. AMN107 (nilotinib): a novel and selective inhibitor of BCR-ABL. Br J Cancer. 2006;94:1765–9.
35. Keller G, Schafhausen P, Brummendorf TH. Bosutinib: a dual SRC/ABL kinase inhibitor for the treatment of chronic myeloid leukemia. Expert Rev Hematol. 2009;2:489–97.
36. Jabbour E, Branford S, Saglio G, Jones D, Cortes JE, Kantarjian HM. Practical advice for determining the role of BCR-ABL mutations in guiding tyrosine kinase inhibitor therapy in patients with chronic myeloid leukemia. Cancer. 2010;117(9):1800–11.
37. Rosti G, Palandri F, Castagnetti F, et al. Nilotinib for the frontline treatment of Ph(+) chronic myeloid leukemia. Blood. 2009;114:4933–8.
38. Cortes JE, Jones D, O'Brien S, et al. Nilotinib as front-line treatment for patients with chronic myeloid leukemia in early chronic phase. J Clin Oncol. 2010;28:392–7.
39. Cortes JE, Jones D, O'Brien S, et al. Results of dasatinib therapy in patients with early chronic-phase chronic myeloid leukemia. J Clin Oncol. 2010;28:398–404.
40. Saglio G, Kim DW, Issaragrisil S, et al. Nilotinib versus imatinib for newly diagnosed chronic myeloid leukemia. N Engl J Med. 2010;362:2251–9.
41. Saglio G, Hughes TP, Clark RE, Nakamae H, Kim DW, Jootar S, Etienne G, Flinn I, Lipton JH, Pasquini R, Moiraghi B, Kemp C, Fan X, Menssen HD, Kantarjian HM, Larson RA. ENESTnd Update: Nilotinib (NIL) Vs Imatinib (IM) in patients (pts) with newly diagnosed chronic myeloid leukemia in chronic phase (CML-CP) and the impact of Early Molecular Response (EMR) and Sokal risk at diagnosis on long-term outcomes. Blood. 2013;122:92.
42. Kantarjian H, Shah NP, Hochhaus A, et al. Dasatinib versus imatinib in newly diagnosed chronic-phase chronic myeloid leukemia. N Engl J Med. 2010;362:2260–70.
43. Cortes J SG, Shah N, et al. Final study results of DASISION (Dasatinib versus Imatinib in newly diagnosed chronic Myeloid Leukemia in Chronic Phase CML). European School of Hematology meeting. Philadelphia, 2014.
44. Radich JP, Kopecky KJ, Appelbaum FR, et al. A randomized trial of dasatinib 100 mg versus imatinib 400 mg in newly diagnosed chronic-phase chronic myeloid leukemia. Blood. 2012;120:3898–905.
45. Cortes JE, Kim DW, Kantarjian HM, et al. Bosutinib versus imatinib in newly diagnosed chronic-phase chronic myeloid leukemia: results from the BELA trial. J Clin Oncol. 2012;30:3486–92.
46. Giles FJ, Mauro MJ, Hong F, et al. Rates of peripheral arterial occlusive disease in patients with chronic myeloid leukemia in the chronic phase treated with imatinib, nilotinib, or non-tyrosine kinase therapy: a retrospective cohort analysis. Leukemia. 2013;27:1310–5.
47. Marin D, Ibrahim AR, Lucas C, et al. Assessment of BCR-ABL1 transcript levels at 3 months is the only requirement for predicting outcome for patients with chronic myeloid leukemia treated with tyrosine kinase inhibitors. J Clin Oncol. 2012;30:232–8.
48. Bradord S, Yeung DT, Parker WT, et al. Prognosis for patients with CML and >10% BCR-ABL1 after 3 months of imatinib depends on the rate of BCR-ABL1 decline. Blood. 2014;124:511–8.

49. Hanfstein B, Shlyakhto V, Lauseker M, et al. Velocity of early BCR-ABL1 transcript elimination as an optimized predictor of outcome in chronic myeloid leukemia (CML) patients in chronic phase on treatment with imatinib. Leukemia. 2014;28:1988–92.
50. Fava C, Rege-Cambrin G, Saglio G. The choice of first-line chronic myelogenous leukemia treatment. Ann Hematol. 2015;94 Suppl 2:123–31.
51. Morotti A, Fava C, Saglio G. Milestones and monitoring. Curr Hematol Malig Rep. 2015;10 (2):167–72.

# Chapter 9
# The Role of New TKIs and Combinations with Interferon-α for the Treatment of CML

**Franck E. Nicolini, Marie Balsat, Hélène Labussière-Wallet, Mohamad Sobh, Arthur Bert, and Maël Heiblig**

**Abstract** Despite the remarkable success of tyrosine kinase inhibitors (TKIs) in the treatment of CML, patients that do not respond or do not tolerate well these agents accumulate, and new options have to be found to avoid these situations. In this chapter, we discuss the importance of ponatinib, a third-generation TKI, and omacetaxine mepesuccinate, an untargeted therapy for such patients, and the use of combinations of TKI and interferon-α front line in order to prevent the onset of disease resistance.

**Keywords** CML • Ponatinib • Pegylated interferon • Omacetaxine

## 9.1 Introduction

Approximately 40 % of chronic myelogenous leukemia (CML) patients fail to respond or to tolerate properly imatinib mesylate in the long term [1, 2], and it is estimated that ~50 % of them are adequately rescued by second-generation tyrosine kinase inhibitors (TKIs). However, a number of patients that have failed these two generations of inhibitors accumulate with time and represent nowadays substantial cohorts worldwide. Recently [3, 4], ponatinib, a third-generation tyrosine kinase inhibitor, represents a new option able to induce and maintain responses over time but is limited by a significant toxicity. In patients remaining in chronic or accelerated phase, unfit to this therapeutic option or for allogeneic stem cell transplanta-

F.E. Nicolini, MD, PhD (✉)
Hematology Department 1G, Centre Hospitalier Lyon Sud, Lyon, France

INSERM U1052, Centre de Recherche en Cancérologie de Lyon, Lyon, France

French group of CML (Fi-LMC Group), Laboratory of Hematology, Hôpital Haut Lévêque, Pessac, France
e-mail: franck-emmanuel.nicolini@chu-lyon.fr

M. Balsat • H. Labussière-Wallet • M. Sobh • A. Bert • M. Heiblig
Hematology Department 1G, Centre Hospitalier Lyon Sud, Lyon, France

 
M. Kizaki (ed.), *Molecular Pathogenesis and Treatment of Chronic Myelogenous Leukemia*, DOI 10.1007/978-4-431-55714-2_9

tion, omacetaxine mepesuccinate (OMA), a subcutaneously bioavailable form of homoharringtonine, can be used successfully as a third- or fourth-line therapy for chronic phase and sometimes accelerated phase.

Looking at the problem through another angle, a majority of patients currently still fail in achieving deep molecular responses on imatinib, dasatinib, or nilotinib, presumably because a pool of uncycling $Ph^+$ stem cells persist, sustaining the disease over time and not depending on BCR-ABL for its survival [5]. Therefore, this compartment is not hit by TKI. Interferon-α can induce long-term disease control [6, 7] and exerts different biological activities on leukemic (stem) cells, differing from that of TKI. Thus, interferon-α combined to TKI for improvements in responses represents a promising approach and should avoid further TKI resistance by contributing to reduce the $Ph^+$ stem cell reservoir.

## 9.2 Ponatinib

Ponatinib (Iclusig®, ARIAD) is a third-generation TKI active against unmutated and mutated BCR-ABL, including the threonine-to-isoleucine ABL mutation at position 315 (T315I), which is present in up to 20 % of patients with TKI-resistant disease and confers resistance to all other approved BCR-ABL TKIs [8–13]. In an initial phase 1 study [3], ponatinib showed substantial antileukemic activity in patients with $Ph^+$ diseases (i.e., CML and $Ph^+$ ALL) resistant or significantly intolerant from previous TKI. This activity has been confirmed in the phase 2 PACE (Ponatinib $Ph^+$ ALL and CML Evaluation) clinical trial for chronic phase, accelerated phase, and blast phase CML or Ph-positive ALL either intolerant or resistant to nilotinib and dasatinib or harboring a T315I mutation.

### *9.2.1 Ponatinib in Chronic Phase CML Patients*

Four hundred and forty-nine patients have been enrolled in this multicentric international trial with 270 patients in chronic phase at the time of entry assigned to receive 45 mg of ponatinib once daily. The median age was 60 (18–94) years, and the majority of these patients have been heavily pretreated (median time since CML diagnosis, 7 years; 93 % of patients had $\geq$2 TKI and 60 % $\geq$3 TKI). The last update has been presented lately [14] with a median follow-up of 38 months and with a median of 32 months of ponatinib. Only 45 % of patients were still on core treatment. The rate of responses observed at any time point is very high considering such a poor prognosis population, with 59 % of patients in major cytogenetic response (MCyR), 53 % in complete cytogenetic response (CCyR), and 39 % in major molecular response (MMR) in the total CP CML populations. Even deep molecular responses (MR4 and MR4.5) are observed in a significant proportion of patients (27 and 22 %, respectively) (Fig. 9.1). The T315I group of patients seems

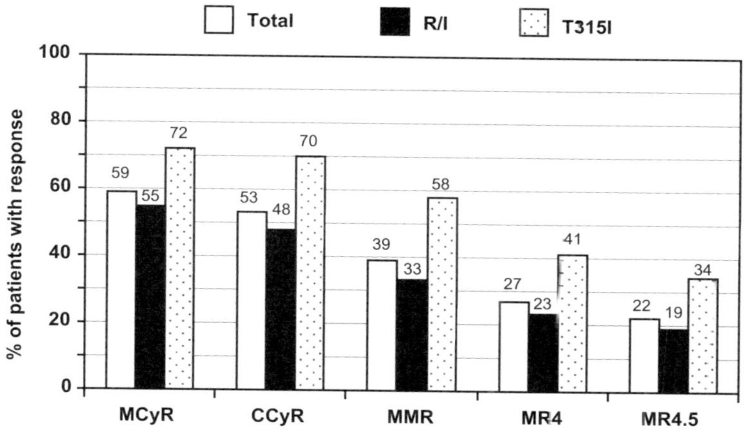


**Fig. 9.1** Overall cytogenetic and molecular response rates of chronic phase CML to ponatinib within the PACE trial [14]. MCyR states for major cytogenetic response, CCyR for complete cytogenetic response, MMR for major molecular response, MR4 for molecular response 4 logs, MR4.5 for molecular response 4.5 logs, R/I for resistant/intolerant

to experience higher responses related to less advanced diseases, when compared with patients with ≥2–3 lines of TKIs, as imatinib-resistant first-line patients with a T315I mutation could be enrolled. The cytogenetic responses seem stable over time with 83 % of patients remaining in MCyR, at 36 months. The progression-free survival and overall survival rates are outstanding in the fraction of patients still on treatment (61 % and 82 % at 36 months, respectively). However, these enthusiastic results are tempered by the onset of significant adverse events, even in chronic phase patients. Common hematologic adverse events are seen, as usual in patients with an important load of $Ph^+$ cells in their marrow (35 % thrombocytopenia, 17 % neutropenia, 9 % anemia grades 3–4), but some worrying severe thrombotic cardiovascular events – mostly arterial – were unexpected (22 % severe, of the chronic phase populations, + 29 % non-severe arterial thrombotic adverse events, total 51 %), associated with a significant percentage of ponatinib-induced hypertensions. The onset of these cardiovascular events (severe and non-severe, including hypertension) has been shown to occur quite early in an academic study performed in a small series of chronic phase CML patients (Fig. 9.2) [15]. The physiopathology of these events remains unclear, but it generally occurs in patients with cardiovascular risk factors (but sometimes not) and is dose dependent [14]. Neither glucose nor blood lipid levels vary on ponatinib. Considering that the median age of diagnosis of CML is – outside of clinical trials – 62 years [16], this is a significant problem, and the phase 3 first-line clinical trial for chronic phase CML patients comparing imatinib with ponatinib has been abrogated by the FDA because of these unacceptable events in first-line patients. Thus, it is unlikely that this drug will be developed further as a first-line option.

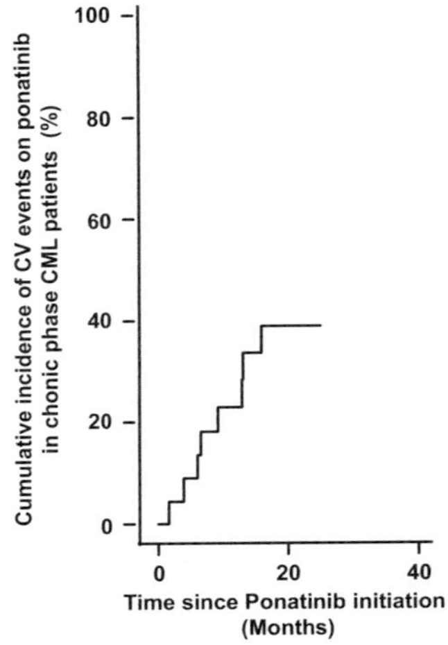


**Fig. 9.2** Cumulative incidence of overall cardiovascular events on ponatinib in chronic phase CML patients as defined in [15]. *CV* states for cardiovascular

### *9.2.2 Ponatinib in Advanced Phases CML and Ph + ALL Patients*

Ponatinib retains a significant activity in patients in accelerated phase at enrolment within the PACE trial [4, 14] with 59 % of living patients after 36 months of median follow-up [14]. Conversely, the activity of this compound as monotherapy in blast crisis patients and refractory $Ph^{+}$ ALL remains unusual with catastrophic overall survival after a median follow-up of 36 months: 9 % and 16 %, respectively [14]. However, this compound can be useful as a therapeutic bridge or a debulking agent prepared for allogeneic stem cell transplantation.

## 9.3 Omacetaxine (OMA)

OMA (Synribo®, Teva) is a protein inhibitor synthesis without any tyrosine kinase activity first tested in solid tumors. Before the TKI era, OMA – formerly known as homoharringtonine – was then used as second-line therapy for chronic phase patients failing interferon-α [17, 18]. The demonstration that OMA retains activity on leukemic stem cells in murine models (90 % of the leukemic stem cells (LSCs) die after in vitro OMA exposure versus 9 % after imatinib) promoted the revival of this almost forgotten compound. Recently, it became a suitable option for the treatment of resistant CML in the CGX-635-CML-203 trial with 12.8 % of major cytogenetic responses (MCyR) and 69 % of major hematologic responses (MaHR), for chronic phase patients [19]. Interestingly, OMA exerts a specific activity on ABL mutated clones – particularly T315I – through an unknown mechanism and is

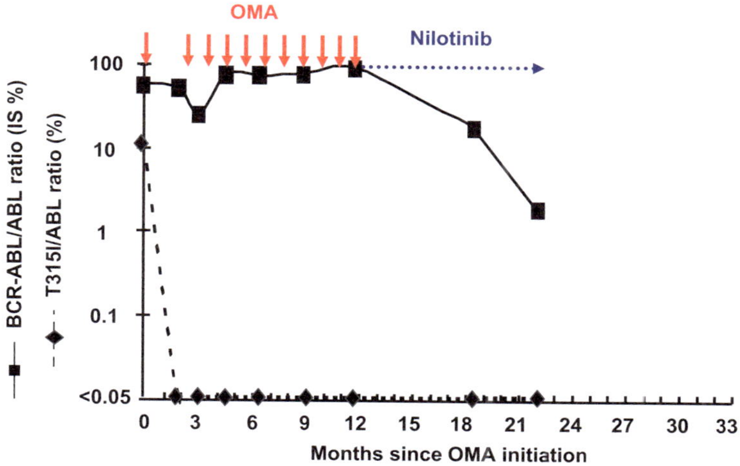


**Fig. 9.3** Overall molecular and T315I mutated transcript response rates of a chronic phase T315I+ CML patient treated with several courses of OMA (*top arrows*) followed by a nilotinib rechallenge (*dashed arrow*). Published in part in [20]. *OMA* states for omacetaxine mepesuccinate

able to retard or abrogate disease progression in such patients and allow TKI rechallenge (Fig. 9.3.) [20, 21].

### 9.3.1 *Omacetaxine in Chronic Phase CML Patients*

In 1995, O'Brien et al. demonstrated some activity in late chronic phase CML patients as monotherapy with a daily dose of 2.5 mg/m$^2$ for 14 days (CHR = 72 %, overall cytogenetic response = 31 %, CCyR = 7 %, MCyR = 15 %) [17]. The same authors went on exploring the combination of OMA + IFN-α for early chronic phase, initially as a sequential schedule: 90 patients with 2.5 mg/m$^2$ daily as a continuous infusion for 14 days, followed by maintenance for 7 days a month. Overall cytogenetic response rates to OMA were 66 %, twice the response rates in late chronic phase with interferon-α alone, and CCyR rates were 23 % (see a summary of the responses described in the literature in Table 9.1). When administrated simultaneously, a further improvement in the CHR rates, overall cytogenetic response rates, and MCyR rates was seen with 84 %, 69 %, and 52 %, respectively, in patients with early chronic phase and 80 %, 50 %, and 40 %, respectively, in late chronic phase. The estimated 2-year survival rate was 90 % (Table 9.1) [22]. In 2002, preliminary in vitro results suggested that imatinib resistance was not generally associated with resistance to Ara-C, daunorubicin, and OMA and may be synergistic to imatinib [23]. Furthermore, because OMA retains some activity on Ph$^+$ cells via different cellular pathways than TKI, D. Marin et al. hypothesized that OMA would reduce the level of residual disease in patients with CML in

**Table 9.1** Overall response rates and survival in chronic and accelerated phase CML patients receiving omacetaxine mepesuccinate (OMA) for TKI resistance

| Trials | Drug | *N* | CHR (%) | MCyR (%) | CCyR (%) | Overall CyR (%) | OS/PFS (months) | BCR-ABL (%) |
|---|---|---|---|---|---|---|---|---|
| *T315I negative* | | | | | | | | |
| O'Brien et al. (1995) [17] | OMA 2.5 mg/$m^2$ | 71 | 72 | 15 | 7 | 31 | 30/NA | NA |
| O'Brien et al. (1999) [41] | OMA 2.5 mg/$m^2$ + IFN 5MUI/$m^2$ | 90 | 92 | 44 | 23 | 66 | NR | NA |
| Kantarjian et al. (2000) [42] | OMA 2.5 mg/$m^2$ + Ara-C 2.5 mg/$m^2$ | 105 | 72 | 15 | 5 | 32 | 55 % at 4 years | NA |
| O'Brien et al. (2002) [22] | OMA 2.5 mg/$m^2$ + IFN 5MUI/$m^2$ | 47 | 84 | 52 | 21 | 66 | 90 % at 2 years | NA |
| Cortes et al. (2013) [19] | OMA 1.25 mg/$m^2$ | 81 | 69 | 20 | 10 | NA | 34/9.6 | NA |
| Nicolini et al. (2013) (Accelerated phase) [27] | OMA 1.25 mg/$m^2$ | 41 | 24 | 0 | 0 | 15 | 16/4.7 | NA |
| *T315I positive* | | | | | | | | |
| Nicolini et al. (2010) [20] | OMA 1.25 mg/$m^2$ ± nilotinib 800 mg/j | 8 | 100 | / | 37.5 | / | / | <0.1 % in 50 % of patients |
| Cortes et al. (2012) [30] | OMA 1.25 mg/$m^2$ | 62 | 77 | 23 | 16 | 44 | NR/7.7 | <0.1 % in 15 % of patients |
| *Case reports T315I in chronic phase CML* | | | | | | | | |
| Legros et al. (2007) [21] | OMA 2.5 mg/$m^2$ | 1 | 5.5 months | / | / | NR | Alive | <0.1 % (5.5 months) |
| de Lavallade et al. (2007) [28] | OMA 1.25 mg/$m^2$ | 1 | 5 months | / | Reached | / | Alive | 27 to 100 % |
| Coude et al. (2012) [29] | OMA 1.25 mg/$m^2$ + nilotinib 800 mg/j | 1 | / | / | Reached | / | Alive | <0.1 % (30 months) |

*N* states for number of patients, *MCyR* for major cytogenetic response, *CCyR* for complete cytogenetic response, *CyR* for cytogenetic response, *OS* for overall survival, and *PFS* for progression-free survival

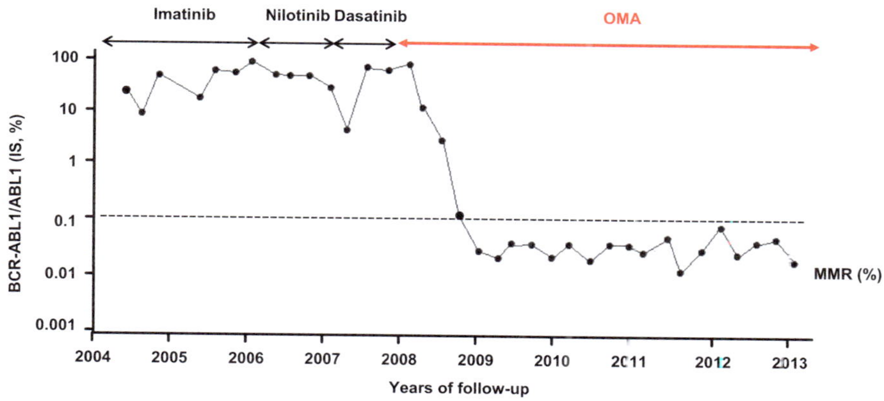


**Fig. 9.4** Long-term molecular follow-up of an interferon-α- and unmutated multi-TKI-resistant chronic phase CML patient treated with OMA

suboptimal cytogenetic response to imatinib with a molecular response observed the majority of patients [24]. In a combination sequence including imatinib + OMA, 63 % of patients reached the CCyR state (versus 20 % without imatinib) and 76 % the MCyR state (versus 46 % without imatinib). The estimated 5-year OS rate was 88 % in this study (Table 9.1) [25]. In a phase 1/2 trial, regardless of the ABL mutational status, Cortes et al. explored the safety and efficacy of OMA in first-line imatinib failure patients. All patients obtained at least a CHR and just 1 a CCyR, with undetectable BCR-ABL transcripts [26]. In our center, OMA demonstrated impressive and long-lasting (>5 years) major molecular response in interferon-α- and multi-TKI-resistant chronic phase CML patient (Fig. 9.4). Recently, data were pooled from 2 phase 2 trials conducted on 122 OMA CML patients (81 in CP, 41 in AP) regardless of the mutation status previously been treated with two or more TKIs introduced OMA as a valuable option for TKI-resistant CML: 20 % of patients in CP achieved a major MCyR (CCyR = 10 %, PCyR = 10 %) with a median duration of MCyR of 18 months. The median overall survival was 34 months [26, 27].

In addition, and interestingly, OMA demonstrated some significant activity in anecdotic observations in patients with a T315I mutation as suspected by us and others [21, 28, 29]. The formal demonstration of its activity was provided by the results of a phase 2 international trial of OMA in 62 chronic phase CML patients harboring the T315I mutation [30]. Complete hematologic response was observed in 48 (77 %) patients, and the median response duration was 9.1 months. Fourteen (23 %) patients achieved MCyR including CCyR in 10 (16 %). The median progression-free survival was 7.7 months (Table 9.1).

### 9.3.2 Omacetaxine in Advanced Phase CML Patients

In accelerated phase resistant to TKI, OMA was able to induce 27 % of major hematologic response and 14 % any cytogenetic response (but no CCyR) for a median duration of 9 months [27], and the median overall survival was 16 months (Table 9.1). Despite poor response rates in this setting, OMA can serve as a bridge toward allogeneic stem cell transplantation, which remains the best option for long-term survival in patients with advanced phase CML (Table 9.1). In blast crisis, OMA does not show any activity in lymphoid blast crisis and very little activity in myeloid blast crisis [31].

## 9.4 Combination of TKI and Interferon-α

### 9.4.1 Imatinib and Interferon-α

Preliminary studies combining high doses of imatinib and pegylated interferon-α have demonstrated its feasibility and showed some restricted activity in this setting [32]. In the long term, imatinib alone fails to control the disease because of resistance or significant intolerance [1, 2], and because interferon-α retains activity on Ph + cells through different means that TKIs do, it was hypothesized that a combination of these two categories of compounds might be successful in the first-line setting. In this perspective, we [33] and others [34, 35] have launched trials combining a 40-kD-branched polyethylene glycol interferon-α improving its tolerability and half-life (Peg-interferon-α-2a Pegasys®, Roche, or Peg-interferon-α-2b ViraferonPeg®, Merck) and imatinib 400 mg/day in first-line patients. These trials demonstrated significant improvements in molecular responses despite increasing toxicities and limitation of progressions but no impact on survival. In one study [34], the improvement was uncertain, even after 5 years [36], due to poor compliance to Peg-interferon-α-2b. A summary of the responses and survival is presented in Table 9.2.

### 9.4.2 TKI2 and Interferon-α

Second-generation TKI (TKI2) such as nilotinib (Tasigna®, Novartis) or dasatinib (Sprycel®, BMS) has shown significantly superior activity to imatinib in randomized trials [37, 38] for cytogenetic responses, major molecular responses (MMR), and deep molecular responses (MR 4 logs (MR4), 4.5 logs (MR4.5), and 5 logs (MR5) [39]) and for nilotinib, a significant limitation of progression. We conducted a national prospective phase 2 trial (NiloPeg trial), combining nilotinib and Peg-interferon-α-2a to evaluate the feasibility, safety, and efficacy of this

**Table 9.2** Overall response rates and survival in chronic phase CML patients receiving a combination of Peg-interferon-α and imatinib first line

| Trials | Drug | *N* | CHR (%) | MCyR (%) | CCyR (%) | OS/PFS (months) | MMR | $MR^{4.5}$ | Median follow-up (months) |
|---|---|---|---|---|---|---|---|---|---|
| Baccarani et al. (2003) [34][a] | IM + Peg 2b | 76 | 99 | 83 | 70 | 98.7/ 97.4 | 48 % | NA | ≥12 |
| Palandri et al. (2008) [36][a] | IM + Peg 2b | 76 | NA | NA | 82 | 96/95 | 65 | 19 | 48 |
| Preudhomme et al. (2010) [33] | IM + Peg 2a | 159 | 91 | NA | 66 | NA/97 | 64 | 16 | 18 |
| Simonsson et al. (2011) [35][b] | IM + Peg 2b | 56 | 100 | NA | 91.1 | 100/100 | 82 | NA | NA |

*N* states for number of patients, *CHR* for complete hematologic response, *MCyR* for major cytogenetic response, *CCyR* for complete cytogenetic response, *OS* for overall survival, *PFS* for progression-free survival, *MMR* for major molecular response, and *MR4.5* for molecular response 4.5 logs

[a]Some cohort of patients with different follow-up

[b]All low Sokal score patients

**Table 9.3** Molecular response rates at 24 months in chronic phase CML patients receiving imatinib, imatinib + Peg-interferon-α, or TKI2 alone or combined to Peg-interferon-α-2a

| Molecular response | French spirit [33] | | DASISION [38] | ENESTnd [37] | NiloPeg [40] |
|---|---|---|---|---|---|
| | IM 400 | IM 400 + Peg-IFN-α-2a | Dasatinib 100 | Nilotinib 600 | Nilo 600 + Peg-IFN-α-2a |
| MMR | 43 % | NA | 64 % | 71 % | 76 % |
| MR4.5 | 21 % | 91 % | NA | 39 % | 49 % |
| MR5 | NA | NA | 17 % | 25 % | 34 % |

Please consider that these results should not be compared one by one.
*MMR* states for major molecular response, *MR4.5* for molecular response 4.5 logs, and MR5 for molecular response 5 logs

combination [40]. Despite additional toxicity, this trial demonstrated the feasibility of this combination and provided extremely high molecular response rates at 1 year, especially deep molecular responses: 72.5 % for MMR, 51 % for MR4, 17 % of MR4.5, and 7 % of MR5, higher than that observed with nilotinib or dasatinib alone or imatinib combined with Peg-interferon-α (see comparison in Table 9.3). Other phase 2 or phase 3 trials combining second-generation TKI and pegylated interferon-α are currently running in France, Germany, and the USA. Such combinations might increase the number of patients eligible for cessation strategies [41].

## 9.5 Conclusion

Despite the considerable success obtained with TKI in the treatment of CML over the past decade, some patients still do not respond optimally to these compounds and new options have to be found: new compounds such as ponatinib, old compounds such as OMA, or new combinations of old and current compounds such as TKI and interferon-α. However we still have to keep in mind for our patients that allogeneic stem cell transplantation remains an attractive alternative in case of failure of these last strategies, in eligible patients.

**Acknowledgments** FEN thanks Barbara White-Meunier, for proofreading this book chapter and the association "Regarde un jour le monde" for their constant support.

## References

1. de Lavallade H, Apperley JF, Khorashad JS, Milojkovic D, Reid AG, Bua M, et al. Imatinib for newly diagnosed patients with chronic myeloid leukemia: incidence of sustained responses in an intention-to-treat analysis. J Clin Oncol. 2008;26(20):3358–63.
2. Deininger M, O'Brien SG, Guilhot F. International randomized study of interferon vs STI571 (IRIS) 8-year follow up: sustained survival and low risk for progression or events in patients

with newly diagnosed chronic myeloid leukemia in chronic phase (CML-CP) treated with imatinib. Blood. 2009;114(22):1126.
3. Cortes JE, Kantarjian H, Shah NP, Bixby D, Mauro MJ, Flinn I, et al. Ponatinib in refractory Philadelphia chromosome-positive leukemias. N Engl J Med. 2012;367(22):2075–88.
4. Cortes JE, Kim DW, Pinilla-Ibarz J, le Coutre P, Paquette R, Chuah C, et al. A phase 2 trial of ponatinib in Philadelphia chromosome-positive leukemias. N Engl J Med. 2013;369(19):1783–96.
5. Hamilton A, Helgason GV, Schemionek M, Zhang B, Myssina S, Allan EK, et al. Chronic myeloid leukemia stem cells are not dependent on Bcr-Abl kinase activity for their survival. Blood. 2012;119(6):1501–10.
6. Talpaz M, McCredie KB, Mavligit GM, Gutterman JU. Leukocyte interferon-induced myeloid cytoreduction in chronic myelogenous leukemia. Blood. 1983;62(3):689–92.
7. Bonifazi F, de Vivo A, Rosti G, Guilhot F, Guilhot J, Trabacchi E, et al. Chronic myeloid leukemia and interferon-alpha: a study of complete cytogenetic responders. Blood. 2001;98(10):3074–81.
8. Cortes J, Jabbour E, Kantarjian H, Yin CC, Shan J, O'Brien S, et al. Dynamics of BCR-ABL kinase domain mutations in chronic myeloid leukemia after sequential treatment with multiple tyrosine kinase inhibitors. Blood. 2007;110(12):4005–11.
9. Nicolini FE, Corm S, Le QH, Sorel N, Hayette S, Bories D, et al. Mutation status and clinical outcome of 89 imatinib mesylate-resistant chronic myelogenous leukemia patients: a retrospective analysis from the French intergroup of CML (Fi(j)-LMC group). Leukemia. 2006;20(6):1061–6.
10. Nicolini FE, Ibrahim AR, Soverini S, Martinelli G, Muller MC, Hochhaus A, et al. The BCR-ABLT315I mutation compromises survival in chronic phase chronic myelogenous leukemia patients resistant to tyrosine kinase inhibitors, in a matched pair analysis. Haematologica. 2013;98(10):1510–6.
11. Soverini S, Colarossi S, Gnani A, Rosti G, Castagnetti F, Poerio A, et al. Contribution of ABL kinase domain mutations to imatinib resistance in different subsets of Philadelphia-positive patients: by the GIMEMA Working Party on Chronic Myeloid Leukemia. Clin Cancer Res. 2006;12(24):7374–9.
12. Nicolini FE, Basak GW, Soverini S, Martinelli G, Mauro MJ, Muller MC, et al. Allogeneic stem cell transplantation for patients harboring T315I BCR-ABL mutated leukemias. Blood. 2011;118(20):5697–700.
13. Nicolini FE, Corm S, Le QH, Roche-Lestienne C, Preudhomme C. The prognosis impact of BCR-ABL P-loop mutations: worse or not worse? Leukemia. 2007;21(2):193–4.
14. Cortes JE, Kim DW, Pinilla-Ibarz J, Le Coutre P, Paquette R, Chuah C, et al. Long-term follow-up of ponatinib efficacy and safety in the Phase 2 PACE Trial. Blood. 2014;124(21): Abstract 3135.
15. Nicolini FE, Gagnieu MC, Heiblig M, Blond E, Legros L, Guillermin Y. Cardio-vascular events occurring on ponatinib In chronic phase Chronic Myeloid Leukemia patients, preliminary analysis of a multicenter cohort. Blood. 2013;122(21): Abstract 4020.
16. Corm S, Roche L, Micol JB, Coiteux V, Bossard N, Nicolini FE, et al. Changes in the dynamics of the excess mortality rate in chronic phase-chronic myeloid leukemia over 1990-2007: a population study. Blood. 2011;118(16):4331–7.
17. O'Brien S, Kantarjian H, Keating M, Beran M, Koller C, Robertson LE, et al. Homoharringtonine therapy induces responses in patients with chronic myelogenous leukemia in late chronic phase. Blood. 1995;86(9):3322–6
18. Kantarjian HM, Talpaz M, Santini V, Murgo A, Cheson B, O'Brien SM. Homoharringtonine: history, current research, and future direction. Cancer. 2001;92(6):1591–605.
19. Cortes J, Digumarti R, Parikh PM, Wetzler M, Lipton JH, Hochhaus A, et al. Phase 2 study of subcutaneous omacetaxine mepesuccinate for chronic-phase chronic myeloid leukemia patients resistant to or intolerant of tyrosine kinase inhibitors. Am J Hematol. 2013;88(5):350–4.

20. Nicolini FE, Chomel JC, Roy L, Legros L, Chabane K, Ducastelle S, et al. The durable clearance of the T315I BCR-ABL mutated clone in chronic phase chronic myelogenous leukemia patients on omacetaxine allows tyrosine kinase inhibitor rechallenge. Clin Lymphoma Myeloma Leuk. 2010;10(5):394–9.
21. Legros L, Hayette S, Nicolini FE, Raynaud S, Chabane K, Magaud JP, et al. BCR-ABL(T315I) transcript disappearance in an imatinib-resistant CML patient treated with homoharringtonine: a new therapeutic challenge? Leukemia. 2007;21(10):2204–6.
22. O'Brien S, Talpaz M, Cortes J, Shan J, Giles FJ, Faderl S, et al. Simultaneous homoharringtonine and interferon-alpha in the treatment of patients with chronic-phase chronic myelogenous leukemia. Cancer. 2002;94(7):2024–32.
23. Burton C, Ranger A, Nadal E. Semi-synthetic homoharringtonine (MyelostatVR) for chronic myeloid leukemia in accelerated phase after imatinib failure. Blood. 2003;102(908): Abstract.
24. Marin D, Kaeda JS, Andreasson C, Saunders SM, Bua M, Olavarria E, et al. Phase I/II trial of adding semisynthetic homoharringtonine in chronic myeloid leukemia patients who have achieved partial or complete cytogenetic response on imatinib. Cancer. 2005;103(9):1850–5.
25. O'Brien S, Giles F, Talpaz M, Cortes J, Rios MB, Shan J, et al. Results of triple therapy with interferon-alpha, cytarabine, and homoharringtonine, and the impact of adding imatinib to the treatment sequence in patients with Philadelphia chromosome-positive chronic myelogenous leukemia in early chronic phase. Cancer. 2003;98(5):888–93.
26. Cortes JE, Nicolini FE, Wetzler M, Lipton JH, Akard L, Craig A, et al. Subcutaneous omacetaxine mepesuccinate in patients with chronic-phase chronic myeloid leukemia previously treated with 2 or more tyrosine kinase inhibitors including imatinib. Clin Lymphoma Myeloma Leuk. 2013;13(5):584–91.
27. Nicolini FE, Khoury HJ, Akard L, Rea D, Kantarjian H, Baccarani M, et al. Omacetaxine mepesuccinate for patients with accelerated phase chronic myeloid leukemia with resistance or intolerance to two or more tyrosine kinase inhibitors. Haematologica. 2013;98(7):78–9.
28. de Lavallade H, Khorashad JS, Davis HP, Milojkovic D, Kaeda JS, Goldman JM, et al. Interferon-alpha or homoharringtonine as salvage treatment for chronic myeloid leukemia patients who acquire the T315I BCR-ABL mutation. Blood. 2007;110(7):2779–80.
29. Coude MM, Luycx O, Cariou ME, Maarek O, Dombret H, Cayuela JM, et al. Undetectable molecular residual disease after omacetaxine and nilotinib combination therapy in an imatinib-resistant chronic myeloid leukaemia patient harbouring the BCR-ABL1 T315I gatekeeper mutation. Br J Haematol. 2012;157(3):407–10.
30. Cortes J, Lipton JH, Rea D, Digumarti R, Chuah C, Nanda N, et al. Phase 2 study of subcutaneous omacetaxine mepesuccinate after TKI failure in patients with chronic-phase CML with T315I mutation. Blood. 2012;120(13):2573–80.
31. Khoury HJ, Cortes J, Baccarani M, Wetzler M, Masszi T, Digumarti R, et al. Omacetaxine mepesuccinate in patients with advanced chronic myeloid leukemia with resistance or intolerance to tyrosine kinase inhibitors. Leuk Lymphoma. 2015;56(1):120–7.
32. Nicolini FE, Hayette S, Legros L, Rousselot P, Maloisel F, Tulliez M, et al. Pegylated IFN-alpha2a combined to imatinib mesylate 600mg daily can induce complete cytogenetic and molecular responses in a subset of chronic phase CML patients refractory to IFN alone or to imatinib 600mg daily alone. Leuk Res. 2011;35(1):80–6.
33. Preudhomme C, Guilhot J, Nicolini FE, Guerci-Bresler A, Rigal-Huguet F, Maloisel F, et al. Imatinib plus peginterferon alfa-2a in chronic myeloid leukemia. N Engl J Med. 2010;363(26):2511–21.
34. Baccarani M, Martinelli G, Rosti G, Trabacchi E, Testoni N, Bassi S, et al. Imatinib and pegylated human recombinant interferon-alpha2b in early chronic-phase chronic myeloid leukemia. Blood. 2004;104(13):4245–51.
35. Simonsson B, Gedde-Dahl T, Markevarn B, Remes K, Stentoft J, Almqvist A, et al. Combination of pegylated IFN-alpha2b with imatinib increases molecular response rates in patients with low- or intermediate-risk chronic myeloid leukemia. Blood. 2011;118 (12):3228–35.

36. Palandri F, Iacobucci I, Castagnetti F, Testoni N, Poerio A, Amabile M, et al. Front-line treatment of Philadelphia positive chronic myeloid leukemia with imatinib and interferon-alpha: 5-year outcome. Haematologica. 2008;93(5):770–4.
37. Kantarjian HM, Hochhaus A, Saglio G, De Souza C, Flinn IW, Stenke L, et al. Nilotinib versus imatinib for the treatment of patients with newly diagnosed chronic phase, Philadelphia chromosome-positive, chronic myeloid leukaemia: 24-month minimum follow-up of the phase 3 randomised ENESTnd trial. Lancet Oncol. 2011;12(9):841–51.
38. Kantarjian HM, Shah NP, Cortes JE, Baccarani M, Agarwal MB, Undurraga MS, et al. Dasatinib or imatinib in newly diagnosed chronic-phase chronic myeloid leukemia: 2-year follow-up from a randomized phase 3 trial (DASISION). Blood. 2012;119(5):1123–9.
39. Cross NC, White HE, Muller MC, Saglio G, Hochhaus A. Standardized definitions of molecular response in chronic myeloid leukemia. Leukemia. 2012;26(10):2172–5.
40. Nicolini FE, Etienne G, Dubruille V, Roy L, Huguet F, Legros L, et al. Nilotinib and peginterferon alfa-2a for newly diagnosed chronic-phase chronic myeloid leukaemia (NiloPeg): a multicentre, non-randomised, open-label phase 2 study. Lancet Haematol. 2015;2(1):37–46.
41. O'Brien S, Kantarjian H, Koller C, Feldman E, Beran M, Andreeff M, et al. Sequential homoharringtonine and interferon-alpha in the treatment of early chronic phase chronic myelogenous leukemia. Blood. 1999;93(12):4149–53.
42. Kantarjian HM, Talpaz M, Smith TL, Cortes J, Giles FJ, Rios MB, et al. Homoharringtonine and low-dose cytarabine in the management of late chronic-phase chronic myelogenous leukemia. J Clin Oncol. 2000;18(20):3513–21.
43. Rea D, Nicolini FE, Tulliez M, Rousselot P, Guilhot F, Gardembas M, et al. Dasatinib or nilotinib discontinuation in chronic phase (CP)-Chronic Myeloid Leukemia (CML) patients (pts) with durably undetectable BCR-ABL transcripts: Interim analysis of the STOP 2G-TKI study with a minimum follow-up of 12 months – on behalf of the French CML Group Filmc. Blood. 2014;124(21): Abstract 811.

# Chapter 10
# Safety Profiles of First-Line TKIs and Managing Adverse Effects

**Gianantonio Rosti, Fausto Castagnetti, Gabriele Gugliotta, and Michele Baccarani**

**Abstract** The treatment armamentarium of chronic myeloid leukemia (CML) is based on at least five TKIs, employed either in first-line CP (imatinib, dasatinib, and nilotinib) and in second and third line (dasatinib, nilotinib, bosutinib, and ponatinib). These drugs share the same target of interest (BCR-ABL) but have profound different off-target effects. In turn, the general spectrum of adverse events experienced by the treated patients, either clinical symptoms, biochemical abnormalities, or severe AEs (or "complications"), varies considerably. SAEs are more frequent with second- and third-generation TKIs, and from this point of view, imatinib remains the safest drug. The early identification of CML patient candidates to experience more frequently SAEs with second (and third)-generation TKIs is of course part of the treatment decision process where the right balance between risk and benefit should be accomplished. Second-generation TKIs, nilotinib and dasatinib, are considered generally to be better tolerated than imatinib. However, two types of complications are described more frequently with nilotinib and ponatinib (cardiovascular, in general, and PAOD in particular) and with dasatinib (pleural effusions and pulmonary hypertension) if compared with imatinib. These two types of complications deserve a particular attention.

**Keywords** TKIs for CML • Toxicity • Management

The treatment armamentarium of chronic myeloid leukemia (CML) is based on at least five TKIs, employed either in first-line CP (imatinib, dasatinib, and nilotinib) and in second and third line (dasatinib, nilotinib, bosutinib, and ponatinib) [1–3]. These drugs share the same target of interest (BCR-ABL) but have profound different off-target effects (Table 10.1). In turn, the general spectrum of adverse events experienced by the treated patients, either clinical symptoms, biochemical abnormalities, or severe AEs (or "complications"), varies considerably. SAEs are

G. Rosti (✉) • F. Castagnetti • G. Gugliotta • M. Baccarani
Ematologia e Oncologia Medica "Seràgnoli", St. Orsola University Hospital – Pavillon 8, Via Massarenti, 9, 40138 Bologna, Italy
e-mail: gianantonio.rosti@unibo.it



M. Kizaki (ed.), *Molecular Pathogenesis and Treatment of Chronic Myelogenous Leukemia*, DOI 10.1007/978-4-431-55714-2_10

**Table 10.1** TKIs employed in CML treatment in first and further lines

| | Imatinib | Nilotinib | Dasatinib | Bosutinib | Ponatinib |
|---|---|---|---|---|---|
| First line, approved dose | 400 mg OD | 300 mg BID | 100 mg OD | NA | NA |
| Second line, approved dose | 300–400 mg BID | 400 mg BID | 70 mg BID or 140 mg OD | 500 mg OD | 45 mg OD |
| Plasma half-life | ~20 h | ~15 h | ~5 h | ~24 h | ~19 h |
| Plasma concentration, peak | 4202 ± 1272 | 2329 ± 772 | 133 ± 74 | ~392 | 145 ± 73 |
| Plasma concentration, through | 2062 ± 1334 | 1923 ± 1233 | 5.5 ± 1.4 | ~268 | 64 ± 29 |
| IC50, BCR-ABL1 | 260–679 | 10–25 | 0.8–1.8 | 42 | 0.5 |
| IC50, PDGFRα | 72 | 75 | 2.9 | 3.0 | 1.1 |
| IC50, c-Kit | 99 | 209 | 18 | 10,000 | 12 |
| IC50, Src | >1000 | >1000 | 0.1 | 3.0 | 5.4 |
| IC50, VEGFR2 | 10,000 | 3720 | NA | NA | 1.5 |
| IC50, BTK | >5000 | NA | 1.1 | 2.5 | 849 |

more frequent with second- and third-generation TKIs (Table 10.1), and from this point of view, imatinib remains the safest drug. The early identification of CML patient candidates to experience more frequently SAEs with second (and third)-generation TKIs is of course part of the treatment decision process where the right balance between risk and benefit should be accomplished. Second-generation TKIs, nilotinib and dasatinib, are considered generally to be better tolerated than imatinib. However, two types of complications are described more frequently with nilotinib and ponatinib (cardiovascular, in general, and PAOD in particular) and with dasatinib (pleural effusions and pulmonary hypertension) if compared with imatinib. These two types of complications deserve a particular attention.

Cardiovascular events leading to ischemic heart disease (IHD), ischemic cerebrovascular events (ICVE), or peripheral artery occlusive disease (PAOD) are an emerging type of toxicity in CML patients treated with nilotinib or ponatinib. The incidence of PAOD ranges between 1.2 and 16.7 % with a potential increase frequency over time. When ankle-brachial index (ABI) has been used prospectively to screen for asymptomatic PAOD (and Doppler US for confirmation), an incidence of >10 % of asymptomatic arterial disease was found [4, 5] (significantly higher with nilotinib as compared to imatinib). Besides PAOD, other reports revealed an increase incidence of IHD and ICVE with nilotinib (rep. in six). The ENESTnd at 72 months revealed an incidence of 12.9 % for all cardiovascular events and of 5.8 %, 2.3 %, and 3.8 % for IHD, ICVE, and PAOD, respectively [7].

Similarly, ponatinib employed in second-line treatment (45 mg OAD) is associated with an increased risk for vascular events (arterial and venous): the latest update (at 3 years) showed a 22 % rate for all cardiovascular events [8]. With ponatinib, the importance of dose intensity is evident [9]. In contrast, there are no data suggesting a higher risk of cardiovascular events in patients treated with imatinib, bosutinib, or dasatinib [10–15]. All these data suggest that arterial events are not a class effect of all the TKIs employed to treat CML (any line of treatment) but specific toxicities related to nilotinib and ponatinib. Both in nilotinib and ponatinib trials, patients developing vascular complications mostly had preexisting CV risk factors [6]. So far, nilotinib (and ponatinib) seemingly determines an increase risk of arterial events exacerbating a preexisting atherosclerotic condition (however, there are reports even in patients without CV risk factor baseline). Early [16, 17] and later [7] trials showed the capacity of nilotinib to promote an increase in fasting blood glucose. Hypercholesterolemia, a well-recognized risk factor for atherosclerosis, has also been observed, even if not constantly, with nilotinib [4] possibly secondary to hyperglycemia. Other possible mechanisms include a pro-inflammatory condition under nilotinib and genetic predisposition [18], direct pro-atherogenic and anti-angiogenic effects on vascular endothelial cells, and the induction of hyperhomocysteinemia. The proper screening of patient candidate to receive nilotinib (and ponatinib) is pivotal, including either ABI or duplex ultrasonography in all newly diagnosed patients with CML and cardiovascular risk factors or positive claudication questionnaire. Moreover, the chemistry profile (baseline and every 4–6 months) should include fasting glucose, HbA1c, lipids (cholesterol, LDL, HDL, and triglycerides), C-reactive protein, and creatinine. Moreover, the calculation of the CV risk score should be done for any new CML patient based on national or international guidelines.

The risk of effusions exists with all the TKIs currently indicated for CML in first line but is much most commonly seen with dasatinib. In second-line treatment with dasatinib, the median time of appearance is 5–11 months [19, 20], but it could be delayed until 2 years. In first-line treatment, time to pleural effusion was 10 months, and most effusions (89 %) occurred more than 8 weeks into treatment [21]. The overall cumulative incidence in first and second line treatment can reach 25–30 % of all the patients treated with dasatinib 100 mg OAD. Although the risk diminished with time, PE can occur along all the treatment. In second-line treatment, previous or concomitant cardiac disease and hypertension seem to be the more common predisposing conditions [22, 23]. Also, BID schedule [22], advanced phases, hypercholesterolemia, a previous history of autoimmune disorders, and skin rashes experienced during imatinib therapy have been identified as risk factors [23]. Older age is also associated with PE [19], and in patients older than 60 years, the presence of concomitant pulmonary disease, initial daily dose of dasatinib (140 mg vs 100 mg), and higher comorbidity index were associated with PE. Apart from knowing the conditions which could increase the risk of PE, patients and doctors must be vigilant on the presence of cough, dyspnea, or chest pain. Physical exam must include auscultation, and it is prudent but not mandatory to order an X-ray exam every year.

However, to the scope of this brief commentary, it is more relevant to look to the future as far as the burden of adverse events, not severe by definition but central to determine compliance of the patients and QOL. In fact, the evaluation of the response for many years (all the past decade) attracted of course the attention of researchers; on the other hand, while collection of the incidence and rate of biochemical and laboratory abnormalities, recorded objectively, continued to determine the overall safety profile of different TKIs, providing useful instruments of management, the incidence of other, and clinical side effects (the majority of AEs referred by the patients) continued to be based on CTC grading system. This way to collect symptoms is, once more, useful to indicate the generic level of toxicity and consequent TKI treatment optimization but not ideal to understand to what extent the patients QOL is affected. This aspect is of particular interest, in general and because QOL perception affects, in turn, compliance and adherence: a lower than ideal adherence may easily jeopardize treatment results, inducing refractoriness to the treatment itself [24]. All available TKIs for first-line therapy, that is, imatinib (i.e., first-generation TKIs) and dasatinib or nilotinib (i.e., second-generation TKIs), have side effects that should be considered when deciding which therapy is best for the individual patient. Imatinib was, since 2001, and remains the golden standard for many patients with CML. While survival of patients who respond to imatinib is not different from that of the general population, it is important to consider that these patients require lifelong therapy that affects their health-related quality of life [25, 26]. The most frequently reported long-term, chronic adverse effects of imatinib therapy include edema, nausea, muscle cramps, and musculoskeletal pain. More recently, "second-generation" tyrosine kinase inhibitors (i.e., dasatinib and nilotinib) have been approved for first-line use in CML patients, based on results from two large randomized trials. This makes the choice of tyrosine kinase inhibitor to be used as first-line therapy a major challenge. While imatinib, dasatinib, and nilotinib have different toxicity profiles, they have been reported to produce similar outcomes in terms of progression-free survival and overall survival. In most studies, recording and assessing the type, the intensity, and the duration of the side effects are not planned, apart from formal reference to some internationally recognized scoring systems (e.g., NCI, SWOG). The data obtained with this methodology can be very different, even in company-sponsored, registrative studies. For example, the incidence of any grade fatigue, muscle pain, and joint/bone pain with imatinib varied in published experience (only RCTs considered) between 8 and 54 %, 34 and 95 %, 0 and 28 %, respectively [27]. It has, therefore, been suggested that, regardless of which drug is used as first-line therapy, timely management of side effects, changing the tyrosine kinase inhibitor when required, is a critical factor for optimal management of patients. In this scenario, close monitoring of relevant symptoms experienced by patients is pivotal to facilitate a timely switch to other available tyrosine kinase inhibitors. Instrumental to the physician's ability to consider alternative treatment strategies, however, is an accurate estimation of symptom severity and overall health status of their patients. Experience in solid tumors has shown that physicians tend to rate symptoms as being less severe than their patients do. Also, patients' self-reported symptoms have been shown to reflect daily health status better than physician-reported symptoms do. Following these considerations, the National Cancer Institute sponsored initiative to create a version of the Institute's Common Terminology Criteria for Adverse Events (PRO-CTCAE) that can be completed by patients themselves [28–30], providing direct feedback from patients on their symptom experience during treatment. These instruments will be of particular value in observational studies and randomized clinical trials (RCTs). Another important area of application of PRO instruments would be their implementation in routine practice, facilitating the discussion of health problems between patients and physicians and supporting the early identification of those CML patients for whom a given therapy is particularly burdensome.

## References


1. Baccarani M, Deininger MW, Rosti G, et al. European LeukemiaNet recommendations for the management of chronic myeloid leukemia. Blood. 2013;122(6):872–84.
2. O'Brien S, Abboud CN, Akhtari M, et al. Clinical practice guidelines in oncology. Chronic myelogenous leukemia, Version 3, National Comprehensive Cancer Network (NCCN). 2014. http://www.nccn.org.
3. Baccarani M, Saglio G, Goldman J, et al. Evolving concepts in the management of chronic myeloid leukemia: recommendations from an expert panel on behalf of the European LeukemiaNet. Blood. 2006;108:1809–20.
4. Kim TD, Rea D, Schwarz M, et al. Peripheral artery occlusive disease in chronic phase chronic myeloid leukemia patients treated with nilotinib or imatinib. Leukemia. 2013;27:1316–21.
5. Labussiere-Wallet H, Guillermin Y, Etienne M, et al. Analysis of clinical arterial and metabolic parameters in chronic phase CML patients on nilotinib in a single center cohort. ASH Annu Meet Abstr. 2012;120:3756.
6. Rea D, Mirault T, Raffoux E, et al. Usefulness of the 2012 European CVD risk assessment model to identify patients at high risk of cardiovascular events during nilotinib therapy in chronic myeloid leukemia. Leukemia. 2015;29(5):1206–9.
7. Larson RA, Kim DW, Issaragrilsil S, Coutre PL, Dorlhiac Llacer PE, G Etienne, Clark RE, Flinn I, Nakamae H, Hochhaus A, Saglio G, Kantarjian HM, Donohue B, Deng W, Menssen HD, Hughes TP. Efficacy and safety of nilotinib (NIL) vs imatinib (IM) in patients (pts) with newly diagnosed chronic myeloid leukemia in chronic phase (CML-CP): long-term follow-up (f/u) of ENESTnd [Clinically relevant abstract] program: oral and poster abstracts. Presented at ASH 2015. 2014 abstract no. 4541.
8. Cortes JE, Kim D-W, Pinilla-Ibarz J, Le Coutre P, Paquette R, Chuah C, Nicolini FE, Apperley JF, Khoury HJ, Talpaz M, DiPersio JF, DeAngelo DJ, Abruzzese E, Rea D, Baccarani M, Müller MC, Gambacorti-Passerini C, Lustgarten S, Rivera VM, Clackson T, Turner CD, Haluska FG, Guilhot F, Deininger MW, Hochhaus A, Hughes TP, Shah NP, Kantarjian HM. Long-term follow-up of ponatinib efficacy and safety in the phase 2 PACE trial [Clinically relevant abstract]. Program: Oral and poster abstracts session: 632. Chronic myeloid leukemia: therapy: poster II. West Building, Level 1 (Moscone Center); 2014:Abstract 3135.
9. Knickerbocker R, Dorer DJ, Haluska FG, Baccarani M, Cortes JE, Hochhaus A, Talpaz M. Impact of dose intensity of ponatinib on selected adverse events: multivariate analyses from a pooled population of clinical trial patients [Clinically relevant abstract] program: oral and poster abstracts. ASH 2014. 2014 abstract no. 4546.
10. Cortes JE, Kim DW, Pinilla-Ibarz J, Coutre PL, Paquette R, Chuah C, Nicolini FE, Apperley JF, Jean Khoury H, Talpaz M, DiPersio JF, DeAngelo DJ, Abruzzese E, Rea D, Baccarani M, Müller MC, Gambacorti-Passerini C, Lustgarten S, Rivera VM, Clackson T, Turner CD, Haluska FG, Guilhot F, Deininger MW, Hochhaus A, Hughes TP, Shah NP, Kantarjian HM. 3135 Long-term follow-up of ponatinib efficacy and safety in the phase 2 PACE trial [Clinically relevant abstract] program: oral and poster abstracts. ASH abstract: Blood. 2013;122(21):1482.
11. Cortes J, Saglio G, Baccarani M, Kantarjian HM, Mayer J, Boqué C, Shah NP, Chuah C, Casanova L, Narayanan G, Bradley-Garelik B, Manos G, Hochhaus A. Final study results of the phase 3 dasatinib versus imatinib in newly diagnosed chronic myeloid leukemia in chronic phase (CML-CP) trial (DASISION, CA180-056) [Clinically relevant abstract] program: oral and poster abstracts. ASH 2014. 2014 abstract no. 152.
12. Gambacorti-Passerini C, Antolini L, Mahon FX, et al. Multicenter independent assessment of outcomes in chronic myeloid leukemia patients treated with imatinib. J Natl Cancer Inst. 2011;103:553–61.
13. Gambacorti-Passerini C, Cortes JE, Lipton JH, et al. Safety of bosutinib versus imatinib in the phase 3 BELA trial in newly diagnosed chronic phase chronic myeloid leukemia. Am J Hematol. 2014;89:947–53.

14. Hochhaus A, O'Brien SG, Guilhot F, et al. Six-year follow-up of patients receiving imatinib for the first-line treatment of chronic myeloid leukemia. Leukemia. 2009;23:1054–61.
15. Kantarjian H, Shah NP, Hochhaus A, et al. Dasatinib versus imatinib in newly diagnosed chronic-phase chronic myeloid leukemia. N Engl J Med. 2010;362:2260–70.
16. Kantarjian HM, Giles F, Gattermann N, et al. Nilotinib (formerly AMN107), a highly selective BCR-ABL tyrosine kinase inhibitor, is effective in patients with Philadelphia chromosome-positive chronic myelogenous leukemia in chronic phase following imatinib resistance and intolerance. Blood. 2007;110:3540–6.
17. le Coutre P, Ottmann OG, Giles F, et al. Nilotinib (formerly AMN107), a highly selective BCR-ABL tyrosine kinase inhibitor, is active in patients with imatinib-resistant or -intolerant accelerated-phase chronic myelogenous leukemia. Blood. 2008;111:1834–9.
18. Aprile L, Puccetti L, Galimberti S, et al. Atherothrombotic risk and TKIs treatment in chronic myeloid leukemia patients: a role for genetic predisposition and pro-inflammatory/pro-oxidative status? Blood. 2013;122(21):1482.
19. Porkka K, Khoury HJ, Paquette RL, Matloub Y, Sinha R, Cortes JE. Dasatinib 100 mg once daily minimizes the occurrence of pleural effusion in patients with chronic myeloid leukemia in chronic phase and efficacy is unaffected in patients who develop pleural effusion. Cancer. 2010;116(2):377–86.
20. Latagliata R, Breccia M, Fava C, Stagno F, Tiribelli M, Luciano L, et al. Incidence, risk factors and management of pleural effusions during dasatinib treatment in unselected elderly patients with chronic myelogenous leukaemia. Hematol Oncol. 2013;31(2):363–9.
21. Porkka K, Baccarani M, Cortes J, Hochhaus A, Kantarjian H, Shah N, et al. Pleural effusion in patients with chronic-phase chronic myeloid leukemia (CML-CP) who received first-line dasatinib in the DASISION trial: patient characteristics, management, and outcomes. Haematologica. 16th Congress of the EHA. 2011. p. 692.
22. Quintas-Cardama A, Kantarjian H, O'Brien S, Borthakur G, Bruzzi J, Munden R, et al. Pleural effusion in patients with chronic myelogenous leukemia treated with dasatinib after imatinib failure. J Clin Oncol. 2007;25(25):3908–14.
23. de Lavallade H, Punnialingam S, Milojkovic D, Bua M, Khorashad JS, Gabriel IH, et al. Pleural effusions in patients with chronic myeloid leukaemia treated with dasatinib may have an immune-mediated pathogenesis. Br J Haematol. 2008;141(5):745–7.
24. Marin D. Initial choice of therapy among plenty for newly diagnosed chronic myeloid leukemia. Hematol Am Soc Hematol Educ Prog. 2012;2012:115–21.
25. Efficace F, Cardoni A, Cottone F, et al. Tyrosine-kinase inhibitors and patient-reported outcomes in chronic myeloid leukemia: a systematic review. Leuk Res. 2013;37:206–13.
26. Efficace F, Baccarani M, Breccia M, et al. Health-related quality of life in chronic myeloid leukemia patients receiving long-term therapy with imatinib compared with the general population. Blood. 2011;118:4554–60.
27. Baccarani M, Efficace F, Rosti G. Moving towards patient-centered decision-making in chronic myeloid leukemia: assessment of quality of life and symptom burden. Haematologica. 2014;99(2):205–8.
28. Williams LA, Gonzalez AG, Ault P, et al. Measuring the symptom burden associated with the treatment of chronic myeloid leukemia. Blood. 2013;122:641–7.
29. Efficace F, Baccarani M, Breccia M, et al. International development of an EORTC questionnaire for assessing health-related quality of life in chronic myeloid leukemia patients: the EORTC QLQ-CML24. Qual Life Res. 2014a;23(3):825–36.
30. Efficace F, Rosti G, Aaronson N, et al. Patient versus physician symptom and health status reporting in chronic myeloid leukemia. Haematologica. 2014b;99(4):788–93.

# Chapter 11
# Molecular Mechanism of TKI Resistance and Potential Approaches to Overcome Resistance

**Hein Than, Charles Chuah, and S. Tiong Ong**

**Abstract** There has been a remarkable improvement in the survival of patients with chronic myeloid leukaemia (CML) in chronic phase since the introduction of tyrosine kinase inhibitors (TKIs). However there are a significant proportion of patients with CML who are resistant to TKIs and are at risk of subsequent transformation to the accelerated and blast phases of CML, which are associated with poor survival. Further, while substantial response heterogeneity exists among patients treated with TKIs, almost all patients, including those with complete molecular remission, will continue to harbour quiescent leukaemic stem cells (LSCs). Although ABL1-kinase domain mutations that impair TKI activity have been linked to drug resistance and blastic transformation, more recent work has highlighted several genetic and epigenetic mechanisms dependent and independent of BCR-ABL1. Interesting interplays between LSCs and intracellular signalling pathways, as well as important contributions from the bone marrow microenvironment, have also been recently described. Several preclinical and clinical studies on

H. Than
Department of Haematology, Singapore General Hospital, 20 College Road, Singapore 169856, Singapore

C. Chuah
Department of Haematology, Singapore General Hospital, 20 College Road, Singapore 169856, Singapore

Program for Cancer and Stem Cell Biology, Duke-NUS Graduate Medical School, 8 College Road, Singapore 169857, Singapore

S.T. Ong (✉)
Department of Haematology, Singapore General Hospital, 20 College Road, Singapore 169856, Singapore

Program for Cancer and Stem Cell Biology, Duke-NUS Graduate Medical School, 8 College Road, Singapore 169857, Singapore

Department of Medical Oncology, National Cancer Centre, 11 Hospital Drive, Singapore 169610, Singapore

Department of Medicine, Duke University Medical Center, Durham, NC, USA
e-mail: sintiong.ong@duke-nus.edu.sg



M. Kizaki (ed.), *Molecular Pathogenesis and Treatment of Chronic Myelogenous Leukemia*, DOI 10.1007/978-4-431-55714-2_11

combining new therapeutic targets with tyrosine kinase inhibitors are underway in efforts to overcome the problem of TKI resistance in CML.

**Keywords** CML • Resistance • TKI

## 11.1 Introduction

Chronic myeloid leukaemia (CML) is a myeloproliferative disorder defined by the presence of the Philadelphia chromosome (Ph), which is as a result of the t(9; 22) reciprocal chromosomal translocation that in turn generates the BCR-ABL1 fusion protein. Tyrosine kinase inhibitors (TKIs) targeting the constitutive kinase activity of BCR-ABL1 have revolutionized the treatment of CML and have turned a previously deadly disease into a chronic condition [1]. Furthermore, patients with chronic phase (CP) CML who achieve deeper responses [complete cytogenetic response (CCyR) or major molecular response (MMR)] with TKIs have a superior progression-free and overall survival compared with those who do not [2, 3]. However about 5–10 % of patients on imatinib remain at risk of transformation to accelerated phase (AP) or blast crisis (BC) with poor survival rates [4].

## 11.2 Resistance to TKIs

Resistance to TKIs can be defined as failure to achieve an optimal level of BCR-ABL1 transcript at defined time points or loss of MMR, CCyR, or complete haematological response (CHR) at any time, as mentioned in the European LeukemiaNet (ELN) recommendations in 2013 [5]. Further, current clinical guidelines define a set of time-dependent milestones to be reached in evaluating TKI response since optimal molecular response as early as 3 months has been shown to be predictive of long-term outcome and survival of CML patients on imatinib and nilotinib [6, 7].

Clinically, resistance can also be divided into primary resistance and secondary resistance. The former is a failure to achieve a significant haematological or cytogenetic or molecular response following initiation of therapy, whereas the latter is the progressive loss of an initial response to TKIs [8, 9]. Here it is important to emphasize that primary and secondary resistance are clinical definitions and do not imply that a particular resistance mechanism is at play, e.g. secondary resistance can be due to germ line as well as acquired resistance mechanisms [10].

The molecular mechanisms that cause TKI resistance and progression to BC have been extensively studied and can be divided into those that depend on BCR-ABL1 reactivation and those that occur independently of BCR-ABL1. Among the former are mutations in the ABL kinase domain that impair binding of TKIs to their target and amplification of the *BCR-ABL1* gene resulting in overexpression of the oncoprotein [11–22]. Several other resistance-conferring mechanisms independent of BCR-ABL1 have also been described and include those that alter intracellular concentrations of TKIs and activation of alternative transforming pathways [8, 9, 23–27]. With respect to persistence of LSCs, factors that are intrinsic to the LSCs, as well as those that are extrinsic and arising from the microenvironment, have also been recently implicated.

## *11.2.1* BCR-ABL1-*Dependent Mechanisms*

### 11.2.1.1 *ABL1*-Kinase Domain Mutations

The emergence of clones with point mutations in the *ABL*1-kinase domain is the most frequently described mechanism of resistance in patients treated with TKIs. *ABL1*-kinase mutations are detected in about 50 % of patients who fail TKIs and experience disease progression [13, 16, 28–30]. Interestingly, clinically relevant mutations have been detected in patients who have never been exposed to TKIs, suggesting that such clones arise stochastically and expand only when the selective pressure of TKI therapy is applied [14]. Consistent with this notion, the probability of detecting mutant clones in patients with low disease burden is less than those with high disease burden [17, 20, 31]. In addition, the ability of TKIs to cause selective expansion of clones bearing specific mutation suggests that different mutants confer differential levels of fitness, a conclusion that is consistent with cellular and biochemical data [32].

Mutations can be categorized into four types involving the (1) TKI-binding site, (2) ATP binding site (P loop), (3) activation (A) loop, and (4) catalytic (C) domain.

One of the first mutations detected in TKI-resistant patients was the T315I mutation, resulting from substitution of the amino acid threonine with isoleucine at position 315 of the ABL moiety. This substitution reduces the affinity for TKIs in two ways. Firstly, the lack of threonine 315 residue at the gatekeeping position of the nucleotide-binding site interferes with a crucial hydrogen bond between TKIs and BCR-ABL1. Secondly, isoleucine allosterically blocks TKI binding by an extra hydrocarbon group on its side chain. The T315I mutation is one of the most frequent mutations that confer resistance to first- and second-generation TKIs, associated with poor outcome [29].

Mutations that cluster within the ATP-binding site (phosphate or P-loop) can be found in up to 50 % of imatinib-resistant patients [11, 33]. This mutation modifies the flexibility of the P-loop and destabilizes the conformation required for imatinib binding. P-loop mutations have been shown to have a worse prognosis than non-P-loop mutations in some reports [33].

The activation (A) loop of the kinase can adopt a closed (inactive) or an open (active) conformation. Mutations in the A loop can disturb the energetic balance for stabilization of the closed conformation, favouring the open, active conformation and thereby inhibiting imatinib binding [11]. Mutations in the catalytic (C) domain that have a close topologic relation to the base of the activation loop can also influence the binding of imatinib [11].

Recent reports suggested that compound mutations in BCR-ABL1 alleles at 12 key positions, particularly T315I mutants, conferred varying resistance to TKIs including ponatinib [34].

#### 11.2.1.2 *BCR-ABL1* Amplification

Overexpression of the BCR-ABL1 protein due to genomic amplification has been seen in a relatively small proportion of imatinib-resistant patients. It was first reported in a study of 3 out of 11 patients with BP CML with secondary resistance to imatinib when multiple copies of the *BCR-ABL1* gene were detected by fluorescence in situ hybridization (FISH) [12]. Similar genomic amplification of *BCR-ABL1* was also observed in in vitro studies with nilotinib resistance, which reflected excess target protein needed for inhibition at therapeutic drug doses. A transient amplification of *BCR-ABL1* may also precede the emergence of a dominant mutant clone, as suggested by kinetic studies in cell lines [27, 29]. In addition, overexpression of *BCR-ABL1* transcripts and protein has been described to occur independently of *BCR-ABL1* gene amplification [35] and appears to be a consistent feature of BC cells. Whether overexpression is transcriptionally or post-transcriptionally driven remains to be determined, but it is likely that several mechanisms are at play, including the possibility of a general upregulation of cap-dependent mRNA translation [36–40].

### *11.2.2* BCR-ABL1-*Independent Mechanisms*

#### 11.2.2.1 Drug Pumps

Imatinib and other TKIs are substrates of ATP-binding cassette transporter family (ABCB1) and multidrug resistance *MDR1* gene product P-glycoprotein, an efflux pump at the cell surface [41]. Overexpression of ABCB1 results in the reduction of intracellular drug uptake by CML cells through active efflux and leads to ineffective drug concentration in the cells, hence resistance to imatinib in cell line studies [23, 42, 43]. Another drug transporter, breast cancer resistance protein ABCG2, was also shown to limit the intracellular delivery of dasatinib and nilotinib by active efflux of the drugs [44].

Human organic cation transporter 1 (hOCT1) mediates the active transport of imatinib into cells, and hOCT1 inhibition decreases the intracellular concentration of imatinib, leading to a lower rate of MMR. The higher hOCT1 gene expression was seen in patients who achieved a CCyR with imatinib treatment compared with those who did not [24, 25]. Single nucleotide polymorphism involving genes of drug transporters, ABCB1, ABCG2 and hOCT1, have also been reported in patients with imatinib resistance and have led the call for therapeutic monitoring of imatinib trough levels [44, 45].

#### 11.2.2.2 *BIM* Deletion Polymorphism

A common deletion polymorphism in the second intron of the gene encoding *BCL2-like 11* (*BIM*) has also been described as a mechanism for inferior TKI responses in East Asian patients [10]. BIM is a pro-apoptotic member of the B-cell CLL/lymphoma 2 (BCL2) family of proteins, and its upregulation is required for TKI-mediated induction of apoptosis in a broad range of kinase-driven cancers, including CML [46–50]. Mechanistically, the *BIM* polymorphism results in preferential splicing and expression of BIM isoforms lacking the pro-apoptotic BCL2-homology domain 3 (BH3). This in turn confers intrinsic TKI resistance in CML cell lines and patient samples [10]. The study also demonstrated the possibility of individualized therapy with so-called BH3 mimetics to overcome *BIM* polymorphism-associated TKI resistance. Importantly, biological and clinical validation of the *BIM* deletion as a biomarker of poor response has also been provided through independent studies in another kinase-driven human cancer, epidermal growth factor receptor (EGFR)-mutated non-small-cell lung cancer. Here, four independent groups have found that patients with the *BIM* deletion polymorphism experienced a halving of their progression-free survival while on EGFR TKI therapy compared with patients without the deletion [51–55]. Interestingly, the existence of other TKI resistance-associated polymorphic *BIM* variants has since been described by other groups in European CML populations [56].

#### 11.2.2.3 Activation of *BCR-ABL1*-Independent Transforming Pathways

The activation of alternative pathways to transformation has also been described to mediate TKI resistance in CML [57]. Examples include the JAK-STAT pathway where activation of Lyn occurs in a Janus kinase 2 (JAK2)-dependent manner via a SET-PP2A-SHP1 pathway [58]. In addition, activation of Lyn, a member of the Src family kinases, was observed in imatinib-resistant CML cell lines and in samples from CML patients with resistance to imatinib. Lyn overexpression was also associated with CML patients with failure of nilotinib treatment [26, 59].

Very recent work has also suggested upregulation of Protein Kinase C, PKCeta in a BCR-ABL1-independent manner as an activator of mitogen-activated protein kinase (MAPK) signalling, and that use of mitogen-activated protein extracellular signal-regulated kinase (MEK) inhibitors with TKIs can overcome this form of *BCR-ABL1*-independent TKI resistance [60].

#### 11.2.2.4 Persistence of LSCs

LSCs are known to persist in patients with CML, even when they attain durable complete molecular remissions [61, 62]. Mechanistically, these may be divided into LSC intrinsic or extrinsic causes (e.g. factors dependent on the bone marrow microenvironment). Intrinsic mechanisms include the ability of CML progenitors to enter a state of quiescence in which they appear impervious to TKI-induced apoptosis but sensitive to other drugs including histone deacetylase inhibitors (HDACi) [63–69]. Within the quiescent LSC population, BCR-ABL1 expression but not kinase activity was found to be important for activation of a JAK2/PP2A-Wnt axis and could be targeted with protein phosphatase 2A (PP2A) activators to extinguish LSCs [70]. Meanwhile others have described a tumour necrosis factor (TNF)-α-dependent autocrine loop that supports LSC survival in a BCR-ABL1-kinase-independent manner [71]. Interestingly, others have identified signalling pathways that appear to be restricted to LSCs and include a TGF-β-FOXO pathway that is important for maintaining CML LSCs in vivo [72].

#### 11.2.2.5 Bone Marrow Environment

Several recent studies have described that factors arising from the bone marrow microenvironment and the stem cell niche can play an important role in rendering CML LSCs independent of BCR-ABL1 activity. Inflammatory cytokines including leukotrienes and prostaglandins, respective metabolites of lipoxygenase and cyclo-oxygenase, are upregulated in CML cells and mediate LSC self-renewal [73, 74]. Interestingly, among patients without kinase domain mutations and who were clinically resistant to TKIs, extrinsic fibroblast growth factor 2 (FGF2) signalling from the microenvironment was found to activate MAPK signalling to mediate TKI resistance. Importantly, these investigators also found that treatment with a third-generation TKI, ponatinib, could overcome FGF2-mediated TKI resistance by inhibition of BCR-ABL1 and FGF2 concurrently [75].

Recent studies from our group have also identified physiologic hypoxia, which occurs in the bone marrow microenvironment, as an important mediator of BCR-ABL1-independent TKI resistance and LSC maintenance [76]. Physiologic hypoxia was found to enhance the activation of hypoxia-inducible factor (HIF)-dependent signalling resulting in the transactivation of a set of hypoxia-induced genes in CML but not normal progenitors. These data demonstrate that CML LSCs respond differentially to hypoxic stimuli compared to normal counterparts and suggest novel avenues for therapeutic intervention by targeting HIF signalling itself or select genes downstream of HIF.

## 11.3 Overcoming TKI Resistance

Given the better understanding of the mechanisms underlying TKI resistance, either dependent or independent of BCR-ABL1 activity, there have been several strategies proposed to overcome the resistance, including by combining novel agents with TKIs (Table 11.1) [90–92]. Multiple clinical and preclinical studies exploring the effects of targeting downstream signalling pathways, eradicating CML stem cells and epigenetic modifications have shown promising results [58, 79, 87, 93–98].

### *11.3.1 Tackling* ABL1-*Kinase Mutants*

Second-generation TKIs, such as dasatinib and nilotinib, have been approved for first-line therapy for CML as well as second-line therapy for those with imatinib

**Table 11.1** Mechanisms of TKI resistance and treatment strategies/potential targets

| Mechanism of resistance | | Treatment strategies |
|---|---|---|
| BCR-ABL1-dependent | *ABL1*-kinase domain mutations[a] | Second-generation TKIs<br>Ponatinib [77, 78] or allosteric inhibitors |
| | *BCR-ABL1* amplification | |
| BCR-ABL1-independent (intrinsic) | Activation of downstream signalling<br>JAK-STAT pathway<br>PI3K/AKT/mTOR pathway | JAK2 inhibitors (ruxolitinib) with TKIs [58]<br>mTOR inhibitors (rapamycin, everolimus, temsirolimus) with TKIs [79, 80, 81] |
| | Genetic polymorphisms[b] | BH3 mimetics with TKIs [49] |
| | Drug transport pumps[b] | |
| | Epigenetic modification[b] | HDAC inhibitors (panobinostat) [82]<br>miRNA-targeted therapy |
| | Persistence of LSCs<br>Wnt/β-catenin pathway<br>Hedgehog pathway | Autophagy inhibitors (chloroquine, clarithromycin) [83, 84]<br>Apoptosis inducers (17-AAG or tanespimycin) [85, 86]<br>Arsenic trioxide<br>Cyclooxygenase inhibitors (indomethacin) [87]<br>SMO antagonists [88, 89] |
| BCR-ABL1-independent (extrinsic) | Bone marrow environment<br>Cytokines<br>Hypoxia | Anti-HIF1 [76] |

[a]Kinase domain mutations are found in 20 % of chronic phase CML and 75 % of blast crisis
[b]Possible mechanisms of heterogeneity of responses to TKI

failure [5]. Dasatinib, a dual Src/ABL1-kinase inhibitor, is active against many imatinib-resistant mutants except the T315I [8, 90]. Nilotinib, with *N*-methylpiperazine moiety incorporated into imatinib, is a more potent compound against most of the clinically relevant *BCR-ABL1* mutants, except the T315I mutant [8, 90, 91].

Ponatinib is a pan-TKI effective against the T315I mutation and has recently been approved for the treatment of patients who failed previous TKI therapy [5, 77, 78]. However, its use has to be carefully monitored against its toxicity since serious cardiovascular, cerebrovascular and peripheral vascular adverse events have been reported in the study, especially in the presence of risk factors including hypertension, hyperlipidaemia and diabetes [99].

Allosteric inhibitors, such as ABL-001, which target sites on BCR-ABL1 other than the ATP-binding site, have been shown to prevent TKI resistance in preclinical models, and the results of ongoing phase I studies are eagerly awaited [www.clinicaltrials.gov identifier: NCT02081378].

### 11.3.2 Targeting Downstream Signalling Pathways

Combining TKIs with compounds targeted against different downstream signalling pathways has been widely studied in preclinical and clinical studies [57]. JAK2 inhibitors induced apoptosis and decreased survival of CML stem cells in cultures and mouse models, when given together with imatinib [58, 93]. Early-phase clinical trials of ruxolitinib in combination with TKIs in CML with residual disease have been carried out.

Another approach is to combine mammalian target of rapamycin (mTOR) inhibitors with TKIs in treating TKI-resistant mutants [79]. Rapamycin has been shown to be effective in overcoming imatinib resistance in cell lines with *BCR-ABL1* amplification or *ABL1*-kinase mutation [40, 80, 81, 100]. Allosteric mTOR inhibitors, everolimus and temsirolimus, have also been studied in phase 1 trials for CML.

### 11.3.3 Modifying Epigenetic Regulators

Histone deacetylase inhibitors (HDACi), such as suberoylanilide hydroxamic acid (SAHA), suppress *BCR-ABL1* levels in TKI-resistant CML cells in vitro and in vivo [94, 95]. Panobinostat (LBH589) has recently been shown to eliminate quiescent CML LSCs that are otherwise resistant to elimination by imatinib in mouse models. Clinical studies of panobinostat in combination with imatinib are being carried out in CML patients with residual disease [82].

DNA methylation inhibitors (DNMTi) or demethylating agents have also been tested in CML patients with TKI resistance. Early clinical studies of decitabine treatment showed modest response in CML patients who developed resistance to imatinib but are now being tested in combination with TKIs [101, 102].

Therapy based on microRNA (miRNA) may also be another promising epigenetic approach as *BCR-ABL1* regulates miRNA profiles and miRNA has targets on down-stream signalling pathways in CML, such as PI3K/AKT/mTOR pathway [103].

### 11.3.4 Eradicating CML Stem Cells

Wnt/β-catenin pathway can be an attractive novel target for the elimination of CML stem cells [87, 96]. A study in mice showed that indomethacin, a cyclooxygenase inhibitor, reduced β-catenin and inhibited proliferation of LSCs. The hedgehog pathway is another potential target since smoothened (SMO) antagonists are found to effectively decrease replication in CML cell lines in vitro [88, 89].

An alternative approach is the use of arsenic trioxide, which impairs BCR-ABL1 stability and causes depletion of CML LSCs through autophagosomal degradation [104, 105]. Early-phase clinical trials with those small molecules in combination with TKIs for resistant CML patients are being carried out [www.clinicaltrials.gov identifier: NCT00250042 and NCT01397734].

### 11.3.5 Targeting Bone Marrow Environment and Cytokines

Modification of inflammatory cytokines, leukotrienes and prostaglandins by targeting against lipoxygenase and cyclooxygenase pathways in bone marrow environment has been shown to be a feasible approach to suppress proliferation and induces apoptosis of human CML cells and mouse models [73, 74].

Since hypoxia and up-regulated HIF1a in bone marrow environment have been implicated in TKI resistance, targeting HIF1a and associated genes may be a potential strategy to overcome resistance and eliminate CML LSCs [76].

### 11.3.6 Inducing Apoptosis and Inhibiting Autophagy

HSP90, a chaperone molecule for oncoproteins such as BCR-ABL1 can be inhibited by 17-allylamino-17-demethoxygeldanamycin (17-AAG) or tanespimycin [85, 86]. While studies using tanespimycin have been initiated, results of these studies are not publicly available.

Another potential therapeutic approach is inhibition of autophagy. Autophagy is a mechanism used by cancer cells to resist apoptosis and is characterized by intracellular formation of autophagosomes and breakdown/recycling of cell components [106]. CML cells can undergo autophagy to avoid apoptosis induced by TKIs and develop resistance to treatment. Compounds such as chloroquine and clarithromycin inhibit essential autophagy and increase the sensitivity of CML stem cells to treatment with TKIs [83, 84, 107].

## 11.4 Summary

With the advent of TKIs, patients with CML now enjoy increased survival with a reasonable quality of life. However, most patients will likely have to remain on long-term therapy with imatinib and second-generation TKIs. Even among those who achieve durable molecular response with imatinib, cessation of therapy results in recurrent disease in a significant majority. Accordingly, the outcomes of similar studies employing second-generation TKIs are underway.

The next lap of CML research will be directed at eliminating the CML LSCs and providing effective cure for CML off any drug therapy. With the current knowledge and understanding of CML pathogenesis, several targetable pathways have been identified. In practical terms, such studies will have to balance the possibility of long-term cure against toxicity.

## References

1. Hochhaus A. Educational session: managing chronic myeloid leukemia as a chronic disease. Hematology Am Soc Hematol Educ Program. 2011;2011:128–35.
2. Hochhaus A, O'Brien SG, Guilhot F, Druker BJ, Branford S, Foroni L, et al. Six-year follow-up of patients receiving imatinib for the first-line treatment of chronic myeloid leukemia. Leukemia. 2009;23(6):1054–61.
3. Deininger M, O'Brien SG, Guilhot F, Goldman JM, Hochhaus A, Hughes TP, et al. International randomized study of interferon Vs STI571 (IRIS) 8-year follow up: sustained survival and low risk for progression or events in patients with newly diagnosed chronic myeloid leukemia in chronic phase (CML-CP) treated with imatinib [abstract]. Blood (ASH Annual Meeting Abstracts). 2009;114:1126.
4. Druker BJ, Guilhot F, O'Brien SG, Gathmann I, Kantarjian H, Gattermann N, et al. Five-year follow-up of patients receiving imatinib for chronic myeloid leukemia. N Engl J Med. 2006;355(23):2408–17.
5. Baccarani M, Deininger MW, Rosti G, Hochhaus A, Soverini S, Apperley JF, et al. European LeukemiaNet recommendations for the management of chronic myeloid leukemia: 2013. Blood. 2013;122(6):872–84.
6. Marin D, Ibrahim AR, Lucas C, Gerrard G, Wang L, Szydlo RM, et al. Assessment of BCR-ABL1 transcript levels at 3 months is the only requirement for predicting outcome for patients with chronic myeloid leukemia treated with tyrosine kinase inhibitors. J Clin Oncol. 2012;30(3):232–8.
7. Branford S, Kim DW, Soverini S, Haque A, Shou Y, Woodman RC, et al. Initial molecular response at 3 months may predict both response and event-free survival at 24 months in imatinib-resistant or -intolerant patients with Philadelphia chromosome-positive chronic myeloid leukemia in chronic phase treated with nilotinib. J Clin Oncol. 2012;30(35):4323–9.
8. Melo JV, Chuah C. Resistance to imatinib mesylate in chronic myeloid leukaemia. Cancer Lett. 2007;249(2):121–32.

9. Milojkovic D, Apperley J. Mechanisms of resistance to imatinib and second-generation tyrosine inhibitors in chronic myeloid leukemia. Clin Cancer Res. 2009;15(24):7519–27.
10. Ng KP, Hillmer AM, Chuah CTH, Juan WC, Ko TK, Teo ASM, et al. A common BIM deletion polymorphism mediates intrinsic resistance and inferior responses to tyrosine kinase inhibitors in cancer. Nat Med. 2012;18(4):521–8.
11. Mahon FX, Deininger MW, Schultheis B, Chabrol J, Reiffers J, Goldman JM, et al. Selection and characterization of BCR-ABL positive cell lines with differential sensitivity to the tyrosine kinase inhibitor STI571: diverse mechanisms of resistance. Blood. 2000;96 (3):1070–9.
12. Gorre ME, Mohammed M, Ellwood K, Hsu N, Paquette R, Rao PN, et al. Clinical resistance to STI-571 cancer therapy caused by BCR-ABL gene mutation or amplification. Science. 2001;293(5531):876–80.
13. Branford S, Rudzki Z, Walsh S, Grigg A, Arthur C, Taylor K, et al. High frequency of point mutations clustered within the adenosine triphosphate-binding region of BCR/ABL in patients with chronic myeloid leukemia or Ph-positive acute lymphoblastic leukemia who develop imatinib (STI571) resistance. Blood. 2002;99(9):3472–5.
14. Roche-Lestienne C, Soenen-Cornu V, Grardel-Duflos N, Laï JL, Philippe N, Facon T, et al. Several types of mutations of the Abl gene can be found in chronic myeloid leukemia patients resistant to STI571, and they can pre-exist to the onset of treatment. Blood. 2002;100 (3):1014–8.
15. Roumiantsev S, Shah NP, Gorre ME, Nicoll J, Brasher BB, Sawyers CL, et al. Clinical resistance to the kinase inhibitor STI-571 in chronic myeloid leukemia by mutation of Tyr-253 in the Abl kinase domain P-loop. Proc Natl Acad Sci U S A. 2002;99(16):10700–5.
16. Shah NP, Nicoll JM, Nagar B, Gorre ME, Paquette RL, Kuriyan J, et al. Multiple BCR-ABL kinase domain mutations confer polyclonal resistance to the tyrosine kinase inhibitor imatinib (STI571) in chronic phase and blast crisis chronic myeloid leukemia. Cancer Cell. 2002;2 (2):117–25.
17. Corbin AS, La Rosée P, Stoffregen EP, Druker BJ, Deininger MW. Several Bcr-Abl kinase domain mutants associated with imatinib mesylate resistance remain sensitive to imatinib. Blood. 2003;101(11):4611–4.
18. von Bubnoff N, Schneller F, Peschel C, Duyster J. BCR-ABL gene mutations in relation to clinical resistance of Philadelphia-chromosome-positive leukaemia to STI571: a prospective study. Lancet. 2002;359(9305):487–91.
19. Shah NP, Sawyers CL. Mechanisms of resistance to STI571 in Philadelphia chromosome-associated leukemias. Oncogene. 2003;22(47):7389–95.
20. Gambacorti-Passerini CB, Gunby RH, Piazza R, Galietta A, Rostagno R, Scapozza L. Molecular mechanisms of resistance to imatinib in Philadelphia-chromosome-positive leukaemias. Lancet Oncol. 2003;4(2):75–85.
21. Branford S, Rudzki Z, Parkinson I, Grigg A, Taylor K, Seymour JF, et al. Real-time quantitative PCR analysis can be used as a primary screen to identify patients with CML treated with imatinib who have BCR-ABL kinase domain mutations. Blood. 2004;104 (9):2926–32.
22. Chu S, Xu H, Shah NP, Snyder DS, Forman SJ, Sawyers CL, et al. Detection of BCR-ABL kinase mutations in CD34+ cells from chronic myelogenous leukemia patients in complete cytogenetic remission on imatinib mesylate treatment. Blood. 2005;105(5):2093–8.
23. Thomas J, Wang L, Clark RE, Pirmohamed M. Active transport of imatinib into and out of cells: implications for drug resistance. Blood. 2004;104(12):3739–45.
24. Crossman LC, Druker BJ, Deininger MWN, Pirmohamed M, Wang L, Clark RE. hOCT 1 and resistance to imatinib. Blood. 2005;106(3):1133–4; author reply 1134.
25. White DL, Saunders VA, Dang P, Engler J, Zannettino ACW, Cambareri AC, et al. OCT-1-mediated influx is a key determinant of the intracellular uptake of imatinib but not nilotinib (AMN107): reduced OCT-1 activity is the cause of low in vitro sensitivity to imatinib. Blood. 2006;108(2):697–704.

26. Donato NJ, Wu JY, Stapley J, Gallick G, Lin H, Arlinghaus R, et al. BCR-ABL independence and LYN kinase overexpression in chronic myelogenous leukemia cells selected for resistance to STI571. Blood. 2003;101(2):690–8.
27. Hochhaus A, Kreil S, Corbin AS, La Rosée P, Müller MC, Lahaye T, et al. Molecular and chromosomal mechanisms of resistance to imatinib (STI571) therapy. Leukemia. 2002;16 (11):2190–6.
28. Soverini S, Martinelli G, Rosti G, Bassi S, Amabile M, Poerio A, et al. ABL mutations in late chronic phase chronic myeloid leukemia patients with up-front cytogenetic resistance to imatinib are associated with a greater likelihood of progression to blast crisis and shorter survival: a study by the GIMEMA Working Party on Chronic Myeloid Leukemia. J Clin Oncol. 2005;23(18):4100–9.
29. Apperley JF. Part I: mechanisms of resistance to imatinib in chronic myeloid leukaemia. Lancet Oncol. 2007;8(11):1018–29.
30. Parker WT, Ho M, Scott HS, Hughes TP, Branford S. Poor response to second-line kinase inhibitors in chronic myeloid leukemia patients with multiple low-level mutations, irrespective of their resistance profile. Blood. 2012;119(10):2234–8.
31. Nardi V, Azam M, Daley GQ. Mechanisms and implications of imatinib resistance mutations in BCR-ABL. Curr Opin Hematol. 2004;11(1):35–43.
32. Griswold IJ, MacPartlin M, Bumm T, Goss VL, O'Hare T, Lee KA, et al. Kinase domain mutants of Bcr-Abl exhibit altered transformation potency, kinase activity, and substrate utilization, irrespective of sensitivity to imatinib. Mol Cell Biol. 2006;26(16):6082–93.
33. Branford S, Rudzki Z, Walsh S, Parkinson I, Grigg A, Szer J, et al. Detection of BCR-ABL mutations in patients with CML treated with imatinib is virtually always accompanied by clinical resistance, and mutations in the ATP phosphate-binding loop (P-loop) are associated with a poor prognosis. Blood. 2003;102(1):276–83.
34. Zabriskie MS, Eide CA, Tantravahi SK, Vellore NA, Estrada J, Nicolini FE, et al. BCR-ABL1 compound mutations combining key kinase domain positions confer clinical resistance to ponatinib in Ph chromosome-positive leukemia. Cancer Cell. 2014;26(3):428–42.
35. Barnes DJ, Palaiologou D, Panousopoulou E, Schultheis B, Yong ASM, Wong A, et al. Bcr-Abl expression levels determine the rate of development of resistance to imatinib mesylate in chronic myeloid leukemia. Cancer Res. 2005;65(19):8912–9.
36. Carayol N, Vakana E, Sassano A, Kaur S, Goussetis DJ, Glaser H, et al. Critical roles for mTORC2- and rapamycin-insensitive mTORC1-complexes in growth and survival of BCR-ABL-expressing leukemic cells. Proc Natl Acad Sci U S A. 2010;107(28):12469–74.
37. Zhang M, Fu W, Prabhu S, Moore JC, Ko J, Kim JW, et al. Inhibition of polysome assembly enhances imatinib activity against chronic myelogenous leukemia and overcomes imatinib resistance. Mol Cell Biol. 2008;28(20):6496–509.
38. Prabhu S, Saadat D, Zhang M, Halbur L, Fruehauf JP, Ong ST. A novel mechanism for Bcr-Abl action: Bcr-Abl-mediated induction of the eIF4F translation initiation complex and mRNA translation. Oncogene. 2007;26(8):1188–200.
39. Perrotti D, Trotta R, Calabretta B. Altered mRNA translation: possible mechanism for CML disease progression. Cell Cycle. 2003;2(3):177–80.
40. Ly C, Arechiga AF, Melo JV, Walsh CM, Ong ST. Bcr-Abl kinase modulates the translation regulators ribosomal protein S6 and 4E-BP1 in chronic myelogenous leukemia cells via the mammalian target of rapamycin. Cancer Res. 2003;63(18):5716–22.
41. Hegedus T, Orfi L, Seprodi A, Váradi A, Sarkadi B, Kéri G. Interaction of tyrosine kinase inhibitors with the human multidrug transporter proteins, MDR1 and MRP1. Biochim Biophys Acta. 2002;1587(2–3):318–25.
42. Widmer N, Colombo S, Buclin T, Decosterd LA. Functional consequence of MDR1 expression on imatinib intracellular concentrations. Blood. 2003;102(3):1142.
43. Illmer T, Schaich M, Platzbecker U, Freiberg-Richter J, Oelschlägel U, von Bonin M, et al. P-glycoprotein-mediated drug efflux is a resistance mechanism of chronic myelogenous leukemia cells to treatment with imatinib mesylate. Leukemia. 2004;18(3):401–8.

44. Burger H, van Tol H, Brok M, Wiemer EAC, de Bruijn EA, Guetens G, et al. Chronic imatinib mesylate exposure leads to reduced intracellular drug accumulation by induction of the ABCG2 (BCRP) and ABCB1 (MDR1) drug transport pumps. Cancer Biol Ther. 2005;4 (7):747–52.
45. Takahashi N, Miura M, Scott SA, Kagaya H, Kameoka Y, Tagawa H, et al. Influence of CYP3A5 and drug transporter polymorphisms on imatinib trough concentration and clinical response among patients with chronic phase chronic myeloid leukemia. J Hum Genet. 2010;55(11):731–7.
46. Soh S, Ong ST. A novel BIM deletion polymorphism: implications and lessons for cancer targeted therapies. Rinsho Ketsueki. 2013;54(10):1714–9.
47. Gong Y, Somwar R, Politi K, Balak M, Chmielecki J, Jiang X, et al. Induction of BIM is essential for apoptosis triggered by EGFR kinase inhibitors in mutant EGFR-dependent lung adenocarcinomas. PLoS Med. 2007;4(10), e294.
48. Costa DB, Halmos B, Kumar A, Schumer ST, Huberman MS, Boggon TJ, et al. BIM mediates EGFR tyrosine kinase inhibitor-induced apoptosis in lung cancers with oncogenic EGFR mutations. PLoS Med. 2007;4(10):1669–79; discussion 1680.
49. Kuroda J, Puthalakath H, Cragg MS, Kelly PN, Bouillet P, Huang DCS, et al. Bim and Bad mediate imatinib-induced killing of Bcr/Abl+ leukemic cells, and resistance due to their loss is overcome by a BH3 mimetic. Proc Natl Acad Sci U S A. 2006;103(40):14907–12.
50. Gordon PM, Fisher DE. Role for the proapoptotic factor BIM in mediating imatinib-induced apoptosis in a c-KIT-dependent gastrointestinal stromal tumor cell line. J Biol Chem. 2010;285(19):14109–14.
51. Zhao M, Zhang Y, Cai W, Li J, Zhou F, Cheng N, et al. The Bim deletion polymorphism clinical profile and its relation with tyrosine kinase inhibitor resistance in Chinese patients with non-small cell lung cancer. Cancer. 2014;120(15):2299–307.
52. Lee JH, Lin YL, Hsu WH, Chen HY, Chang YC, Yu CJ, et al. Bcl-2-like protein 11 deletion polymorphism predicts survival in advanced non-small-cell lung cancer. J Thorac Oncol. 2014;9(9):1385–92.
53. Isobe K, Hata Y, Tochigi N, Kaburaki K, Kobayashi H, Makino T, et al. Clinical significance of BIM deletion polymorphism in non-small-cell lung cancer with epidermal growth factor receptor mutation. J Thorac Oncol. 2014;9(4):483–7.
54. Lee JK, Shin JY, Kim S, Lee S, Park C, Kim JY, et al. Primary resistance to epidermal growth factor receptor (EGFR) tyrosine kinase inhibitors (TKIs) in patients with non-small-cell lung cancer harboring TKI-sensitive EGFR mutations: an exploratory study. Ann Oncol. 2013;24 (8):2080–7.
55. Ong ST, Chuah CTH, Ko TK, Hillmer AM, Lim WT. Reply: the BIM deletion polymorphism cannot account for intrinsic TKI resistance of Chinese individuals with chronic myeloid leukemia. Nat Med. 2014;20(10):1090–1.
56. Augis V, Airiau K, Josselin M, Turcq B, Mahon FX, Belloc F. A single nucleotide polymorphism in cBIM is associated with a slower achievement of major molecular response in chronic myeloid leukaemia treated with imatinib. PLoS One. 2013;8(11), e78582.
57. Ahmed W, Van Etten RA. Alternative approaches to eradicating the malignant clone in chronic myeloid leukemia: tyrosine-kinase inhibitor combinations and beyond. Hematology Am Soc Hematol Educ Program. 2013;2013:189–200.
58. Samanta AK, Chakraborty SN, Wang Y, Kantarjian H, Sun X, Hood J, et al. Jak2 inhibition deactivates Lyn kinase through the SET-PP2A-SHP1 pathway, causing apoptosis in drug-resistant cells from chronic myelogenous leukemia patients. Oncogene. 2009;28 (14):1669–81.
59. Mahon FX, Hayette S, Lagarde V, Belloc F, Turcq B, Nicolini F, et al. Evidence that resistance to nilotinib may be due to BCR-ABL, Pgp, or Src kinase overexpression. Cancer Res. 2008;68(23):9809–16.
60. Ma L, Shan Y, Bai R, Xue L, Eide CA, Ou J, et al. A therapeutically targetable mechanism of BCR-ABL-independent imatinib resistance in chronic myeloid leukemia. Sci Transl Med. 2014;6(252):252ra121.

61. Mahon FX, Réa D, Guilhot J, Guilhot F, Huguet F, Nicolini F, et al. Discontinuation of imatinib in patients with chronic myeloid leukaemia who have maintained complete molecular remission for at least 2 years: the prospective, multicentre Stop Imatinib (STIM) trial. Lancet Oncol. 2010;11(11):1029–35.
62. Mahon FX. Is going for cure in chronic myeloid leukemia possible and justifiable? Hematology Am Soc Hematol Educ Program. 2012;2012:122–8.
63. Hamilton A, Helgason GV, Schemionek M, Zhang B, Myssina S, Allan EK, et al. Chronic myeloid leukemia stem cells are not dependent on Bcr-Abl kinase activity for their survival. Blood. 2012;119(6):1501–10.
64. Helgason GV, Young GAR, Holyoake TL. Targeting chronic myeloid leukemia stem cells. Curr Hematol Malig Rep. 2010;5(2):81–7.
65. Konig H, Holyoake TL, Bhatia R. Effective and selective inhibition of chronic myeloid leukemia primitive hematopoietic progenitors by the dual Src/Abl kinase inhibitor SKI-606. Blood. 2008;111(4):2329–38.
66. Copland M, Hamilton A, Elrick LJ, Baird JW, Allan EK, Jordanides N, et al. Dasatinib (BMS-354825) targets an earlier progenitor population than imatinib in primary CML but does not eliminate the quiescent fraction. Blood. 2006;107(11):4532–9.
67. Copland M, Pellicano F, Richmond L, Allan EK, Hamilton A, Lee FY, et al. BMS-214662 potently induces apoptosis of chronic myeloid leukemia stem and progenitor cells and synergizes with tyrosine kinase inhibitors. Blood. 2008;111(5):2843–53.
68. Graham SM, Jørgensen HG, Allan E, Pearson C, Alcorn MJ, Richmond L, et al. Primitive, quiescent, Philadelphia-positive stem cells from patients with chronic myeloid leukemia are insensitive to STI571 in vitro. Blood. 2002;99(1):319–25.
69. Zhang B, Strauss AC, Chu S, Li M, Ho Y, Shiang KD, et al. Effective targeting of quiescent chronic myelogenous leukemia stem cells by histone deacetylase inhibitors in combination with imatinib mesylate. Cancer Cell. 2010;17(5):427–42.
70. Neviani P, Harb JG, Oaks JJ, Santhanam R, Walker CJ, Ellis JJ, et al. PP2A-activating drugs selectively eradicate TKI-resistant chronic myeloid leukemic stem cells. J Clin Invest. 2013;123(10):4144–57.
71. Gallipoli P, Pellicano F, Morrison H, Laidlaw K, Allan EK, Bhatia R, et al. Autocrine TNF-α production supports CML stem and progenitor cell survival and enhances their proliferation. Blood. 2013;122(19):3335–9.
72. Naka K, Hoshii T, Muraguchi T, Tadokoro Y, Ooshio T, Kondo Y, et al. TGF-beta-FOXO signalling maintains leukaemia-initiating cells in chronic myeloid leukaemia. Nature. 2010;463(7281):676–80.
73. Chen Y, Hu Y, Zhang H, Peng C, Li S. Loss of the Alox5 gene impairs leukemia stem cells and prevents chronic myeloid leukemia. Nat Genet. 2009;41(7):783–92.
74. Hegde S, Kaushal N, Ravindra KC, Chiaro C, Hafer KT, Gandhi UH, et al. Δ12-prostaglandin J3, an omega-3 fatty acid-derived metabolite, selectively ablates leukemia stem cells in mice. Blood. 2011;118(26):6909–19.
75. Traer E, Javidi-Sharifi N, Agarwal A, Dunlap J, English I, Martinez J, et al. Ponatinib overcomes FGF2-mediated resistance in CML patients without kinase domain mutations. Blood. 2014;123(10):1516–24.
76. Ng KP, Manjeri A, Lee KL, Huang W, Tan SY, Chuah CTH, et al. Physiologic hypoxia promotes maintenance of CML stem cells despite effective BCR-ABL1 inhibition. Blood. 2014;123(21):3316–26.
77. O'Hare T, Shakespeare WC, Zhu X, Eide CA, Rivera VM, Wang F, et al. AP24534, a pan-BCR-ABL inhibitor for chronic myeloid leukemia, potently inhibits the T315I mutant and overcomes mutation-based resistance. Cancer Cell. 2009;16(5):401–12.
78. Cortes JE, Kantarjian H, Shah NP, Bixby D, Mauro MJ, Flinn I, et al. Ponatinib in refractory Philadelphia chromosome-positive leukemias. N Engl J Med. 2012;367(22):2075–88.
79. Janes MR, Limon JJ, So L, Chen J, Lim RJ, Chavez MA, et al. Effective and selective targeting of leukemia cells using a TORC1/2 kinase inhibitor. Nat Med. 2010;16(2):205–13.

80. Mohi MG, Boulton C, Gu TL, Sternberg DW, Neuberg D, Griffin JD, et al. Combination of rapamycin and protein tyrosine kinase (PTK) inhibitors for the treatment of leukemias caused by oncogenic PTKs. Proc Natl Acad Sci U S A. 2004;101(9):3130–5.
81. Sillaber C, Mayerhofer M, Böhm A, Vales A, Gruze A, Aichberger KJ, et al. Evaluation of antileukaemic effects of rapamycin in patients with imatinib-resistant chronic myeloid leukaemia. Eur J Clin Invest. 2008;38(1):43–52.
82. Bhatia R, Snyder D, Lin AEA. A phase I study of the HDAC inhibitor LBH589 in combination with imatinib for patients with CML in cytogenetic remission with residual disease detectable by Q-PCR [abstract]. Blood (ASH Annual Meeting Abstracts). 2009;114 (22):2194.
83. Bellodi C, Lidonnici MR, Hamilton A, Helgason GV, Soliera AR, Ronchetti M, et al. Targeting autophagy potentiates tyrosine kinase inhibitor-induced cell death in Philadelphia chromosome-positive cells, including primary CML stem cells. J Clin Invest. 2009;119(5):1109–23.
84. Carella AM, Beltrami G, Pica G, Carella A, Catania G. Clarithromycin potentiates tyrosine kinase inhibitor treatment in patients with resistant chronic myeloid leukemia. Leuk Lymphoma. 2012;53(7):1409–11.
85. An WG, Schulte TW, Neckers LM. The heat shock protein 90 antagonist geldanamycin alters chaperone association with p210bcr-abl and v-src proteins before their degradation by the proteasome. Cell Growth Differ. 2000;11(7):355–60.
86. Nimmanapalli R, O'Bryan E, Bhalla K. Geldanamycin and its analogue 17-allylamino-17-demethoxygeldanamycin lowers Bcr-Abl levels and induces apoptosis and differentiation of Bcr-Abl-positive human leukemic blasts. Cancer Res. 2001;61(5):1799–804.
87. Heidel FH, Bullinger L, Feng Z, Wang Z, Neff TA, Stein L, et al. Genetic and pharmacologic inhibition of β-catenin targets imatinib-resistant leukemia stem cells in CML. Cell Stem Cell. 2012;10(4):412–24.
88. Zhang B, Irvine D, Ho YEA. Inhibition of chronic myeloid leukemia stem cells by the combination of the Hedgehog pathway inhibitor LDE225 with nilotinib [abstract]. Blood (ASH Annual Meeting Abstracts). 2010;116(21):514.
89. Tauchi T, Katagiri S, Okabe S, Minami Y, Naoe T, Ohyashiki K. Targeting the Hedgehog signaling pathway limits the self-renewal of BCR-ABL1 positive leukemia cells: molecular mechanisms [abstract]. Blood (ASH Annual Meeting Abstracts). 2012;120(21):531.
90. Melo JV, Chuah C. Novel agents in CML therapy: tyrosine kinase inhibitors and beyond. Hematology Am Soc Hematol Educ Program. 2008;1:427–35.
91. Bixby D, Talpaz M. Mechanisms of resistance to tyrosine kinase inhibitors in chronic myeloid leukemia and recent therapeutic strategies to overcome resistance. Hematology Am Soc Hematol Educ Program. 2009;1:461–76.
92. Bixby D, Talpaz M. Seeking the causes and solutions to imatinib-resistance in chronic myeloid leukemia. Leukemia. 2011;25(1):7–22.
93. Chen M, Gallipoli P, DeGeer D, Sloma I, Forrest DL, Chan M, et al. Targeting primitive chronic myeloid leukemia cells by effective inhibition of a new AHI-1-BCR-ABL-JAK2 complex. J Natl Cancer Inst. 2013;105(6):405–23.
94. Fiskus W, Wang Y, Joshi R, Rao R, Yang Y, Chen J, et al. Cotreatment with vorinostat enhances activity of MK-0457 (VX-680) against acute and chronic myelogenous leukemia cells. Clin Cancer Res. 2008;14(19):6106–15.
95. Nimmanapalli R, Fuino L, Stobaugh C, Richon V, Bhalla K. Cotreatment with the histone deacetylase inhibitor suberoylanilide hydroxamic acid (SAHA) enhances imatinib-induced apoptosis of Bcr-Abl-positive human acute leukemia cells. Blood. 2003;101(8):3236–9.
96. Goessling W, North TE, Loewer S, Lord AM, Lee S, Stoick-Cooper CL, et al. Genetic interaction of PGE2 and Wnt signaling regulates developmental specification of stem cells and regeneration. Cell. 2009;136(6):1136–47.
97. Rokah OH, Granot G, Ovcharenko A, Modai S, Pasmanik-Chor M, Toren A, et al. Downregulation of miR-31, miR-155, and miR-564 in chronic myeloid leukemia cells. PLoS One. 2012;7(4), e35501.

98. Bueno MJ, Pérez de Castro I, Gómez de Cedrón M, Santos J, Calin GA, Cigudosa JC, et al. Genetic and epigenetic silencing of microRNA-203 enhances ABL1 and BCR-ABL1 oncogene expression. Cancer Cell. 2008;13(6):496–506.
99. Cortes JE, Kim DW, Pinilla-Ibarz J, le Coutre P, Paquette R, Chuah C, et al. A phase 2 trial of ponatinib in Philadelphia chromosome-positive leukemias. N Engl J Med. 2013;369 (19):1783–96.
100. Mayerhofer M, Aichberger KJ, Florian S, Krauth MT, Hauswirth AW, Derdak S, et al. Identification of mTOR as a novel bifunctional target in chronic myeloid leukemia: dissection of growth-inhibitory and VEGF-suppressive effects of rapamycin in leukemic cells. FASEB J Off Publ Fed Am Soc Exp Biol. 2005;19(8):960–2.
101. Issa JPJ, Kantarjian HM. Targeting DNA methylation. Clin Cancer Res. 2009;15 (12):3938–46.
102. Oki Y, Kantarjian HM, Gharibyan V, Jones D, O'brien S, Verstovsek S, et al. Phase II study of low-dose decitabine in combination with imatinib mesylate in patients with accelerated or myeloid blastic phase of chronic myelogenous leukemia. Cancer. 2007;109(5):899–906.
103. Machova Polakova K, Koblihova J, Stopka T. Role of epigenetics in chronic myeloid leukemia. Curr Hematol Malig Rep. 2013;8(1):28–36.
104. Zhang QY, Mao JH, Liu P, Huang QH, Lu J, Xie YY, et al. A systems biology understanding of the synergistic effects of arsenic sulfide and Imatinib in BCR/ABL-associated leukemia. Proc Natl Acad Sci U S A. 2009;106(9):3378–83.
105. Goussetis DJ, Gounaris E, Wu EJ, Vakana E, Sharma B, Bogyo M, et al. Autophagic degradation of the BCR-ABL oncoprotein and generation of antileukemic responses by arsenic trioxide. Blood. 2012;120(17):3555–62.
106. Amaravadi RK, Thompson CB. The roles of therapy-induced autophagy and necrosis in cancer treatment. Clin Cancer Res. 2007;13(24):7271–9.
107. Schafranek L, Leclercq TM, White DL, Hughes TP. Clarithromycin enhances dasatinib-induced cell death in chronic myeloid leukemia cells, by inhibition of late stage autophagy. Leuk Lymphoma. 2013;54(1):198–201.

# Chapter 12
# Discontinuation of Therapy and Treatment-Free Remission in CML

**David M. Ross and Timothy P. Hughes**

**Abstract** Tyrosine kinase inhibitor (TKI) treatment of chronic myeloid leukaemia (CML) has resulted in a life expectancy comparable to that of the general population for many individuals. This has led patients and clinicians to question whether, after a sustained period of deep molecular response, it might one day be possible to discontinue the TKI. A sustained molecular response without the need for ongoing treatment is referred to as a treatment-free remission (TFR). TFR has many potential advantages: patients in TFR may be free of chronic TKI toxicities that affect quality of life, and they may avoid the potential for late emerging toxicities (e.g. vascular events with nilotinib, pulmonary complications with dasatinib). It is imperative that young women with CML stop TKI prior to pregnancy due to the risk of teratogenesis. This can be achieved most safely for the mother and the baby if TFR has already been established. TFR reduces the considerable economic burden of long-term drug provision and improves the cost-effectiveness of the treatment. In this chapter, we review the clinical and biological data relevant to the topic of treatment discontinuation.

**Keywords** Chronic myeloid leukaemia • Tyrosine kinase inhibitors • Minimal residual disease • Treatment-free remission

---

D.M. Ross
Haematology Directorate, SA Pathology, Adelaide, SA 5000, Australia

School of Medicine, University of Adelaide, Adelaide, SA 5000, Australia

Department of Haematology and Genetic Pathology, Flinders University and Medical Centre, Adelaide, SA 5042, Australia

Cancer Theme, South Australian Health and Medical Research Institute, Adelaide, SA 5000, Australia

T.P. Hughes (✉)
Haematology Directorate, SA Pathology, Adelaide, SA 5000, Australia

School of Medicine, University of Adelaide, Adelaide, SA 5000, Australia

Cancer Theme, South Australian Health and Medical Research Institute, Adelaide, SA 5000, Australia
e-mail: timothy.hughes@health.sa.gov.au


M. Kizaki (ed.), *Molecular Pathogenesis and Treatment of Chronic Myelogenous Leukemia*, DOI 10.1007/978-4-431-55714-2_12

## 12.1 Introduction

Tyrosine kinase inhibitor (TKI) treatment of chronic myeloid leukaemia (CML) has resulted in a life expectancy comparable to that of the general population for many individuals [1]. This has led patients and clinicians to question whether, after a sustained period of deep molecular response, it might one day be possible to discontinue the TKI. A sustained molecular response without the need for ongoing treatment is referred to as a treatment-free remission (TFR). TFR has many potential advantages: patients in TFR may be free of chronic TKI toxicities that affect quality of life [2], and they may avoid the potential for late emerging toxicities (e.g. vascular events with nilotinib, pulmonary complications with dasatinib) [3–5]. It is imperative that young women with CML stop TKI prior to pregnancy due to the risk of teratogenesis [6]. This can be undertaken most safely for the mother and the baby if TFR has already been established. TFR reduces the considerable economic burden of long-term drug provision and improves the cost-effectiveness of the treatment. In this chapter, we review the clinical and biological data relevant to the topic of treatment discontinuation.

## 12.2 Measuring Deep Molecular Response

Patients who have stopped a TKI shortly after achieving a complete cytogenetic response (CCR) or major molecular response (MMR) virtually always relapse. Untreated CML relapses with a doubling time (based on BCR-ABL mRNA levels) of around 10–14 days [7]. The first patients reported with sustained molecular response had undetectable minimal residual disease (UMRD) at the time of therapy discontinuation [8]. UMRD is not equivalent to the absence of CML, since disease may remain below the limit of detection of the test. Conventional real-time reverse transcriptase quantitative PCR (RQ-PCR) has a detection limit of 4–5 log below the level of BCR-ABL seen at diagnosis. The detection limit will vary between laboratories, and even within a laboratory there will be variation in the sample, RNA degradation, and PCR efficiency. In order to standardize criteria for deeper levels of molecular response, recommendations have been published [9]. For example, MR4.5 is defined as either UMRD in a sample with a detection limit of at least 4.5 log or detectable BCR-ABL at a level below 0.0032 % in a laboratory using the BCR-ABL International Scale. All values discussed in this chapter are expressed on the International Scale, and it is important for each clinician to be aware of the performance characteristics of the BCR-ABL assay in his or her local laboratory. TKI discontinuation may expose the patient to unnecessary risks if high-quality monitoring of CML cannot be provided in a timely manner.

## 12.3 TFR in Different Patient Populations

### 12.3.1 Allogeneic Stem Cell Transplantation

The first treatment for CML to result in deep molecular responses was allogeneic stem cell transplantation. The achievement of UMRD post-transplant is strongly associated with sustained molecular remission [10, 11]. Response to donor lymphocyte infusion for the treatment of relapse after allografting is strong evidence for the sensitivity of CML to immunological control. UMRD after an allograft, and without the need for ongoing immunosuppression, may be considered a form of TFR and is commonly considered to represent a cure for CML. Rare late relapses of CML can occur even in this cohort [12, 13], an observation that emphasizes the need for some degree of long-term follow-up of CML patients, even after highly effective treatment. Goldman and colleagues reviewed the outcomes of more than 1500 patients receiving a sibling allograft in first chronic phase and remaining in remission for at least 5 years: remarkably, even in this good-risk cohort, the cumulative incidence of relapse was 8 % over the succeeding decade [14].

### 12.3.2 Interferon-α

Recombinant interferon-α (IFN-α) entered CML practice in the 1980s and (until the appearance of imatinib) was established as the most effective non-transplant therapy for chronic phase CML [15, 16]. Approximately 20 % of patients treated with IFN achieved a CCR, and a small fraction of these patients achieved an MMR or even UMRD [17]. Mahon reported on the outcome of six patients who stopped IFN in UMRD, five of whom sustained TFR [18]. IFN may promote the entry of CML stem cells into cell cycle, resulting in gradual depletion of the relatively resistant leukemic stem cells [19]. IFN is also associated with the emergence of cytotoxic T lymphocytes (CTLs) reactive against myeloid-associated antigens [20, 21]. A study of IFN maintenance treatment (after the combination of imatinib and IFN) showed a progressive reduction in the level of MRD that was associated with the emergence of CTLs reactive against PR3, an antigen associated with neutrophil granules [22]. These effects of IFN have renewed interest in the drug, especially in combination with TKIs.

### 12.3.3 Imatinib

Several prospective studies of imatinib discontinuation in chronic phase CML have now been reported. The findings between studies have been remarkably consistent. The French STIM (STop IMatinib) study and the Australian TWISTER (Trial of Withdrawing Imatinib in STablE Remission) study both enrolled patients with

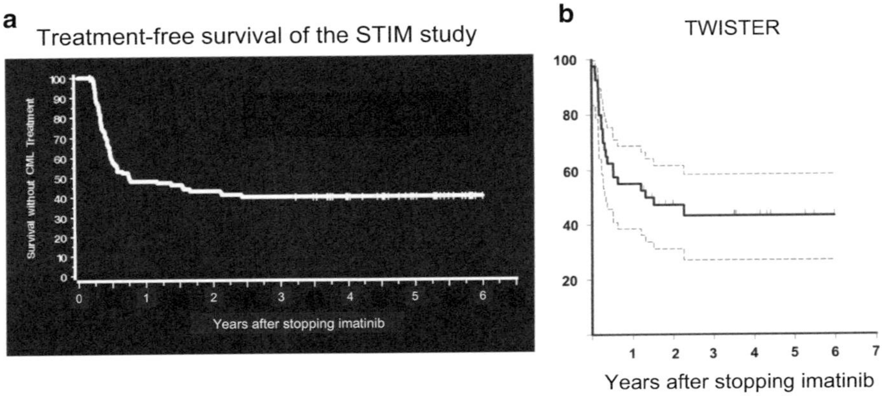


**Fig. 12.1** Rates of treatment-free remission in the (**a**) STIM and (**b**) TWISTER clinical trials. Kaplan-Meier estimates of the proportion of patients free of molecular recurrence after imatinib withdrawal. The *solid line* indicates the Kaplan-Meier estimate of the probability of remaining in TFR. *Dashed lines* (TWISTER) indicate the 95 % confidence interval. Relapse was defined as loss of UMRD confirmed on a second sample (TWISTER) or followed by a onefold rise in BCR-ABL (STIM) (Mahon et al., ASH 2013 [abstract 255]).

UMRD for at least 2 years, and both showed a TFR rate around 40 % with most molecular relapses occurring in the first 6 months (Fig. 12.1) [23, 24]. The first patient in the TWISTER study stopped imatinib in August 2006 and remained in UMRD without the need for treatment at last follow-up, 9 years later. All patients who restarted imatinib treatment in STIM and TWISTER remained sensitive to the TKI, and no patient developed kinase domain mutations. Molecular relapse in these two studies was defined as loss of UMRD. A follow-up study from the French group (A-STIM; according to STIM) tested loss of MMR as a trigger for resumption of imatinib and showed that the rate of TFR (i.e. remaining in MMR without treatment) increased to around 50 % [25]. One patient in that study relapsed, restarted imatinib and again achieved a deep molecular response, but some months later abruptly developed lymphoid blast crisis. No other instance of loss of response has been reported to date among over 500 patients undergoing a trial of TFR.

STIM, A-STIM, and TWISTER enrolled a mixture of patients treated second line with imatinib after interferon and those treated first line. All studies showed a higher rate of TFR in the patients previously treated with IFN (around 50 %) versus first-line patients (around 30 %) [23–25]. This analysis is confounded by the fact that patients who remained on IFN for long enough to switch to imatinib may have had more favourable disease biology to begin with. The heterogeneous patient population also confounds any attempt to identify characteristics that predict successful TFR (see Sect. 12.4). The STIM2 study, which is enrolling only first-line imatinib-treated patients, may help to clarify some of these questions. An interim analysis of STIM2 reported 61 % of patients still in MMR at a median of 12 months after imatinib discontinuation [26]. Interestingly, more than half of the patients in MMR had detectable BCR-ABL transcripts at a low level, and 28 % of patients maintained UMRD, consistent with the earlier studies. Why this persistent disease does not inevitably lead to relapse remains a key unanswered question.

### 12.3.4 Newer TKIs

Prospective multicentre studies of TFR after response to nilotinib and dasatinib are currently underway, but the published experience of withdrawal of second-generation TKIs is currently limited to registry data and small series. Réa and colleagues reported a series of 34 patients with at least 6 months of follow-up, and the probability of stable MMR after 12 months off TKI was 58 % [27]. The limited results available indicate a TFR rate at least equivalent to that seen after imatinib withdrawal. Since deeper molecular responses are seen earlier and more frequently in patients treated with more potent TKIs [3, 28], there is an expectation that the increasing use of second-generation TKIs may result in a larger proportion of patients being eligible for a trial of TFR.

### 12.3.5 Higher-Risk Patients

The STIM study showed a strong association of Sokal score with molecular relapse [23]. It is remarkable that simple clinical markers of risk at diagnosis should still have an impact on the probability of TFR many years later, in spite of deep molecular response. This suggests that previous disease biology remains relevant and cautions us that the hazards of TKI discontinuation may be greater in higher-risk patients. A French study of stopping dasatinib or nilotinib in UMRD reported that the rate of TFR among patients on second-line therapy for poor response was around half of that seen in patients treated first line with dasatinib/nilotinib or second line after imatinib intolerance [27]. Nevertheless, there are rare reports of TFR among patients achieving a deep molecular response following treatment for imatinib-resistant disease with kinase domain mutations or even after blast crisis [29, 30]. It should be noted that most of these patients stopped the TKI due to toxicity concerns. Patients with kinase domain mutations or advanced phase CML are generally excluded from TFR studies, and elective TKI discontinuation is not recommended in this population.

## 12.4 Relapse Definitions

The earliest TFR studies used conservative criteria for restarting TKI therapy, since the safety of drug withdrawal was not known. As the volume of clinical experience has increased, it has become apparent that molecular relapse can be rescued by the

**Table 12.1** Summary of key features of TFR studies reported to date

| | | Relapse criterion | | |
|---|---|---|---|---|
| | Treatment | Loss of UMRD (TWISTER [24]) | Loss of UMRD and tenfold rise in BCR-ABL (STIM [23]) | Loss of MMR (A-STIM [25]) |
| STIM2 [26] | First-line imatinib | | X | |
| HOVON51 [31] | Imatinib + cytarabine | X | | |
| DADI [32] | Dasatinib | X | | |
| ENESTfreedom[a] | Nilotinib | | | X |
| DASfree[a] | Dasatinib | | | X |

[a]These studies are not yet reported. Study details are available at clinicaltrials.gov

reintroduction of the original TKI, that TKI resistance at relapse is not a problem, and that low-level molecular positivity does not inevitably lead to a progressive rise in disease burden. Criteria for restarting TKI in selected TFR studies are shown in Table 12.1. STIM and TWISTER mandated restarting treatment if BCR-ABL mRNA was detectable in two consecutive samples. Some patients were seen in whom intermittent positive samples did not lead to loss of MMR [24]. This observation was examined in A-STIM, where the trigger to restart TKI was loss of MMR. The kinetics of low-level BCR-ABL revealed that around half of patients who lose UMRD will remain in MMR without treatment [25]. Importantly, MMR was maintained with longer follow-up, with very few relapses occurring later than 2 years.

## 12.5 Eligibility for a Trial of TFR

Just as the relapse definitions were conservative in the earliest studies, so too were the inclusion criteria. No detectable BCR-ABL in any sample in the 2 preceding years was required in STIM and TWISTER. Since loss of UMRD does not translate to clinical relapse, it is logical to ask whether less stringent molecular responses can be accepted prior to attempting TFR. A further, and important, motivation to change the inclusion criteria for TFR comes from the difficulty of standardizing UMRD (discussed in Sect. 12.2). Ongoing studies are using sustained MR4.5 or MR4 as qualifying levels of molecular response for a trial of TFR.

The A-STIM trial allowed the enrolment of patients with a less stringent definition of UMRD that allowed occasional low-level positive results within the preceding 2 years. The rate of treatment-free MMR in those patients was identical to patients meeting the stringent UMRD criterion, but the rate of treatment-free UMRD was significantly lower [25]. It remains to be seen whether or not this difference is clinically relevant with longer follow-up.

## 12.6 Biology of TFR

Whereas the achievement and maintenance of deep molecular response appears to be a prerequisite for TFR, a low level of minimal residual disease is not sufficient to guarantee that a patient will sustain TFR. This means that TFR should be thought of as a distinct biological state, the determinants of which remain to be elucidated. There are at least three possible elements that define TFR: the first is the amount of residual CML; the second is the quality of the residual CML clone; and the third comprises factors extrinsic to the CML clone, such as stromal interactions or immunological surveillance [33].

The first studies of TFR included patients with UMRD (based on conventional RQ-PCR) with the simple idea that in some cases the CML clone was completely eradicated and that if only we could identify these patients, we could select those who no longer needed TKI treatment. In fact, it is now clear that most, or even all, patients who remain in TFR still have residual CML cells. A limitation of conventional RQ-PCR for BCR-ABL for very low levels of MRD is the risk of false-positive results that may occur due to cross-contamination between samples processed in the same laboratory or due to rare BCR-ABL transcripts that can be found in normal individuals [34]. An assay for patient-specific BCR-ABL intronic DNA sequences virtually eliminates the risk of false-positive results because each patient's breakpoint is essentially unique, whereas the vast majority of CML patients have one or both of the two common mRNA transcripts [35–37]. Using a semi-quantitative DNA PCR approach, it was shown that all 26 patients tested in the TWISTER study had detectable CML cells on at least one occasion during follow-up. There was no significant difference in the risk of relapse when comparing those with and without detectable BCR-ABL DNA prior to imatinib withdrawal, but the number of patients assessed was too small to draw definitive conclusions on the relationship between depth of response and relapse risk [24]. The nature of the cells that are providing the positive DNA signal was not studied, but in A-STIM, an analysis of three patients with fluctuating low-level BCR-ABL showed that BCR-ABL mRNA transcripts were enriched in the CD15+ myeloid fraction, and not in B cells or T cells [25]. It is possible that there is an MRD threshold (somewhere around MR4.0) above which TFR cannot be achieved. What is not yet clear is whether deeper levels of response (e.g. MR5.0 to MR6.0) are associated with a lower risk of molecular recurrence, since such levels of response are not accurately quantifiable with routine assays.

The association of Sokal score with the risk of molecular recurrence many years later argues that factors intrinsic to the leukemic clone still play an important role in TFR biology. Multiple biological parameters (e.g. OCT-1 activity [38], KIR genotype [39]) have been reported to influence the probability of achieving molecular response, but none has yet emerged as a reliable predictor of TFR after deep molecular response has been achieved. A major obstacle to studying this question is the time elapsed between diagnosis and a trial of TFR: this means that relatively few patients will have available diagnostic material for study.

Immunological function is the best-studied of the CML-extrinsic factors that may be relevant to TFR. It was already mentioned above that cytotoxic T lymphocytes reactive against myeloid antigens are associated with stable or deepening molecular response after TKI withdrawal in patients who continue IFN [22]. NK cell numbers are the only immunological parameter to emerge as a potential predictor of TFR in clinical studies. A Japanese study identified increased CD3-CD56+ NK cell numbers in patients in TFR after imatinib withdrawal, but NK cell numbers were not measured prior to TKI withdrawal so the predictive value of NK cell numbers could not be assessed [40]. IMMUNOSTIM, a scientific substudy of the original STIM trial reported that mean NK cell numbers at study entry were higher in patients who maintained TFR than in those who relapsed [41]. The difference was most striking in the $CD56^{dim}$ population of NK cells that is thought to have the greatest cytotoxic activity. The range of NK cell numbers in the TFR group and the relapse group overlapped considerably. At present, there is no robust immunological predictor of TFR.

## 12.7 Future Directions

The rate of TFR after treatment with imatinib, nilotinib, and dasatinib will be known within the next few years. Long-term follow-up of these patients, especially those in MMR with detectable disease, will be needed to reassure patients that they are not being exposed to a risk of late relapse. In the allograft setting, a relapse risk of 0.5–1 % per annum persists even for patients in long-term remission. It is remarkable that there have so far been no relapses from TFR later than 3 years after TKI withdrawal. Whether this will prove true with larger numbers and longer follow-up remains to be seen. Patients may have anxieties concerning TKI toxicity from continuing therapy and conversely may have anxieties about relapse risk associated with TFR. Patient education and counselling regarding these issues will assume increasing importance if TFR is to become a major aim of CML treatment.

## References

1. Bjorkholm M, Ohm L, Eloranta S, et al. Success story of targeted therapy in chronic myeloid leukemia: a population-based study of patients diagnosed in Sweden from 1973 to 2008. J Clin Oncol. 2011;29(18):2514–20.
2. Efficace F, Baccarani M, Breccia M, et al. Health-related quality of life in chronic myeloid leukemia patients receiving long-term therapy with imatinib compared with the general population. Blood. 2011;118(17):4554–60.
3. Jabbour E, Kantarjian HM, Saglio G, et al. Early response with dasatinib or imatinib in chronic myeloid leukemia: 3-year follow-up from a randomized phase 3 trial (DASISION). Blood. 2014;123(4):494–500.

4. Aichberger KJ, Herndlhofer S, Schernthaner GH, et al. Progressive peripheral arterial occlusive disease and other vascular events during nilotinib therapy in CML. Am J Hematol. 2011;86(7):533–9.
5. Montani D, Bergot E, Gunther S, et al. Pulmonary arterial hypertension in patients treated by dasatinib. Circulation. 2012;125(17):2128–37.
6. Ault P, Kantarjian H, O'Brien S, et al. Pregnancy among patients with chronic myeloid leukemia treated with imatinib. J Clin Oncol. 2006;24(7):1204–8.
7. Branford S, Yeung DT, Prime JA, et al. BCR-ABL1 doubling times more reliably assess the dynamics of CML relapse compared with the BCR-ABL1 fold rise: implications for monitoring and management. Blood. 2012;119(18):4264–71.
8. Rousselot P, Huguet F, Rea D, et al. Imatinib mesylate discontinuation in patients with chronic myelogenous leukemia in complete molecular remission for more than 2 years. Blood. 2007;109(1):58–60.
9. Cross NC, White HE, Muller MC, Saglio G, Hochhaus A. Standardized definitions of molecular response in chronic myeloid leukemia. Leukemia. 2012;26(10):2172–5.
10. Mughal TI, Yong A, Szydlo RM, et al. Molecular studies in patients with chronic myeloid leukaemia in remission 5 years after allogeneic stem cell transplant define the risk of subsequent relapse. Br J Haematol. 2001;115(3):569–74.
11. Radich JP, Gehly G, Gooley T, et al. Polymerase chain reaction detection of the BCR-ABL fusion transcript after allogeneic marrow transplantation for chronic myeloid leukemia: results and implications in 346 patients. Blood. 1995;85(9):2632–8.
12. van Rhee F, Lin F, Cross NC, et al. Detection of residual leukaemia more than 10 years after allogeneic bone marrow transplantation for chronic myelogenous leukaemia. Bone Marrow Transplant. 1994;14(4):609–12.
13. Norkin M, Uberti JP, Schiffer CA. Very late recurrences of leukemia: why does leukemia awake after many years of dormancy? Leuk Res. 2011;35(2):139–44.
14. Goldman JM, Majhail NS, Klein JP, et al. Relapse and late mortality in 5-year survivors of myeloablative allogeneic hematopoietic cell transplantation for chronic myeloid leukemia in first chronic phase. J Clin Oncol. 2010;28(11):1888–95.
15. Guilhot F, Chastang C, Michallet M, et al. Interferon alfa-2b combined with cytarabine versus interferon alone in chronic myelogenous leukemia. French Chronic Myeloid Leukemia Study Group. N Engl J Med. 1997;337(4):223–9.
16. Hehlmann R, Berger U, Pfirrmann M, et al. Drug treatment is superior to allografting as first-line therapy in chronic myeloid leukemia. Blood. 2007;109(11):4686–92.
17. Muller MC, Gattermann N, Lahaye T, et al. Dynamics of BCR-ABL mRNA expression in first-line therapy of chronic myelogenous leukemia patients with imatinib or interferon alpha/ara-C. Leukemia. 2003;17(12):2392–400.
18. Mahon FX, Delbrel X, Cony-Makhoul P, et al. Follow-up of complete cytogenetic remission in patients with chronic myeloid leukemia after cessation of interferon alfa. J Clin Oncol. 2002;20(1):214–20.
19. Essers MA, Offner S, Blanco-Bose WE, et al. IFNalpha activates dormant haematopoietic stem cells in vivo. Nature. 2009;458(7240):904–8.
20. Kanodia S, Wieder E, Lu S, et al. PR1-specific T cells are associated with unmaintained cytogenetic remission of chronic myelogenous leukemia after interferon withdrawal. PLoS One. 2010;5(7), e11770.
21. Burchert A, Wolfl S, Schmidt M, et al. Interferon-alpha but not the ABL-kinase inhibitor imatinib (STI571), induces expression of myeloblastin and a specific T-cell response in chronic myeloid leukemia. Blood. 2003;101(1):259–64.
22. Burchert A, Muller MC, Kostrewa P, et al. Sustained molecular response with interferon alfa maintenance after induction therapy with imatinib plus interferon alfa in patients with chronic myeloid leukemia. J Clin Oncol. 2010;28(8):1429–35.

23. Mahon FX, Rea D, Guilhot J, et al. Discontinuation of imatinib in patients with chronic myeloid leukaemia who have maintained complete molecular remission for at least 2 years: the prospective, multicentre Stop Imatinib (STIM) trial. Lancet Oncol. 2010;11(11):1029–35.
24. Ross DM, Branford S, Seymour JF, et al. Safety and efficacy of imatinib cessation for CML patients with stable undetectable minimal residual disease: results from the TWISTER study. Blood. 2013;122(4):515–22.
25. Rousselot P, Charbonnier A, Cony-Makhoul P, et al. Loss of major molecular response as a trigger for restarting tyrosine kinase inhibitor therapy in patients with chronic-phase chronic myelogenous leukemia who have stopped imatinib after durable undetectable disease. J Clin Oncol. 2014;32(5):424–30.
26. Mahon FX, Nicolini FE, Noël MP, et al. Preliminary report of the STIM2 study: a multicenter stop imatinib trial for chronic phase chronic myeloid leukemia de novo patients on imatinib. Blood. 2013;122(21):Abstract 654.
27. Rea D, Rousselot P, Guilhot F, et al. Discontinuation of second generation (2G) tyrosine kinase inhibitors (TKI) in chronic phase (CP)-chronic myeloid leukemia (CML) patients with stable undetectable BCR-ABL transcripts. Blood. 2012;120(21):Abstract 916.
28. Larson RA, Hochhaus A, Hughes TP, et al. Nilotinib vs imatinib in patients with newly diagnosed Philadelphia chromosome-positive chronic myeloid leukemia in chronic phase: ENESTnd 3-year follow-up. Leukemia. 2012;26(10):2197–203.
29. Ross DM, Bartley PA, Goyne J, Morley AA, Seymour JF, Grigg AP. Durable complete molecular remission of chronic myeloid leukemia following dasatinib cessation, despite adverse disease features. Haematologica. 2011;96(11):1720–2.
30. Hill BG, Shen AQ, El Rassi F, Khoury HJ. Sustained complete molecular remission after discontinuation of tyrosine kinase inhibitors in blast-phase chronic myeloid leukemia. J Clin Oncol. 2014;32, doi 10.1200/JCO.2013.50.1221.
31. Thielen N, van der Holt B, Cornelissen JJ, et al. Imatinib discontinuation in chronic phase myeloid leukaemia patients in sustained complete molecular response: a randomised trial of the Dutch-Belgian Cooperative Trial for Haemato-Oncology (HOVON). Eur J Cancer. 2013;49(15):3242–6.
32. Tanaka H, Imagawa J, Okada M, et al. Discontinuation of dasatinib in patients with CML who have maintained complete molecular response for at least one year: results from a prospective discontinuation (DADI) trial blood. 2013;122(21):Abstract 3998.
33. Melo JV, Ross DM. Minimal residual disease and discontinuation of therapy in chronic myeloid leukemia: can we aim at a cure? Hematology Am Soc Hematol Educ Program. 2011;2011:136–42.
34. Bose S, Deininger M, Gora-Tybor J, Goldman JM, Melo JV. The presence of typical and atypical BCR-ABL fusion genes in leukocytes of normal individuals: biologic significance and implications for the assessment of minimal residual disease. Blood. 1998;92(9):3362–7.
35. Ross DM, Branford S, Seymour JF, et al. Patients with chronic myeloid leukemia who maintain a complete molecular response after stopping imatinib treatment have evidence of persistent leukemia by DNA PCR. Leukemia. 2010;24(10):1719–24.
36. Ross DM, O'Hely M, Bartley PA, et al. Distribution of genomic breakpoints in chronic myeloid leukemia: analysis of 308 patients. Leukemia. 2013;27(10):2105–7.
37. Sobrinho-Simoes M, Wilczek V, Score J, Cross NC, Apperley JF, Melo JV. In search of the original leukemic clone in chronic myeloid leukemia patients in complete molecular remission after stem cell transplantation or imatinib. Blood. 2010;116(8):1329–35.
38. White DL, Dang P, Engler J, et al. Functional activity of the OCT-1 protein is predictive of long-term outcome in patients with chronic-phase chronic myeloid leukemia treated with imatinib. J Clin Oncol. 2010;28(16):2761–7.
39. Marin D, Gabriel IH, Ahmad S, et al. KIR2DS1 genotype predicts for complete cytogenetic response and survival in newly diagnosed chronic myeloid leukemia patients treated with imatinib. Leukemia. 2011;26(2):296–302.

40. Ohyashiki K, Katagiri S, Tauchi T, et al. Increased natural killer cells and decreased CD3(+) CD8(+)CD62L(+) T cells in CML patients who sustained complete molecular remission after discontinuation of imatinib. Br J Haematol. 2012;157(2):254–6.
41. Rea D, Dulphy N, Henry G, et al. Low natural killer (NK) cell counts and functionality are associated with molecular relapse after imatinib discontinuation in patients (pts) with chronic phase (CP)-chronic myeloid leukemia (CML) with undetectable BCR-ABL transcripts for at least 2 years: preliminary results from immunostim, on behalf Of STIM investigators. Blood. 2013;122(21):Abstract 856.

MIX
Papier aus verantwortungsvollen Quellen
Paper from responsible sources
FSC® C105338

If you have any concerns about our products,
you can contact us on
**ProductSafety@springernature.com**

In case Publisher is established outside the EU,
the EU authorized representative is:
**Springer Nature Customer Service Center GmbH**
**Europaplatz 3, 69115 Heidelberg, Germany**

Printed by Libri Plureos GmbH
in Hamburg, Germany